Bone Health Beyond the Scan: A Multifaceted Approach to Osteoporosis

Faris

Copyright © 2024 by Faris

All rights reserved. No part of this book may be reproduced in any manner whatsoever without written permission except in the case of brief quotations embodied in critical articles and reviews.
First Printing, 2024

Contents

Chapter 1

Introduction

1.1 Motivation

Bone fracture is a social health problem with increasing magnitude because of its prevalence in aged population due to osteoporosis [1, 2, 3]. Osteoporosis is a bone disease characterized by a decrease of bone mineral density (BMD), which makes bone structure more brittle, and it is associated to a reduction of cortical shell thickness and an increase of cancellous bone voids. Those effects are results of metabolic changes which affect bone resorption and formation within bone remodeling process. There are 8.9 million fractures per year worldwide due to osteoporosis [4], where hip, vertebra, wrist and rib fractures are the most common. Besides, patients suffering from an osteoporotic fracture have a 86 % probability of experiencing a second fracture [5]. Therefore, an early diagnosis of osteoporosis is important to prevent subsequent fractures. In addition, osteoporosis is highly prevalent in post-menopausal aged women, whose fractures lead to disability and pain [5].

The gold standard to predict osteoporosis is based on BMD measurements using dual-energy X-ray absorptiometry (DXA). However, some studies in the literature claim that this technique cannot predict 40% of non-traumatic fractures [6] and BMD values of individuals with and without bone fractures overlap [7]. A possible reason is that DXA provides a mean value of the density, but gives no further information about bone microstructure, which has been proved to influence bone strength [8, 9, 10, 11]. These facts highlight that BMD alone is not able to perform accurate predictions so there is a need of other methodologies to evaluate the mechanical competence of bone. Many efforts have been made to propose a better procedure to assess bone quality where imaging techniques like DXA, computed tomography (CT), multi-detector computed tomography (MDCT), peripheral quantitative computed tomography (HR-qQCT), magnetic resonance imaging (MRI) or micro-computed tomography have been studied. Specifically, due to radiation issues, micro-CT is used for *ex vivo* investigations and permits to estimate cancellous bone properties in a spatial resolution of micrometers, offering a great contrast between bone and the tissues surrounding it [12, 13], while CT, MDCT, HR-qQCT and MRI induce lower levels of radiation and have been used to investigate bone *in vivo*. The above mentioned techniques may be understood as an image of bone state in a certain moment, so they do not take into account other continuum phenomena like bone remodeling. It is accepted that fracture risk assessment not only depends on bone density but also on the quality of its underlying microstructure which can be quantified by image analysis [8, 9, 10, 11]. Hence, a thorough understanding of bone biomechanics and its relationship to microarchitecture is required.

The use of numerical methods like the finite element (FE) method permits to simulate multiple situations, evaluate clinical treatments or characterize the mechanical performance of bone saving resources, because biological tissues degrade over time and only admit a single destructive testing. Thus, from some decades ago, FE models have been widely used to reproduce cancellous bone mechanical response and to relate it to microstructure. Other applications include to design and evaluate implants used in orthopedic surgeries and preoperative planning. On the other hand, the highly hierarchical structure of bone makes it necessary to study each level separately to provide information about how bone behaves at each scale and how it affects to the next level. Homogenization through scales enables to account for the characteristics observed at each dimension in multiscale models in order to better predict fracture and healing. Moreover, the study of the influence of homogenization on the results at the macroscale has research interest, and the study of bone fracture at different scales has not been entirely solved in the literature. Complex models have been reported, but their experimental validation is difficult and a simple failure model for fracture risk assessment is interesting because it may improve diagnosis and treatment evaluation.

Cancellous bone biomechanical characterization through its different scales and the relationship with morphometry may be used to improve diagnosis and evaluate treatments for diseases, resulting in a better bone fracture prevention.

1.2 Aims

The main objective of this book is to characterize cancellous bone tissue. It is accomplished from two points of view: mechanical and morphometric. The mechanical characterization is achieved from the following approaches: experimental testing, finite element modeling and digital image correlation. The morphometric characterization is carried out by analyzing micro-CT images result from cancellous bone samples scanning. On the other hand, other objective emerged from a research stage which is the case of the study of the evaluation of spine fixation techniques.

The secondary objectives of this book, divided in topics, are:

- Mechanical characterization

  - To study the mechanical behavior of cancellous bone tissue at the macro- and microscales.

  - To investigate failure models for cancellous bone tissue.

  - To estimate the apparent elastic behavior of a heterogeneous structure like cancellous bone through the homogenization of its microscale.

  - To analyze how microarchitecture is related to biomechanics.

  - To estimate tissue mechanical properties of cancellous bone.

  - To analyze the capabilities of digital image correlation technique to estimate full-field strain measurements in cancellous bone-like structures.

- Image analysis

  - To study and apply micro-computed tomography (μCT) to characterize cancellous bone morphometry.

  - To analyze the influence of segmentation threshold variation on the morphometry.

  - To study and implement the assessment of morphometric parameters.

  - To investigate relationships between mechanical performance and morphometry in cancellous bone tissue.

- To investigate the performance of different phantoms used to estimate compression stiffness as function of bone mineral density (BMD) in μCT acquisitions.

- Evaluation of spine fixation systems using bone failure models

    - To evaluate differences on load bearing between pedicle screws and sublaminar tape fixation configurations.

    - To generate density-based finite element models at clinical CT resolution to evaluate fixation constructs.

    - To investigate a simple model to estimate the pull-out strength of an implant inserted in a vertebra.

    - To analyze the influence of volume of interest size on the pull-out strength prediction.

    - To study the influence of implant insertion depth on the pull-out strength estimation.

    - To propose relationships between morphometry of cancellous bone surrounding the implant and the pull-out strength.

1.3 book organization

This book is organized as follows:

Chapter 1 deals with the introduction to the topics studied, the motivation to investigate them and the presentation of the objectives of the book. Bone tissue is presented from biological and mechanical perspectives. Then, a review of the state of the art of cancellous bone characterization is performed.

Chapter 2 deals with cancellous bone characterization from a morphological perspective. High resolution imaging bone imaging is described, followed by the segmentation procedure and the morphometry estimations. Furthermore, an analysis of the influence of segmentation threshold variation on the morphometry and elastic properties is presented

Chapter 3 presents cancellous bone experimental characterization by means of testing and digital image correlation, and its numerical characterization through finite element modeling.

Chapter 4 contains the study of trabecular bone surrogates of different densities. The methodology to characterize cancellous bone is also tested on surrogates.

Chapter 5 is the result of the research stay at Technique University of Eindhoven (TU/e) with professor B. van Rietbergen and summarizes our investigations about the estimation of the pull-out strength of an implant inserted in a vertebra using the FE method.

The book conclusions and its original contributions are stated in chapter 6.

Finally, the future work are presented in chapter 7.

1.4   Bone tissue

Bone tissue is the main component of vertebrates skeleton. Its functions include: to support body weight and daily loadings, to protect vital organs, to provide sites for tendons and muscles attachment, store ions like calcium and phosphorus and to trap dangerous materials such as lead [14, 15]. Bone is considered a great biomaterial: its microstructure is optimized as a function of its location and boundary conditions which makes it a high strength but lightweight material. It adapts to the external load history (following the so-called Wolff's law) and self-repairs. Bone adapts to high loads adding material while it is removed in low loaded locations. At the organ level, bones can be categorized as long, flat, short or irregular bones.

From a material point of view, bone is considered as a porous, heterogeneous, composite material made up of organic and inorganic constituents [10]. Specifically, the inorganic part consists of a mineral phase, which is mostly hydroxyapatite, and water, while the organic matrix is mainly composed by collagen, proteoglycans and a low percentage of noncollagenous proteins [14, 16]. The inorganic components provide compression stiffness and strength, whereas the organic components are responsible for the tension properties. Bone composition varies with species, age, sex, location and disease [16].

Depending on the degree of porosity and density, we distinguish between cortical bone (also called compact bone, high density and low porosity, 5-10%) and cancellous bone (also called spongy bone, low density and high porosity, 50-90%). Cortical bone is the main component of the skeleton with around

80% in weight of the total and it can be found at the cortex of bones, while cancellous bone is found near the joints and inside vertebrae. Cancellous bone has a higher surface area to volume ratio than cortical bone, which makes it more suitable for metabolic activities. Thus, cancellous bone is highly vascular and contains red and yellow marrow. The combination of compact and spongy bones forms a sandwich structure, which has optimal structural properties. Fig. 1.1, shows a micro-CT image of a long bone (human femur) where cortical bone, cancellous bone, bone marrow and medullary cavity are pointed out.

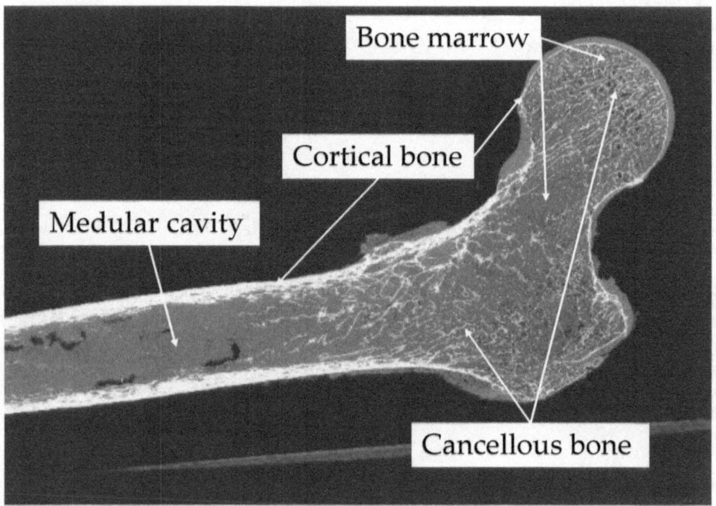

Figure 1.1: Long bone micro-CT image of 60 μm resolution representing cancellous bone, cortical bone, bone marrow and medullary cavity. Original picture, CENIEH, Burgos, Spain.

At the microscale, cancellous bone is composed of a combination of plates and rods that forms its microarchitecture [10, 17, 18]. Fig. 1.2 shows images taken using Field Emission Scanning Electron Microscopy (FESEM) of a porcine vertebral cancellous bone, where rod like and plate like structures may be seen. Changes in the amount of plates and rods produce changes on the mechanical performance of cancellous bone tissue, due to bone adaptation, remodeling or damage events. A highly loaded area will result in a dense plate-like structure, whereas low loading conditions (as in case of astronauts) will result in bone resorption, producing a rod-like structure.

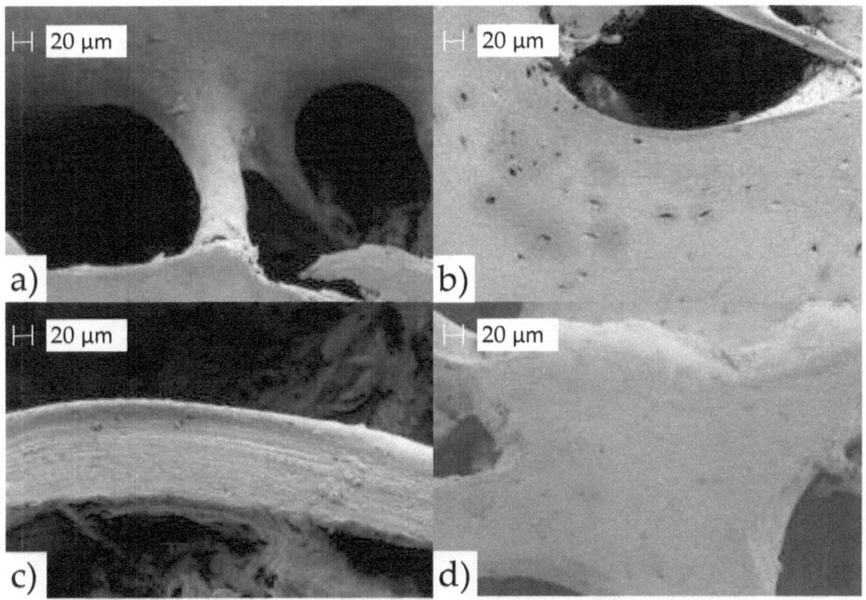

Figure 1.2: Field Emission Scanning Electron Microscopy (FESEM) images of a cancellous bone specimen obtained in this book: a) rod like trabeculae, b) cancellous bone microporosity (lacunae), c) lamellar distribution and d) plate like structure. Original pictures, UPV microscopy service.

The microstructure of a porcine vertebral cancellous bone specimen is presented (Fig. 1.3). The images were taken using a petrographic microscope (Microphot, Nikon, UPV microscopy service). A preferred trabecular orientation is depicted with connecting transversal rods, resulting from bone adaptation, which optimizes its microarchitecture depending on the external loads. The individual structures could be defined as double tapered struts and curved plates aligned to the main loading direction. Some level of ice can also be found, due to an incomplete specimen thawing.

Bone has a highly hierarchical structure that makes it necessary to study its different length scales in order to get knowledge about how each one affects to the next level [14, 15, 19]. Fig. 1.4, presents a hierarchical description of different scales of bone tissue from [15]. The number of hierarchical levels is user-dependent, as stated by Currey [19], but usually it varies from 4 to 7 levels. In this explanation, we will consider the work of Rho JY et al. [15], where the authors account for 5 hierarchical levels, presented in Fig. 1.4: (1) macrostructure (cortical and cancellous bone can be distinguished), (2) microstructure (10-500 μm, Haversian system in compact bone and trabeculae in cancellous bone), (3) sub-microstructure (lamellae), (4) nanostructure (mineral embedded in fibrillar collagen) and (5) sub-nanostructure (organic and inorganic components).

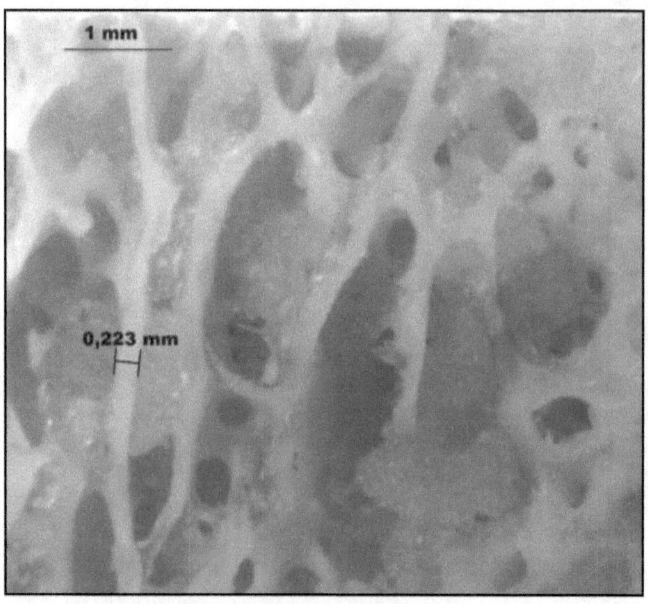

Figure 1.3: Detail of a porcine vertebral cancellous bone specimen acquired using a petrographic microscope (Fig. 1.5 a) marking the thickness of a trabecula. Due to the incomplete thawing of specimens, some ice can be distinguished. Original picture, UPV microscopy service.

At the microstructure, the Haversian system is the basic unit of cortical bone, which is composed by cylindrical arrangement of lamellar tissue around the Haversian canals, forming the so-called osteon, which is surrounded by a weak interface named cement line. In case of cancellous bone, the main structure at this scale is the trabeculae, which is also composed of lamellar tissue, but its distribution is different than in cortical bone, because of its higher porosity. We obtained images of cancellous bone plates and rods and cancellous bone tissue lamellar arrangement organization of a porcine vertebral cancellous bone specimen using Field Emission Scanning Electron Microscopy (FESEM) technology (ZEISS ULTRA 55 model, EHT=3.00 kV, ESB Grid=800 V, UPV Microscopy Service (Fig. 1.5 b)). Fig. 1.2 shows some of the images acquired, where different cancellous bone structures can be distinguished: rod like structure a), plate like structures b,d) and lamellar arrangement aligned to the microstructure c). Further, cancellous bone microporosity (the so-called lacunae) and some microcracks can be found.

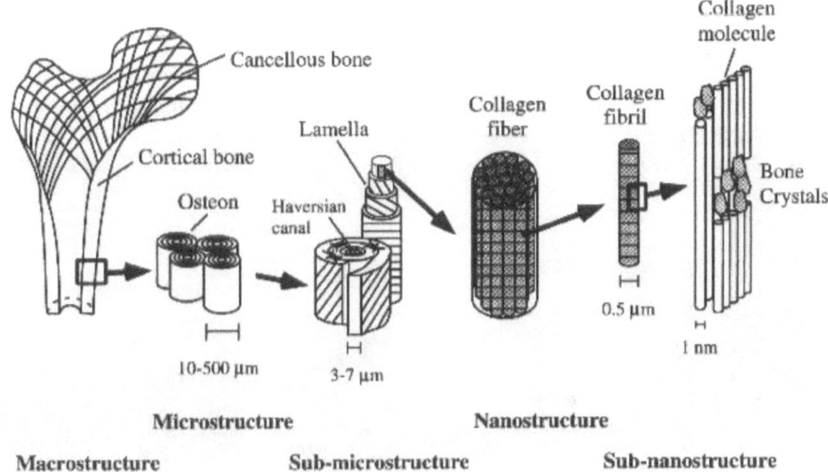

Figure 1.4: Hierarchical structure of bone from macro to sub-nano length scales, from [15].

At a lower level (sub-microstructure) lamellae (3-7 μm thick) are the basic units and they are composed of arrays of mineralized collagen fibrils. The arrangement of collagen fibers differs between cancellous and cortical cases. In case of osteons, the orientation of the lamellae is rotated forming a plywood-like structure [20]. In case of trabeculae, the arrangement orientation seems to differ across its thickness.

A recent study of Georgiadis et al. [21], presents an investigation of the 3D ultrastructure organization in relation to local trabecular direction using 3D scanning small-angle X-ray scattering (sSAXS). They analyzed single trabeculae from human vertebral cancellous bone with different structure types and directions from 4 different subjects. Their results are presented as a function of the distance to trabecular surface. Their results state that bone ultrastructure is mostly aligned to trabecular microstructure near trabecular surface. However, when going towards trabecular core, the ultrastructure alignment decreases to around 40%. Georgiadis et al. [21] hypothesize that it may be result from the highly optimized bone structure, because the cortex of the trabeculae suffer from greater tensile stresses, needing a more oriented ultrastructure. From our point of view, the more oriented ultrastructure near specimen surface results from the plain stress state (2D) at the surface, while at the core of the trabeculae a more complex 3D stress state occurs.

At nanostructural scale, bone is composed of mineralized collagen fibrils (type-I), which are a periodic arrangement of tropocollagen molecules and hydroxyapatite minerals that constitute, together with other noncollagenous proteins and water, the sub-nano scale.

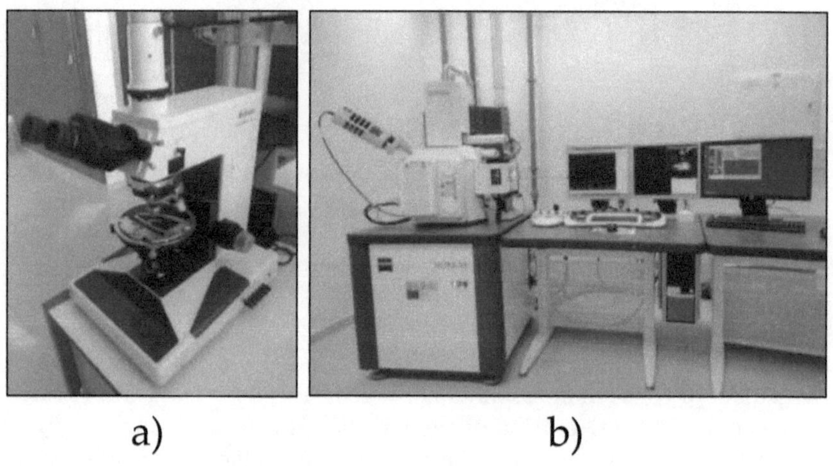

Figure 1.5: Petrographic microscope a) and Field Emission Scanning Electron Microscope used to obtain Figs. 1.3 and 1.2 from the microscopy service at the Universitat Politècnica de València (UPV).

1.5 State of the art: cancellous bone characterization

The review of the state of the art about cancellous bone characterization is accomplished in this section. It is divided in the following topics, which are investigated in this book:

- Mechanical behavior of cancellous bone.

- Experimental tests.

- Elastic properties estimation.

- Failure of cancellous bone.

- Strength properties estimation.

- Bone imaging and segmentation.

- Morphometric characterization.

- Numerical modeling of cancellous bone tissue.

- Cancellous bone surrogates.

- Pull-out strength of an implant inserted in a vertebra.

1.5.1 Mechanical behavior of cancellous bone

Cancellous bone is a porous, heterogeneous, anisotropic and composite material, whose properties are highly influenced by its hierarchical structure. Before failure, bone behaves as a viscoelastic material, that may be considered elastic at low strain rates. The viscous response results from the fluids in bone matrix, which cause the loss of some elastic energy during deformation [22].

In quasi-static analysis, a perfectly elastic behavior is assumed until the yield point [23, 24], which defines a boundary from where permanent damage occur. Therefore, deformations are reversible within the elastic domain and until the yield point. The elastic domain is characterized by the slope of the force-displacement response, the so-called rigidity or stiffness, which is also directly related to as the relationship between the stress and strain: the elastic modulus. At the apparent level, it is influenced by the tissue material elastic properties (Young's modulus), density and microarchitecture.

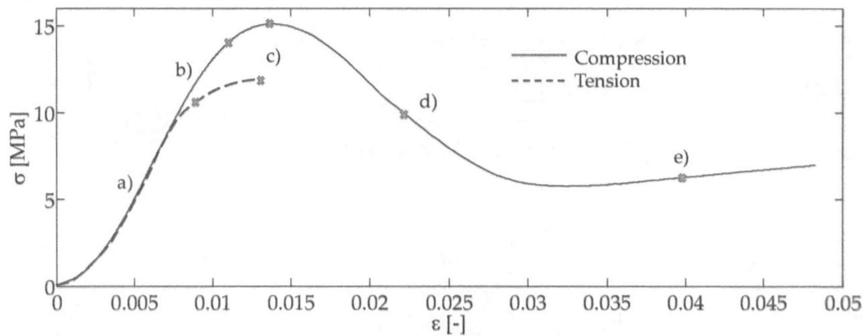

Figure 1.6: Axial mechanical behavior of cancellous bone under quasi-static tension and compression conditions. a) A linear response with reversible deformations is expected until b) the yield point. Lower yielding values occur for tension, with a more brittle response than in compression. c) The ultimate point is defined as the maximum stress, which is followed, in compression, by d) a material softening and e) densification. Original contribution.

From that point, post-yielding behavior is considered, diffuse microcracks appear in the so-called elastic-continuum damage mechanics domain, followed by the fracture mechanics domain, where fracture surfaces are developed if load continues [25]. Under tensile loads, cancellous bone behaves more brittle and yields and fractures at a lower stress level [10, 26], Fig 1.6. Under compression conditions, its response is more ductile and the material at the fractured areas tend to densify until it starts to re-carrying load, in the so-called post-yielding (or plastic domain). Fig. 1.6 depicts the different phases of cancellous bone mechanical behavior at low strain rates in axial direction.

The strain rate affects to cancellous bone stiffness and strength properties [27, 28]. Higher stiffness, yielding and ultimate stresses result from higher strain rates due to cancellous bone viscoelasticity, but no significant dependence is reported regarding yielding and ultimate strains [27, 28].

Cancellous bone presents time-dependent failure behavior [10]. Creep deformation produces permanent deformation in bone due to sustained load, and varies with loading type and local mechanical properties [29, 30]. It is characterized by three stages: in the first one, creep rate decreases and some relaxation occurs, the secondary creep is characterized by a steady state creep rate, while the last one is associated to increasing creep rate and damage accumulation that produces failure if load is sustained [29]. Furthermore, it is considered that creep contributes to damage accumulation in fatigue loading [31].

Cancellous bone cyclic loading results in stiffness loss, attributed to microcracking at different length scales [22], and accumulation of creep deformation [10]. Non-traumatic vertebral failure is believed to depend on damage accumulation due to cyclic loading [32]. Three regions can be distinguished in cancellous bone fatigue behavior: the first one is characterized by a rapid loss of stiffness and the formation of microcracks, which tend to appear localized rather than spread and for a low number of cycles [33]. In the second region, toughening mechanisms like bridging, crack deflection or plasticity increase fatigue life, while microcracks grow without significant loss of stiffness. Finally, in the third region, the coalescence of cracks produce a rapid decrease of stiffness resulting in bone fracture. Furthermore, it has been reported that fatigue failure mechanisms occur at the ultrastructure rather than at higher scales, leading to similar fatigue strain accumulation between locations [34]. Due to bone remodeling, it can be considered that fatigue life measured through cyclic testing is a lower bound of its real value [10].

Cancellous bone anisotropy results both from its architecture and ultrastructural organization. Several works have addressed the study of anisotropy, which varies upon location because it is influenced by bone adaptation to external loads [14]. Keaveny et al. [10] proposed the term strength-to-anisotropy ratio (SAR) and showed that strength was different depending on the loading direction. This was observed for axial and shearing loading modes. Strength properties asymmetry are reported under tension-compression conditions, with higher values for the latter one [10].

On the other hand, hydration plays an important role on bone mechanical properties. A dried sample presents higher modulus and strength than a wet one, but its toughness decreases. So, dried bone absorbs less strain energy and is more brittle than wet bone [22].

In the following sections, the concepts introduced here will be further developed. First, we will present experimental techniques used to characterize the mechanical behavior of cancellous bone. We will review elastic properties reported in the literature and, then, we will present the failure mechanisms of bone at its hierarchical structure and the estimation of its failure properties.

1.5.2 Experimental tests

Testing cancellous bone specimens provides valuable information about its mechanical properties under different loading conditions at each length scale. The determination of those mechanical properties defines bone integrity as a function of age, disease or pharmacological treatment [35]. We will first review the importance of the length scale of analysis and the most common techniques used at each scale. Then, we will describe the preparation of cancellous bone specimens and its storage and, finally, we will present different testing techniques and their applications.

Bone tissue mechanical properties depend on composition, structural, microstructural and nanostructural organization [36] so, depending on the length scale of testing, the highly hierarchical structure of bone conditions both the type of testing and its outcome [35]. We can distinguish between testing at the organ level, mesoscale, microscale or nanoscale. At the organ level and the mesoscale, the most commonly used experimental tests are axial, bending or torsion in either monotonic or cyclic loading. Besides, fracture toughness tests are used to measure the resistance to fracture through the introduction of a sharp notch on the sample [35]. At the organ level, the experiments are influenced by the geometry of the sample and its composition. Each bone is usually tested according to its *in vivo* loading conditions: for example, vertebral bodies are tested under compression, whereas long bones are tested under bending or axial conditions.

Testing bone at the mesoscale (cortical or cancellous) includes the contribution of microarchitecture, density and bone volume fraction [35]. Quasi-static tests are the most common in the literature and characterize the apparent modulus, yield and ultimate stresses and strains and work of fracture. Regarding fatigue testing, stress amplitude to cycles to failure (S-N) or crack growth resistance (R) curves are used to define the fatigue strength.

At the micro level, testing single trabeculae or micro-indentation tests have been reported. Testing single trabeculae provides local failure information [37], which is more difficult to assess at other scales of analysis. Micro-indentation provides tissue hardness and modulus, through measuring the contact area after the indentation and calculating the slope of the indentation curve, respectively [35].

At the nanoscale, nanoindentation, atomic force microscopy and scratch testing are the most common techniques. Nanoindentation gives information about hardness and elastic modulus in lamellar and interlamellar regions, while scratch testing is used to measure *in situ* toughness [35].

Sample preparation has a major importance on the measurements. In whole bone testing, it usually implies the elimination of other tissues than bone and, depending on the testing conditions, keeping it moist or dried. We will focus on the preparation of cancellous bone samples to be tested at the mesoscale, because of the book framework. In the literature, some works deal with the preparation and storage of cancellous bone samples [36, 38, 39, 40, 41]. In some cases, cylindrical-shaped specimens are prepared, extracted using a trephine, to test them along its principal or transversal directions [41, 42, 43, 44, 45]. In other cases, parallelepiped-shaped samples are machined using precision band saws, aiming to test the samples along their three main directions [46, 47, 48, 49]. Bone marrow is often eliminated using an ultrasonic bath or by water jet, and the samples are dried or kept moist using saline solution. Some works report the assessment of the bone volume fraction using Archimedes principle, to use it as a criterion parameter to segment the subsequent micro-CT images [40, 50].

Storage influences the mechanical properties measured [38, 39]. Linde and Sorensen[39] analyzed the effect of different storage methods: ethanol or freezing at -20°C. The elastic properties of the samples were not significantly affected even for 100 days stored [38, 39]. Further thawing and refreezing neither produced significant changes in the elastic properties [38]. However, the viscoelastic properties show small but significant variation after the 100 days storage in ethanol or frozen [39].

Axial testing, under compression or tension conditions, has been used to characterize cancellous bone anisotropic and asymmetric behavior [10, 14]. Tensile tests imply griping the specimens, which is susceptible to induce damage, but embedding the sample end-caps minimize this undesirable effect [26]. Compression testing is the most common experimental procedure to estimate bone mechanical properties due to its simplicity in contrast to other experiments [22]. Those properties represent the overall behavior of the sample, but do not reflect the local inhomogeneities present in cancellous bone [51], which act as strain concentrators and are responsible of failure initiation. Some conditions must be fulfilled in order to minimize experimental artifacts that may affect the measurements, which will be discussed in the following.

Some years ago, there was some controversy about the elastic response of cancellous bone under compression. Some works reported a toe region (see Fig. 1.6) in the initial response, which they assumed to correspond to a real nonlinear behavior [52]. However, it was then identified as an experimental artifact and a fully linear behavior was observed, with equal tensile and compressive apparent modulus [23]. This experimental artifacts were defined as side-artifacts result from damaging specimens during machining, which produce a disruption on the trabecular connectivity [23, 43, 53, 54]. The effect of side-artifacts on the underestimation of the Young's modulus was quantified to be over 50 %, with a mean value of 27 %, by comparing parametric simulations, considering varying volume of analysis size, and compression testing results [53]. Indeed, these side-artifacts are higher for low bone volume fraction samples and also affect to yield strength estimation about 20 to 32 % [55].

In order to minimize those artifacts, some procedures were proposed, like embedding the ends of the samples in PMMA, increasing the aspect ratio of the samples, lubricating the platens to reduce friction at the sample-platens interface or performing preconditioning cycles [30, 23, 52, 56]. Preconditioning cycles to up to 0.5 % apparent strain do not produce modulus degradation [52, 56, 57]

Other experimental artifacts are related to the parallelism of opposite faces [22]. If this condition is not properly fulfilled, high stressed regions at the contact between compression platen and specimen may produce the fracture of the sample in that part. The use of a pivoting compression platen has been proposed to solve this problem [22].

Generally, quasi-static tests are performed, which aim to estimate the elastic properties at the apparent or tissue level. Dynamic tests have been used to determine the effect of increasing strain rate [27, 28] or to assess fatigue properties [33, 32].

Microindentation has been used to assess directional elastic properties [58], which permitted to draw some conclusions about cancellous bone elastic properties for different locations, ages, genders and directions. For example, a higher modulus (between 5 to 12 %) was found at the core than at the cortex of a trabecula. In addition, the axial direction presented higher values than the transversal (between 18 to 27 % higher). It is interesting to remark that no statistical differences were found regarding age or gender, which highlights that the loss of macroscopic mechanical competence due to age is factor of changes in the microarchitecture rather than decreasing material properties [58].

Nanoindentation is a technique that permits the estimation of the elastic modulus and hardness in surface layers with a depth indentation reduced to the submicron range [36]. Hardness is estimated by measuring the contact area for the maximum applied load, while the elastic modulus is measured from the unloading region of the load-displacement curve and using the relationship between contact stiffness and elastic modulus presented in Eq. 1.1 [36]. In Eq. 1.1, other assumptions like elasticity with time-independent plasticity constitutive behavior or known Poisson's ratio are needed.

$$\frac{\mathrm{d}P}{\mathrm{d}h} = \beta \frac{2}{\sqrt{\pi}} \sqrt{A} E_{\mathrm{r}} \tag{1.1}$$

where β is the indenter shape factor, P is the applied load, h, the depth of indentation, A is the contact area and E_{r} is the reduced modulus, defined in Eq. 1.2, which depends on the elastic modulus and the Poisson's ratio of the sample and the indenter (E_{s}, ν_{s}, E_{i}, ν_{i}, respectively).

$$\frac{1}{E_{\mathrm{r}}} = \frac{(1 - \nu_{\mathrm{s}})^2}{E_{\mathrm{s}}} + \frac{(1 - \nu_{\mathrm{i}})^2}{E_{\mathrm{i}}} \tag{1.2}$$

Zysset et al. [36] found a correlation between the elastic modulus and hardness in human femur, both in cortical and cancellous bone. The authors measured lower values for cancellous than for cortical bone, as depicted in Fig. 1.7, which contradicted the assumption that both are made of the same tissue. Indeed, the authors explained those results because of the differences on the canalicular porosity, mineralization and orientation of the collagen distribution between the bone types [36].

Norman et al. [59] developed an interesting work about nanoindentation on human cancellous bone from the intertrochanteric region to investigate micromechanical properties from different spicules of different donors. They found elastic modulus and hardness variations within a single spicule revealing higher values in the inner part compared to outer areas (14.22 and 12.25 GPa regarding elastic modulus and 0.9 and 0.68 GPa in hardness). They attribute the measurement variations to differences in composition, mineral and collagen, and the arrangement of bone ultrastructure. As the rate of turnover within remodeling is greater at the surfaces, the results reported

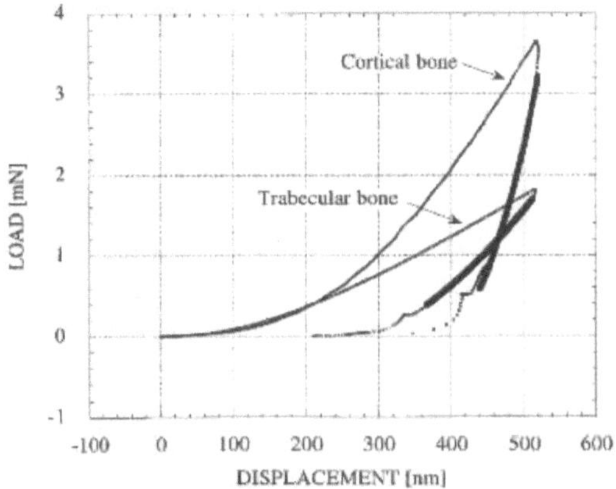

Figure 1.7: Load-displacement curve from nanoindentation tests in cortical and trabecular human femoral bone. The elastic modulus is measured in the unloading part of the test (taken from [36]).

are in line with those observations. Further, the authors give an explanation based on bone adaptation to loading: lamellae near the surface are subjected to greater strains due to bending, so more remodeling occurs in there. Those variations could also be functional, because those high strained areas near the surfaces of lower elastic properties imply less brittle behavior, so it would increase fracture toughness [59].

On the other hand, some of the aforementioned testing techniques can be used in combination with imaging techniques, such as micro-computed tomography (micro-CT) or taking photographs during the experiment. This combination gives insight into local situations that, without them, cannot be measured and may be used to validate fracture models experimentally, which has not been fully solved in the literature. For example, taking photographs or performing micro-CT during testing (and applying digital volume correlation technique (DVC)) provides information about how bone deforms or breaks locally. Nevertheless, visual inspections of the images have not enough accuracy, while micro-CT involves high economic and time costs and must be applied only under quasi-static conditions. However, the application of digital image correlation (DIC) to images acquired during testing is a rapid and cheap solution that makes it possible to estimate strains and deformation mechanisms at lower scales than the test one.

To measure displacements in biological materials, the most common techniques are displacement gauges (for example to measure displacements between compression platens), loading platen transducers, extensometers attached to specimens, strain gauges or optical systems [22]. Digital image correlation (DIC), as an optical technique, has some advantages over the other mentioned options. To begin with, it is a non-contact technique, so it avoids any damage induced to specimens due to measurement system attachment. In addition, DIC measures the local displacement at the specimen's surface, which avoids compliance effects related to other measurement systems. In case of cancellous bone, its microstructure may act itself as the pattern of reference (instead of speckle) which is used to estimate displacement fields [51].

Since DIC was introduced in the 80s [60, 61], the accuracy of the method has been notably improved [62, 63], which has promoted an increasing use in many applications to measure displacements in a wide range of materials. A thorough review of DIC biomechanical applications, potential and limitations was published recently by Palanca et al [64]. Some works have used DIC to further characterize fracture at the organ level [65, 66, 67]. However, little work has been done about its application to study cancellous bone failure onset and propagation.

One limitation of DIC method is that it only provides surface measurements, so if failure does not occur on the visible surface the method is not capable to properly characterize it. However, an averaging of what happens at the subsurfaces along specimen thickness is performed, but it does not permit to distinguish the fractured areas at those subsurfaces clearly [51]. This limitation motivated the use of DVC, which permit to scan by micro-CT a sample during quasi-static testing but, as mentioned, can be used only under quasi-static conditions.

Ultrasonic tests permit to calculate the elastic modulus from the measurement of the velocity of sound waves through an specimen of known density [22]. Depending on the transducer vibration direction with respect to the ultrasound wave propagation, longitudinal or shear waves are produced, which permit the calculation of both longitudinal (E) and shear (G) modulus, using Eqs. 1.3 and 1.4:

$$E = \rho v^2 \tag{1.3}$$

$$G = \rho v_s^2 \tag{1.4}$$

Ultrasonic tests permit multiple non-destructive measurements and are relatively cheap, so constitute a reliable tool to estimate elastic properties. However, strength cannot be measured directly and must be inferred using regressions to the elastic properties [22].

1.5.3   Elastic properties of cancellous bone

The estimation of the elastic properties of cancellous bone a has major importance to determine its mechanical competence and for detailed mechanical analysis of bone, bone healing or bone-implant interaction. Among the elastic properties, we consider the apparent Young's modulus, E_{app}, and the tissue-level Young's modulus, E. The first is related to the stiffness at the macro level, while the second is the elastic modulus at the microscale, the trabecular level. Both parameters are related, because tissue-level Young's modulus with combination of the lattice architecture conditions the apparent stiffness.

In the previous section, we reviewed testing procedures for cancellous bone and its applications. In this section, elastic properties of cancellous bone from different species (but focused on humans), locations and methodologies are reported. Table 1.1 summarizes apparent elastic properties of human cancellous bone from different locations reported in the literature, measured along the main trabecular orientation direction. Commonly, the apparent properties are assessed from axial testing under quasi-static conditions. In some cases, the experiments are combined with the use of optical extensometers, finite elements or nanoindentation. For example, Odgaard and Linde [54] compared the estimations from compression testing and the use of an optical extensometer and obtained higher values for the latter method, which results from lower displacement measurement. On the other hand, Chevalier et al. [40] compared the performance of compression tests and a combination of micro-CT based finite element models whose properties were defined from nanoindentation. The authors obtained similar estimations but the FE models tended to overestimate the elastic modulus.

The apparent modulus values reported in the literature present a wide scattering, because they depend on specimen conditions and location, see Table 1.1. Most of the measurements reported in Table 1.1 correspond to experiments under wet conditions and no obvious distinction can be done comparing to the dry ones. Theoretically, higher modulus values would be expected from the measurements under dry conditions [22].

Li and Aspden [68] reported metrics from osteoarthritic, normal and osteoporotic cancellous bone and, as expected, higher values were obtained for the osteoarthritic, followed by the normal and osteoporotic samples. Among elastic modulus reports, higher values were found for the femoral specimens, while the lowest values were found for vertebral samples. For any comparison, it is important to refer the results to the volume fraction or apparent density of the samples, because it strongly influences the apparent properties [10, 14]. The low value reported by [46] is due to the low value of the bone volume fraction of the samples analyzed (between 6.8 to 10.4 %). This tendency is observed also in the values reported by Morgan and Keaveny [45] for different locations: the lowest apparent density was found for the vertebral specimens, which correlates to the apparent modulus, while the highest was found for the femoral neck, that presents the highest modulus values.

Table 1.1: Elastic apparent modulus (E_{app}) values reported in the literature for cancellous bone from different testing methods, loading modes, species and sites. Mean and standard deviation values are presented when reported.

E_{app} [MPa]	Test method	Specie	Site	Conditions	Ref.
1538 ± 674	Compression	Human*	Femoral head	Wet	[42]
3230 ± 936	Compression	Human	Femoral neck	Wet	[45]
2700 ± 772	Tension				
356		Human**			
310	Compression	Human***	Femoral head	Wet	[68]
247		Human*			
1359.6 ± 1135.7	Compression	Human	Femur	Dry	[40]
1493.7 ± 1226.4	Nanoindentation - FE				
622 ± 302	Compression	Human	Trochanter	Wet	[45]
597 ± 330	Tension				
344 ± 148	Compression	Human	Vertebra	Wet	[45]
349 ± 133	Tension				
99 ± 38.5	Compression	Human	Vertebra	Wet	[46]
276	Tension	Human	Vertebra	Wet	[41]
231	Compression				
1091 ± 634	Compression	Human	Tibia	Wet	[45]
1068 ± 840	Tension				
428 ± 227.8	Compression	Human	Tibia	Dry	[43]
689 ± 438	Compression	Human	Tibia	Wet	[54]
871 ± 581	Optical extensometer				

* Osteoporotic.
** Osteoarthritis.
*** Normal.

A recent review of Young's modulus of trabecular bone at the tissue level by Wu et al. [69], described different methods used for that purpose and summarizes the estimations sorted by methods. They distinguished between:

micro-mechanical testing of single trabeculae, ultrasonic testing, nanoindentation and combination of macro-level mechanical testing and numerical models based on μCT images. In their review, Wu et al. [69] reported tissue elastic modulus ranging between 1.2 to 22.3 GPa, but few of the references are close to the lower bound.

Table 1.2: Elastic modulus at the tissue level (E) reported in the literature for cancellous bone from different testing methods, loading modes, species and sites. Mean and standard deviation values are presented.

Tissue level Young's modulus (E) [GPa]	Test method	Specie	Site	Conditions	Ref.
14.22 ± 1.07 12.25 ± 1.01	Nanoindentation	Human	Femur (inner trabeculae) Femur (outer trabeculae)	Dry	[59]
11.4 ± 5.6	Nanoindentation	Human	Femoral neck	Wet	[36]
13.5 ± 2.0	Nanoindentation	Human	Vertebra	Dry	[70]
20.95 ± 2.1	Nanoindentation	Human	Femur	Dry	[40]
11.31-15.80	Microindentation	Human	Vertebra	Dry	[58]
12.18 ± 0.8	Attenuation coefficient SR-μCT	Human	Femoral neck	Wet	[71]
18.8 ± 5.2	Compression - FE	Human*	Femoral head	Wet	[42]
18.0 ± 2.8	Compression - FE	Human	Femoral neck	Wet	[50]
6.6 ± 1.07	Compression - FE	Human	Vertebra	Wet	[46]
5.6 ± 0.2	Compression - FE	Whale	Vertebra	Wet	[47]
12.59 ± 2.13	Compression - FE	Human	Femur	-	[44]
18.7 ± 3.4	Axial - FE	Bovine	Tibia	-	[72]
16.24 ± 2.47 16.85 ± 2.1	Tension	Human** Human*	Femur	Dry	[73]
10.4 ± 3.5 14.8 ± 1.4	Microtensile Ultrasound	Human	Tibia	Dry	[74]
2.0 ± 1.0	3-point bending	Bovine	Femur	Wet	[37]
10.09 ± 2.42 11.38 ± 1.42	3-point bending	Human** Human*	Femur	Dry	[73]

* Osteoporotic.

** Normal.

Table 1.2 presents Young's modulus at the tissue level reported in the literature, for different locations, conditions and methods. In our review, the mean values range between 2 to 20.95 GPa, so a wide scattering is also found. We report values from nanoindentation, microindentation, density-based measurements, combination of compression testing and finite element modeling, tension tests, ultrasound and bending testing.

Using nanoindentation, the values range between 11 to 21 GPa and lower metrics are found for wet conditions for the same location (11.4 GPa in contrast to 14 or 21 GPa). On the other hand, the combination of compression testing and image-based FE presents elastic modulus values from 5.6 to 19 GPa. Some authors claim that this methodology tends to underestimate the values because compression testing sometimes involves the presence of side artifacts, but some works have addressed this problem to minimize its effects [52, 30, 56]. Nevertheless, this combination of testing and high resolution imaging permits not only to estimate the elastic properties at the tissue level, but also to analyze stresses and strains locally.

Testing single trabeculae also permits to study local effects, but it involves the difficulty of avoiding damage due to gripping in tension tests, compliance effects during testing or an accurate estimation of the cross-sectional area [22]. In case of ultrasonic tests, a value of around 15 GPa is reported in [74], which is in the upper range of the nanoindentation and compression-FE methodologies. However, the presence of voids tends to attenuate the ultrasonic waves, which makes the application of this technique more complex [69].

1.5.4 Failure of cancellous bone: yielding and post-yielding

Bones are loaded during daily activities. If loads are high enough, bone failure may occur. It is said that bone fragility is related to the unbalance between damage accumulation and remodeling [75]. Failure occurs at each length scale of the hierarchical bone structure and it is claimed that the primary inelastic bone deformation happens near the nanoscale [76]. Trabecular bone strength properties are heterogeneous, anisotropic and asymmetric. Thus, they vary with age, location and depending on the loading direction and mode (tension-compression-shearing) [10]. Regarding the loading mode, larger strength values are found for compression, followed by tension and shearing [10, 26].

In the late 80's, Gibson [17] used simplified trabecular configurations to describe cancellous bone compression failure modes: elastic buckling or plastic hinges. The authors related the failure mechanism to the slenderness or the apparent density: buckling would occur at low apparent densities whereas plastic hinges would happen for high density values.

Zioupos [77] analyzed the different phases of the mechanical behavior of bone in compression (elastic, damage and fracture mechanics) and reviewed approaches to determine the parameters that better characterize each phase. After the elastic response, the author identified the damage mechanics phase, were he postulated that the reduced stiffness within this phase was a consequence of the development of microcracks, and pointed out the importance of toughening mechanisms at each length scale for a biological material. On the other hand, Zioupos identified the fracture mechanics phase and discussed approaches reported in the literature to estimate fracture parameters, and also identified crack deflection and bridging as mechanisms to resist fracture in that phase.

More recently, Launey et al. [76] reviewed the toughening mechanisms of bone at different scales in a very interesting work, which is really valuable to understand how bone breaks (or resists to fracture). They describe fracture as a balance between loads that increase fracture surfaces and intrinsic damage mechanisms ahead the crack tip and extrinsic shielding mechanisms behind the crack tip. Fig 1.8 presents extrinsic and intrinsic bone toughening mechanisms at different length scales which are actually the failure mechanisms contributing to increase fracture resistance. Extrinsic mechanisms are related to crack deflection and bridging and affect to scales ≥ 1 μm, while intrinsic mechanisms are related to plasticity and affect to scales < 1 μm. At the

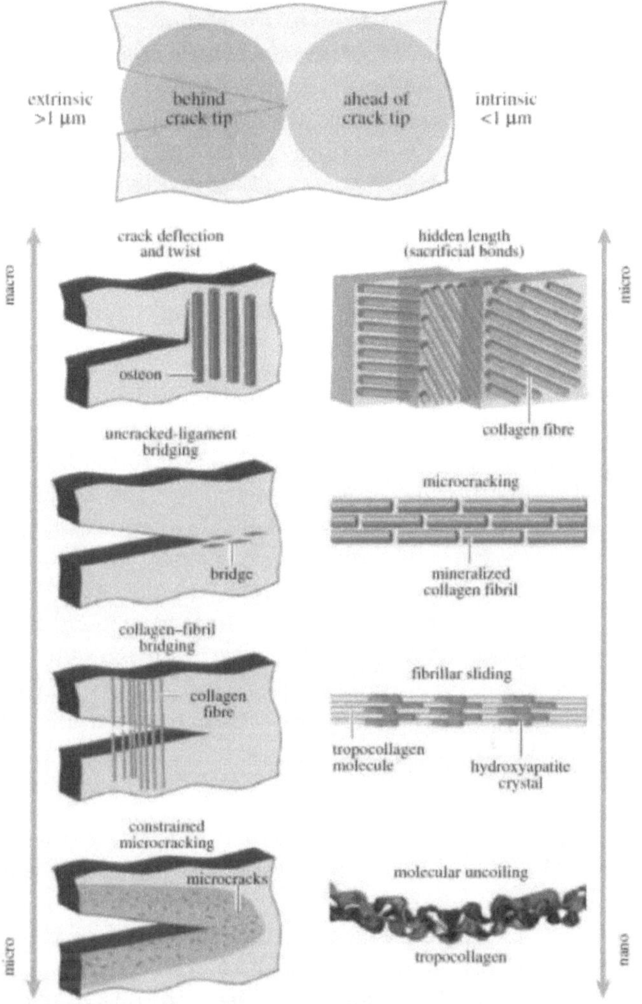

Figure 1.8: Toughening mechanisms of bone at different length scales from [76]. The left side of the figure represents extrinsic shielding mechanisms which occur at higher length scales, while the right side shows intrinsic mechanisms that act at lower length scales.

molecular level (see Fig. 1.8), the basic deformation mechanism of collagen is molecular uncoiling, which results from hydrogen bond breakage. This process also happens in collagen fibrils, where the amount of cross-links determines the ability to dissipate energy: the larger the cross-link density, the more brittle, so it is a factor related to increased fracture risk in elderly population. At the next level, the mineralized collagen fibrils slide as a failure mechanism, where the mineral phase increases the stiffness and energy dissipation. At the micro level, and as a bond between intrinsic and extrinsic toughening mechanisms, microcracking acts as an inelastic deformation but also as crack bridging and deflection mechanism. From micro to macroscale (see Fig. 1.8), the toughening mechanisms are crack deflection and bridging, whose effects have been further studied on osteonal systems rather than on cancellous bone.

Despite all this complexity, bone failure mechanism may be simple. Failure strains are almost independent of specimen density and are relatively constant (for a certain location, age, direction and mode) [10]. Specifically, failure strain shows a low but increasing linear relation to the apparent density in compression, which vanishes in tension [26]. In contrast, Bayraktar et al. [50] observed no dependence of both compressive and tensile yield strains on the apparent density and apparent modulus. On the other hand, a strong linear correlation (other authors report a power law) is found between elastic modulus and yield stress [10, 26, 72, 78]. As strain is stress to modulus ratio for an elastic material under uniaxial loading, this suggests that failure strains are relatively constant. Furthermore, yield strain is isotropic for cancellous bone [10]. This yield strain behavior suggests that bone failure is controlled by strains.

Failure in cancellous bone is more localized in fracture bands rather than generalized [76, 79, 80], see Fig. 1.9 and 1.11. This failure behavior makes bone even a more interesting material, because it tends to concentrate damage (or complete fractures if loading continues increasing) in controlled areas, so remodeling is optimized in there. In that sense, remodeling has been hypothesized to be induced by damage mechanisms due to changes in bone ultrastructure [10, 14, 26].

Failure in cancellous bone has been studied mostly under uniaxial loading conditions, due to its simplicity compared to the multiaxial case. Damage affects the apparent elastic properties of trabecular bone by decreasing them and can propagate if overloaded, increasing fracture risk [79, 81]. Damage affects bone ultrastructure and it has been also hypothesized that disruptions in the canaliculi network may be the stimulus of bone remodeling [79]. It has been observed that damage shows a strong dependence on the applied strain (the greater the applied strain, the more damage [57]), and lower but significant dependence on the loading mode and direction [82]. However, damage cannot be detected in clinical radiography [82].

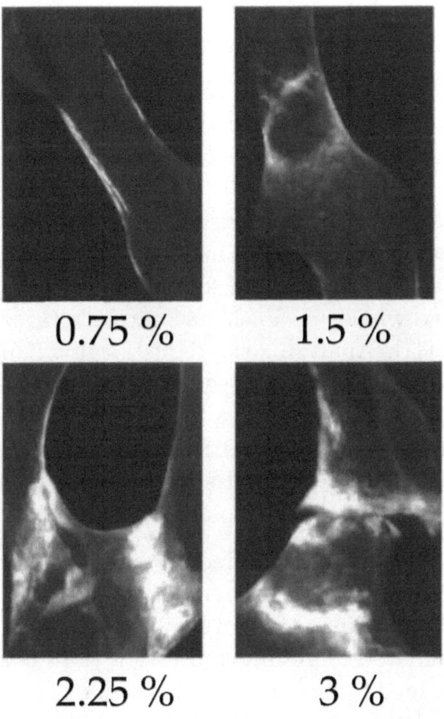

Figure 1.9: Failure histological labeling at different apparent strains, which reveal a transition in failure behavior from short cracks at low apparent strains to multiple microcracks (observed as diffuse damage) and complete fracture as the apparent strain increases. The picture was taken from [75].

Kopperdahl and Keaveny [26] analyzed damage under uniaxial compression and proposed an apparent density threshold transition from compressive yielding to buckling (as the main compressive failure mechanisms), although both mechanisms may co-exist. Buckling dominant failure occurs if its critical stress is lower than the ultimate compressive strength, which occurs for a 0.4 gcm^{-3} apparent density. That density matches the plate to rod-like transition reported in [17].

Nagaraja et al. [79] characterized damage accumulation in bovine cancellous samples under stress relaxation and observed failure localized in bands, while damage depended on the strain level. The development of residual strains under static conditions associated to microdamage may be a reason of increased fracture risk in aged population.

Lambers et al. [41] studied the influence of the loading mode and microstructure on damage accumulation in human vertebral cancellous bone. The authors found greater damage accumulation in tension (3.9% of the total bone volume) than in compression (1.9 %). The asymmetric microdamage behavior may be explained because in tension, tissue fails due to tensile principal strains, which in case of compression involves also compressive yielding, and lower yielding properties are reported for tension mode. Microdamage accumulation and average whole specimen microarchitectural parameters showed subtle relationships [41]. Analyzing the tissue locally, Lambers et al. [41] observed microdamage occurring at trabeculae of thickness greater than average sample values, in contrast to what may be expected, which was explained as follows: thin trabeculae are subjected to unidirectional stresses, while thick trabeculae undergo a more multiaxial stress. This fact suggests that microdamage may occur predominantly in plate-like trabeculae [41].

Wolfram et al. [82] observed different damage accumulation in human vertebral trabecular bone, as a function of loading mode and direction. In case of transverse direction loading, damage accumulation was lower than for axial direction and accumulated more in compression than tension loading modes. The latter, was explained by the amount of bending trabeculae in compression compared to tension loading mode. Further, they found differences of around 5 % between yield strains in compression ($\varepsilon_c^y = 0.0081$) and tension ($\varepsilon_t^y = 0.0072$).

In Hernandez et al. [83], strength and stiffness properties are related to the presence of microdamage under a single compressive overload and subsequent testing. Damage volume fraction was correlated to elastic modulus and yield strength reduction, which had been reported previously in [82]. Furthermore, the authors found that, even for a small fraction of damaged bone volume

($> 1\%$), the modulus reduction ranged [30 - 60 %]. The initial and reload elastic modulus, yield and ultimate strength showed linear correlation to bone volume fraction.

To be able to validate the failure models proposed in the literature, failure detection methodologies are necessary. Damage has been usually detected analyzing histological sections in which staining had been previously applied [57, 75, 41]. However, it is a high time consuming and destructive technique, which has motivated several authors to explore other methodologies. Scanning electron microscopy (SEM) is also commonly used to visualize failure at high magnification [80, 14, 17], so it permits to distinguish microcracks and also different toughening mechanisms, but it only permits to analyze surfaces and very local areas. Other techniques permit to analyze failure on larger areas or even in whole specimens, but obviously, with a lower resolution than SEM. For example, Nagaraja [75] studied microdamage under uniaxial testing conditions by micro-CT, imaged based FEM and histological damage labeling. The authors tested uniaxially cylindrical samples with reduced central region and scanned them at different apparent strain levels, giving insight into the existence of different failure modes depending on the applied strain, see Fig. 1.9. As the apparent strain increases, failure changes from short linear cracks at trabecular surface ($\varepsilon_{app} = 0.75\%$) to long cracks and diffuse damage localized in shear bands ($\varepsilon_{app} = 1.5 - 3\%$). Further, the authors report microdamage initiation strains in the range of [0.0046-0.0063] in compression and [0.0018-0.0024] in tension, calculated from FE analyses.

Some years ago, Nazarian and Müller [84] developed an imaging system that allowed to test a specimen while scanning, which helped to reveal fracture initiation and progression. The authors performed uniaxial compression tests on vertebral whale specimens and micro-CT was applied at each increment load. Their time-lapsed failure imaging showed that failure occurred localized in shear bands, while the remaining structure seemed to not being affected. Within the failure area, trabeculae failed by bending (buckling) followed by a complete fracture [84].

On the other hand, Wang et al. [81] proposed a methodology to detect microdamage using micro-CT, which consisted of labeling the specimens with barium sulfate ($BaSO_4$), which attenuates X-rays more than bone tissue. Then, the images were segmented and microdamage was accurately detected (see Fig. 1.10). However, the technique is not capable of detecting individual cracks, which are visible at higher resolutions [81].

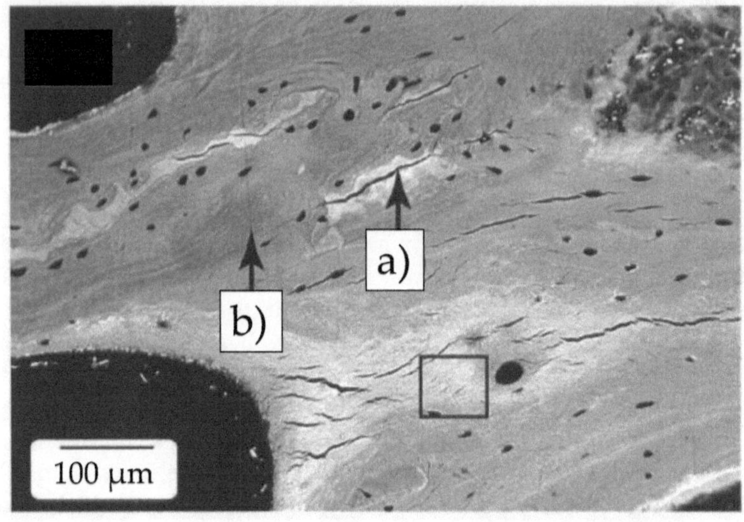

Figure 1.10: SEM image of damaged cancellous bone where microcracks are visible and surrounded by bright intensities due to $BaSO_4$ contrast labeling. In micro-CT images, the microcracks are not visible but the brighter intensities can be thresholded to distinguish damaged areas. Image taken from [81].

Other works have studied the stress whitening effect, which was linked to damage in cancellous bone [24, 37, 80]. Thurner et al. [80] showed that using high-speed photography with high magnification on yielded trabeculae presented whitening, which increased with loading. The authors confirmed damage presence in the whitened areas using SEM, which revealed delamination, numerous microcracks and the concentration of damage in fracture bands, while other trabeculae remained undamaged even for high apparent strains, see Fig. 1.11. Moreover, they succeeded on correlating the whitening effect to microdamage, which appeared far below the apparent yielding point [80]. Time after, Jungmann et al. [37] combined the stress whitening effect from Thurner et al. [80] with digital image correlation (DIC), to estimate local strains, failure onset and fracture strains in single trabeculae submitted to three-point bending tests. The average yield strain was $1 \pm 0.5\%$ while complete failure average strain was $8 \pm 5\%$. Those yielding values estimated through DIC were in the upper bound of values reported in the literature, compared to other methodologies, which may be attributable to lower resolution of DIC compared to FEM.

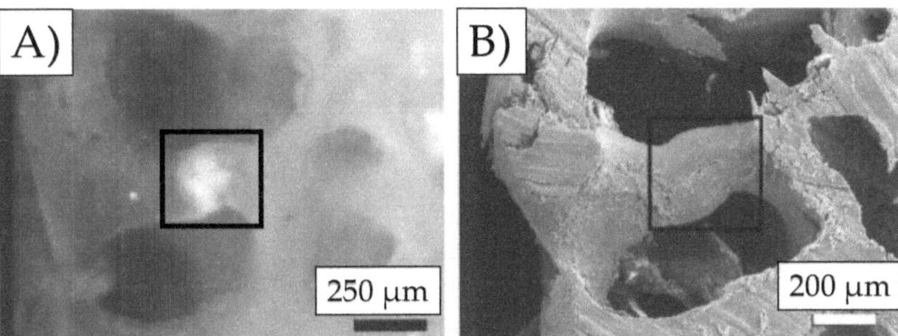

Figure 1.11: Stress whitening effect observed by [80] A) and SEM image of the same trabeculae, where microcracks, delamination and bridging can be distinguished B).

To summarize, bone failure starts by decreasing stiffness within a damage mechanics phase and it is followed by a fracture mechanics phase where fracture surfaces are developed. Failure behavior is conditioned by bone hierarchical microstructure, which provides toughening mechanisms at each length scale: from inelastic deformation resulting from collagen molecules uncoiling or collagen mineralized fibrils gliding at the lower scales, to crack deflection and bridging from micro to macroscales. The deformation mechanisms mentioned occur prior to the apparent yield point and tend to localize failure in the so-called shear bands. Furthermore, the strength properties are heterogeneous, anisotropic and asymmetric. Despite this complexity, yield strains are relatively constant and can be considered isotropic.

1.5.5 Strength properties estimation

The determination of cancellous bone strength properties is clinically important, because they are indicators of bone quality and are necessary to develop numerical models that permit to simulate multiple situations, like implant design and validation, multiaxial loading or disease treatment evaluation. Simulations involve much less costs than experiments, permit to simulate destructive situations and make it possible to model complex loading configurations that are too complicated to be carried out experimentally. In failure modeling, it is important to define appropriate properties according to the failure mode [85]: strength for static failure, fracture toughness for crack growth studies and fatigue strength for fatigue failure. In this book, quasi-static situations are considered, so we focus this review on bone strength properties.

Traditionally, strength properties are assessed through experiments [14], aiming at estimating the apparent strength properties [26, 45] or properties at the microscale, through testing individual trabeculae [24, 37, 73]. The 0.2 % offset method is the most widely used to determine the yield point from experiments, while the fracture point is defined as the maximum stress value within the stress-strain curve. On the other hand, other authors have combined experiments with digital image correlation, to estimate yield properties at the trabecular tissue level [24, 73, 75]. Based on experimental results, many works have attempted to find regressions to estimate strength values. For example, a strong linear correlation between elastic modulus and strength has been reported across a range of bone densities [86], while other authors relate strength to density measurements, which at the end is equivalent [10, 26].

Since the introduction of great advantages in imaging techniques, image-based finite element models have been used to estimate strength properties at different length scales [37, 50, 73, 75]. Those highly discretized models accounting for specimen microstructure permit to estimate local stresses and strains to reproduce trabecular failure at the microscale and also to simulate specimen apparent level yielding and post-yielding [72, 87]. Some of the finite element models have included asymmetric strength properties and non-linear behavior to find tissue yield properties [50, 72]. Further, FE models serve for validating failure parameter values reported in the literature or from own experiments [24].

Commonly, an inverse analysis criterion is used to find the failure properties to be used in finite element models, that is, a parameter calibration that makes the model match the experimental data [37, 73]. The calibration sometimes depends on a single parameter [44], that usually is the yield strain or stress, while other constitutive models need for more parameter calibration [73].

Table 1.3: Failure strains and stresses measurements at the macro (apparent) level reported in the literature, resuming the estimation method, loading mode, species and site.

ε_y [%]	σ_y [MPa]	ε_u [%]	σ_u [MPa]	Method	Loading mode	Species and site	Ref.
0.73	1.48	-	-	0.2 %	Tension	Human -	[41]
0.75	1.19	-	-		Compression	vertebra	
0.81	-	2.5	-	0.2 %	Compression	Human -	[82]
0.72	-	1.57	-		Tension	vertebra	
0.81	-	-	-	0.2 % -	Compression	Human -	[88]
0.33	-	-	-	FE	Tension	1*	
0.77	2.02	-	-		Compression	Human -	
0.70	1.72	-	-		Tension	Vertebra	
0.73	5.83	-	-		Compression	Human -	
0.65	4.50	-	-	0.2 %	Tension	Tibia	[45]
0.70	3.21	-	-		Compression	Human -	
0.61	2.44	-	-		Tension	Trochanter	
0.85	17.45	-	-		Compression	Human -	
0.61	10.93	-	-		Tension	Femur Neck	
0.88	14.37	-	-	0.2 %	Tension	Bovine -	[87]
1.17	21.09	-	-		Compression	Tibia	
0.62	84.9	-	-	0.2 %	Tension	Human -	[50]
1.04	135.3	-	-		Compression	Femur	
0.78	1.75	1.59	2.23	0.2 %	Tension	Human -	[26]
0.84	1.92	1.45	2.23		Compression	Vertebrae	
0.78	14.36	-	-	0.2 % -	Tension	Bovine -	[72]
1.08	20.62	-	-	FE	Compression	Tibia	
0.69	1.1	1.29	1.29	0.2 %	Compression	Human - Vertebrae	[83]
3.01	14.957	3.695	16.113	0.2 %	Compression	Whale - Vertebrae	[84]

1* The study was carried out on different locations: femur, tibia and vertebra.

An interesting contribution from Carretta et al. [73] provided tissue-level failure properties for healthy and osteoporotic human femoral cancellous bone, through single trabeculae testing under tensile and bending conditions, combined with sample imaging and FE analysis. The authors pointed out the difficulties to assess tissue failure properties through testing whole specimens, in contrast to single trabeculae testing, and the importance of the availability of properties at the microscale to be used in simulations. In [73], the volume analyzed is of the order of the element size commonly used in the simulations, so the data set may be meaningful for that purpose.

Bevill et al. [88] used a combination of testing and finite element modeling to analyze the influence of including large deformations on the estimation of the apparent yield values. They concluded that, for low volume fraction samples (<0.2), the effect is quite significant, but vanishes for increasing apparent densities.

Table 1.3 presents failure strains and stresses measurements at the apparent level from the literature, while table 1.4 reports tissue level failure strains and stresses estimations. The tables include yield strains (ε_y) and stresses (σ_y), ultimate strains (ε_u) and stresses (σ_u) values for cancellous bone reported in the literature, including the species, location, calculation method, loading direction, loading mode and reference.

Table 1.4: Failure strains and stresses measurements at the micro or tissue level reported in the literature, including the estimation method, loading mode, specie and site.

ε_y [%]	σ_y [MPa]	ε_u [%]	σ_u [MPa]	Method	Loading mode	Specie and Site	Ref.
0.46-0.63	88-121	-	-	FE	Compression	Bovine -	[75]
0.18-0.24	35-43	-	-		Tension	Tibia	
1.6	-	12	-	σ whitening & DIC	3-point bending[2*]	Bovine - Femur	[37]
0.72	115.43	5.14	166.89	Single trabeculae testing	Tension	Human[3*] -	[73]
1.45	138.67	8.2	204.98		3-p bending	Femur	
0.77	130.28	2.4	164.71		Tension	Human[4*] -	
1.21	135.98	6.01	208.62		3-p bending	Femur	
0.6	-	-	-	FE - testing	Tension	Bovine -	[72]
1.01	-	-	-		Compression	Tibia	
0.41	82.8	-	-	FE - testing	Tension	Human -	[50]
0.83	133.6	-	-		Compression	Femur	

2* Yielding estimation in tension area.
3* Healthy donors.
4* Osteoporotic donors.

The apparent level yield values in Table 1.3 were measured using the 0.2% offset method and, in some cases, combined FE analysis to validate the metrics. As discussed in section 1.5.4, the yield stress values show wide scattering because they depend on the apparent density and the elastic modulus, while yield strains remain almost constant for a certain location, loading mode and direction. Furthermore, higher yield strain values are reported for compression compared to tension values, which take a value for human vertebrae between 0.69 to 0.84 % for compression and between 0.7 to 0.78 % in tension. Bovine tibia and whale vertebrae values are significantly larger than human ones, see Table 1.3. Regarding ultimate strain values, most of the works did not focus on them, but the reported values for human vertebral tissues ranges [1.29-2.5] % in compression and around 1.58 % in tension.

On the other hand, the yield values at the tissue level, given in Table 1.4, were estimated from an inverse calibration of numerical models to match tests, single trabeculae testing or a combination of stress whitening and digital image correlation. The latter method provided the highest values and may be the least accurate. Lower yield strain values were estimated for the tissue than for the apparent level and the combination of a high discretization and testing reveals a good performance on the estimation of failure properties at the microscale.

Other authors have proposed alternative parameters to evaluate the quality of trabecular bone. For example, Roque et al. [89] proposed a mechanical competence parameter (MCP) that included the influence of bone volume fraction, elasticity modulus, connectivity and tortuosity. They used data from micro-CT scanned specimens which were simulated using finite elements to obtain the apparent modulus. A principal competence analysis was performed, which allowed to find MPC. Then, it was applied to both healthy and osteoporotic samples and confirmed that MPC was able to distinguish between groups, so it may be used to determine bone quality. More recently, Filletti and Roque [90] pointed out the time consuming methodology to calculate MPC from image analysis and simulations and proposed an alternative method based on data analysis, using a neural network approach.

1.5.6 Cancellous bone imaging and segmentation

Cancellous bone microarchitecture is a 3D lattice naturally optimized for the applied loads. However, before advances in imaging techniques, its structure was traditionally analyzed studying sections by histomorphometry [91, 92]. Through section analysis, its microstructure was visible and it was presented as a non-repetitive complex structure. Some authors made efforts trying to simplify its structure in their models [17, 18, 93] but the improvements on the non-destructive imaging systems allowed to visualize cancellous microstructure in 3 dimensions at a high resolution.

Analyzing cancellous bone by imaging has some issues to take into account: imaging system, resolution and segmentation. Regarding imaging systems, their physical working principles condition the resulting images, together with the parameters used for scanning. On the other hand, resolution has major importance on the detection and definition of structures at low length scales, while segmentation is critical, because it influences both the estimation of microstructural characteristics and the numerical models developed from the segmented masks.

1.5.6.1 Imaging systems

The high radiation absorption of calcified tissues allows X-ray based systems such as computed tomography (CT) or micro-computed tomography (micro-CT) to present bone tissue at a high sensitivity [8, 12]. In case of other techniques like magnetic resonance imaging (MRI), bone is presented with background intensities due to its working principle: it consists of measuring relaxation times after inducing a magnetic field that changes material spin orientation and, in case of Calcium, the even number of protons and neutrons does not produce magnetic resonance signal because of its lack of spin-angular momentum [6].

Depending on its applicability to clinical practice, bone imaging systems can be divided according to the radiation dose induced to the specimen. For example, MRI does not induce radiation on the specimen, low radiation dose systems are CT, QCT, high-resolution peripheral quantitative tomography (HR-pQCT) or multi-row-detector computed tomography (MDCT), while micro-CT, induces high radiation doses (in general) which are not permissible in clinical practice.

In this book, we use X-ray micro computed tomography (micro-CT or μCT) to scan bone samples, attempting to describe its microstructure with high accuracy (between 13 to 24 μm isotropic resolution). Choosing a high radiation imaging system like micro-CT is justified because of its great per-formance in terms of resolution and contrast achieved for bone. Micro-CT working principle is based on the attenuation of X-rays across the sample scanned, see fig. 1.12. The attenuation of an X-ray beam at a certain distance (x), follows Eq. 1.5, where I_0 is the incident intensity and μ is the attenuation coefficient.

$$I_x = I_0 e^{-\mu x} \tag{1.5}$$

X-rays are emitted from the tube, then are attenuated by crossing the material and finally recorded by the detector. The sample is rotated and the process is repeated after each rotation. Then, the projections are computed to reconstruct the 3D structure scanned. In addition, it is common to use calibration phantoms which permit to relate the attenuation coefficient of micro-CT images to material density. Those phantoms are scanned using the same imaging parameters because, as mentioned above, the image intensity values are dependent on them. The use of calibration phantoms permits to define material properties of the numerical models based on its density, which will be further discussed in section 2.3.

The first use of micro-CT to study cancellous bone was carried out by Feldkamp et al. [12]. The imaging system used was originally designed for defects detection in ceramic materials. Feldkamp et al. [12] stated the procedure to scan and reconstruct images by micro-CT and highlighted the importance of performing image corrections for the 3D reconstruction and in order to measure the attenuation coefficient (μ) with accuracy. They also warned about beam hardening image artifacts and propose corrections for this effect. They achieved a spatial resolution of 70 μm and claimed that lower resolution was possible by improving the detector system and decreasing specimen-X-ray source distance. Their subsequent objective was to evaluate the 3D structure of bone, which was traditionally carried out on 2D histological sections, and they focused on the connectivity and anisotropy analysis, which are true 3D characteristics.

From that time, micro-CT has become a standard tool to analyze cancellous bone microstructure, disease progression and healing, and to generate preclinical models. A recent article from Boerckel et al. [94] reviews applications of this technique in bioengineering, specifically for bone tissue, cartilage and cardiovascular structures, and also presents novel approaches, like phase-contrast micro-CT, which will constitute great advances in micro-CT imaging in the near future.

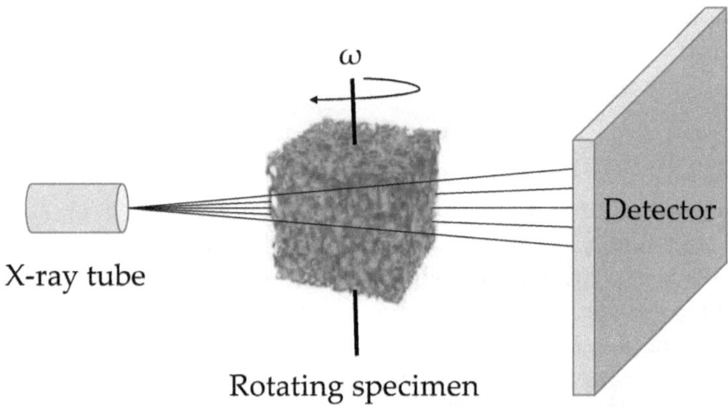

Figure 1.12: Micro-computed tomography working principle: X-rays passing through the sample are attenuated and recorded by the detector. The specimen rotates at a low velocity and a projection is recorded for each rotation angle. Then, those projections are used to reconstruct the images that represent the 3D structure.

1.5.6.2   Image artifacts

Image artifacts are a potential problem that may happen when using imaging systems. Image artifacts can be defined as any discrepancy between imaging reconstruction and material density and geometry expectations [95]. Image artifacts may degrade image quality, which may affect diagnosis or metrics measurements. They usually follow a pattern of bright or dark shadows, rings or distortion and can be categorized as a function of its source: physics-based, patient-based, scanner-based and image reconstruction artifacts [96]. Fig. 1.13 shows some image artifacts: beam hardening, specimen movement artifacts and materials with high differences between absorption coefficients.

Within physics-based artifacts, beam hardening is the most common one, and may be briefly explained as follows: An X-ray beam is composed of pho-

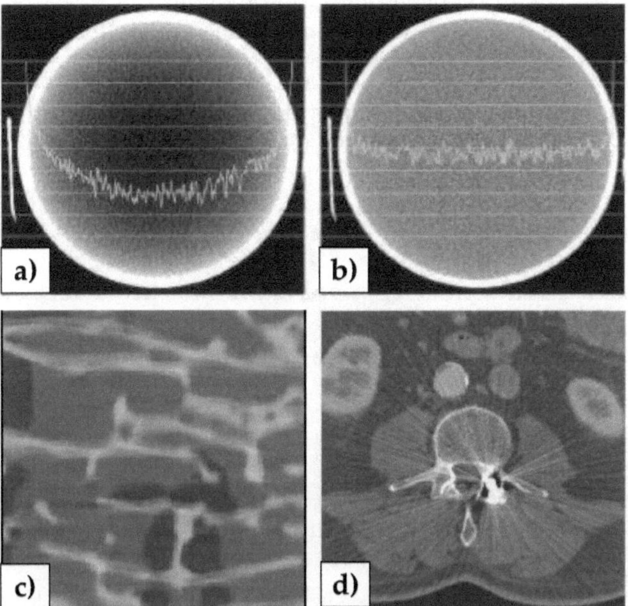

Figure 1.13: Examples of image artifacts: beam hardening together with a representation of the attenuation coefficient (in yellow) in an homogeneous phantom a) and its correction using filtering b), image artifacts due to small movements of specimen c) and image artifacts resulting from the presence of a metallic material. Images a), b) and d) taken from [96].

tons with a range of energies. As the beam crosses a material, the lower-energy photons are absorbed and the mean energy of the beam is increased, which may influence density measurements and morphometric parameters estimation [95]. This effect is seen in cupping artifacts (in a homogeneous material with non-uniform shape, the X-rays in areas of higher thickness are hardened more than in areas of lower thickness) and in streaks and dark bands (it happens at heterogeneous materials with different densities). Beam hardening artifacts are minimized using filters that attenuate the lower-energy components of the beam, or calibration corrections with phantoms. Meganck et al. [95] studied the influence of beam hardening correction using filters to reduce cupping artifacts, aiming to have accurate measurements of bone mineral density. They claim that using filters attenuates beam hardening and provides, together with the use of calibration phantoms, accurate mineral density measurements. However, too much filtering increases noise, decreasing image contrast [95].

Other physics-based artifacts are partial volume, resulting from an off-centered specimen, and photon starvation, which occur in highly attenuating zones (for example, high thickness areas).

Within patient-based artifacts, we may distinguish between specimen motion and metallic materials. Specimen motion is more common in CT acquisitions, but can occur also in micro-CT when a frozen specimen did not thaw completely or if it is not properly gripped. On the other hand, ring artifacts lie on scanner-based category and consist of circular pattern artifacts. However, it can be avoided by re-calibrating the X-ray detector [96].

1.5.6.3 Image segmentation

Image segmentation may be defined as the process through which an image, or set of images, is divided into parts. In case of cancellous bone segmentation, it implies a simple differentiation between bone and background. Segmentation is very susceptible to image features and imaging system. In micro-CT, due to the high differences between the absorption coefficients of bone and surrounding tissues, its segmentation is relatively straightforward. In the literature, several segmentation methods are found, used alone or combined: thresholding, active contours or region growing. However, cancellous bone segmentation problem is usually solved by thresholding, which consist of choosing a gray level intensity (or a range of intensities), corresponding to bone tissue. Often, methodologies include also image pre-processing by means of applying a smoothing filter. Thresholding segmentation techniques differ from each other by how the threshold is chosen: manually, based on density measurement or automatically. Manual procedures are based on image visual inspection, density-based on the use of calibration phantoms during sample imaging, while automatic segmentation depend on the analysis of image features.

Global threshold may be the most used method to segment cancellous bone, due to its simplicity and high performance [12, 13, 41, 95]. It consist of choosing a gray level which separates bone tissue from other tissues. However, a fixed-global threshold may result in loss of thin trabeculae and oversizing thick trabeculae.

On the other hand, adaptive thresholding requires different thresholds for each image or neighborhood. It requires some form of manual intervention, more parameters than global thresholding and it is usually slower. The choice of the local threshold varies between methodologies: intensity gradients or local intensity distribution among them [97].

Among automatic thresholding, Otsu [98] proposed a non-parametric automatic threshold selection method. The method accounts for two (or more) classes within the grayscale of the image and calculates the optimum threshold that minimizes the intra-class variance. Other automatic thresholding techniques have been proposed and evaluated [99].

Other techniques, not based on image thresholding, like active contours or region growing have been also applied to cancellous bone segmentation [100]. Active contours is an iterative method that needs for an initial contour, which evolves through the iterations minimizing a functional that includes internal (contour) and external (image) energies. The method depends on several parameters that define how the contours can evolve and how image features affect them. This method has some disadvantages: it requires several parameters and local functional minimums may condition the solution.

Region growing technique is another iterative method that adds pixels from a seed point if accomplish the criterion chosen, that usually is related to a distance from the seed point and to the difference between its intensity and a threshold. As an iterative method, it is slower than the other methods mentioned and it also depends on the initial seed point.

Some works in the literature have compared segmentation methods. Gómez et al. [99] reviewed segmentation methodologies applied in the literature to cancellous bone and compared different automatic global thresholding approaches. Further, they proposed a simple method to adapt them locally. A recent work of Tassani et al. [100] compares three commonly used segmentation methods (global thresholding, Otsu and active contours) of bone micro-CT images. Their results show that global thresholding and active contours give better accuracy than Otsu's method, with errors larger than 20 % compared to histological images manual segmentation. Furthermore, the low number of parameters of global thresholding compared to active contours and the difficulty to assess them make the first method more suitable to be used as a standard.

1.5.7 Morphometric characterization

The term morphometry refers to measurements of shape and size. Traditionally, when applied to bone tissue, it was commonly called bone histomorphometry, and implied the preparation of histological sections which were analyzed under a microscope. In earlier studies, when there was not consensus about cancellous bone architecture, morphometric measurements allowed to distinguish between different plate- and rod-like structures [101]. Singh [101] analyzed a large number of human bones, pointing the dependence of the microarchitecture on bone location. By that time, the analysis were performed from 2D and 3D measurements, like anisotropy or connectivity, were inferred using principles from stereology [91]. However, those estimations were not fully compatible with the inherent 3D structure of cancellous bone [12]. In 1987, the American Society for Bone and Mineral Research (ASBMR) created an expert committee to standardize the definition, nomenclature and units of bone histomorphometry, to make the communications about this topic more understandable, published in [102].

The advances in bone imaging provide the researchers with of 3D images that quantify bone shape and size and evaluate bone state, pathologies or treatments. In cancellous bone analysis, it is accepted that not only is density important, but also it is architecture [8, 10, 11, 47, 92]. Therefore, many efforts have been made in the literature to find parameters that better describe changes in cancellous microarchitecture, to relate them to pathologies like osteoporosis, or to elucidate how they affect to the mechanical competence of a cancellous bone-like structure.

The most used parameters to characterize cancellous microstructure are volume fraction (BV/TV), surface area to volume ratio (BS/BV), mean trabecular thickness (Tb.Th), mean trabecular separation (Tb.Sp), degree of anisotropy or orientation (DA), fractal dimension (D) and connectivity (Conn). Aiming to explain the variation of the mechanical properties that are not related to bone mineral density, Ulrich et al. [8] explored linear multivariate relationships between mechanical properties derived from finite element simulations and morphometric parameters, such as BV/TV, BS/TV, Tb.Th, Tb.Sp, Tb.N and DA. They concluded that the predictions improved from a correlation coefficient of 53 % to about 90 % when including further parameters than BV/TV. However, the authors pointed out that the regressions obtained did not work for other data sets from different locations, so there is a need for further studies [8].

Similarly, Nazarian et al. [103] evaluated BV/TV ability to describe mechanical properties variations related to osteoporotic and metastatic cancer specimens, which revealed that the amount of bone is sufficient to predict load capacity changes regardless affection. They distinguished between healthy and osteoporotic cancellous bone according to BMD, but it produced an overlapping regarding BV/TV between both groups. This suggests that BMD is not enough to discern between healthy and osteoporotic bone [103].

The degree of orientation, also known as material anisotropy, is fundamental for the characterization of heterogeneous materials. Bone adaptation to external loads conditions the presence of preferred orientations in terms of microarchitecture anisotropy. Within bone histomorphometry, the first study, from Whitehouse [91], was performed in histological sections and introduced the concept of mean intercept length (MIL), which when represented as a polar plot generates an ellipse in 2D and an ellipsoid in 3D, for materials presenting three symmetry planes. MIL method consists in counting the intersections between a grid of lines and bone interface, as a function of the grid lines orientation. Based on MIL principle, other measurements like volume orientation (VO) or star length distribution (SLD) were derived, represented in Fig. 1.14 [92].

Harrigan and Mann [104] presented the use of a second rank tensor to describe anisotropy degree of orthotropic materials, based on the results of MIL from [91]. In 3D, the MIL produces a set of points defining an ellipsoid of a general expression like Eq. 1.6:

$$Ax_1^2 + Bx_2^2 + Cx_3^2 + Dx_1x_2 + Ex_1x_3 + Fx_2x_3 = 1 \qquad (1.6)$$

Eq. 1.6 may be presented as a tensor in the form of Eq. 1.7:

$$[M] = \begin{bmatrix} A & D & E \\ D & B & F \\ E & F & C \end{bmatrix} \qquad (1.7)$$

The tensorial representation shows interesting properties, like major orientation determination from principal axis analysis, or material anisotropic description, which can be included in material definition.

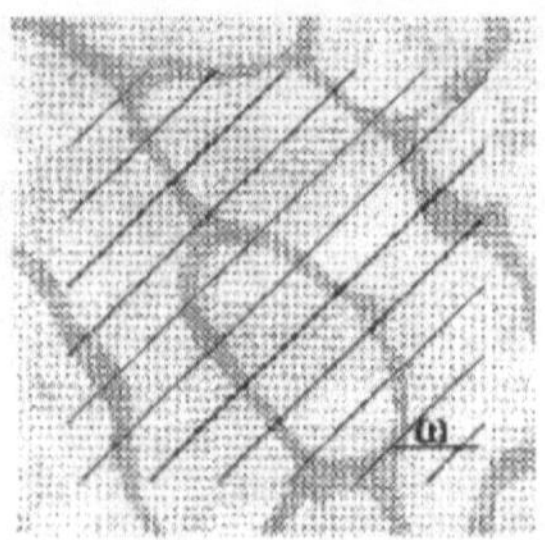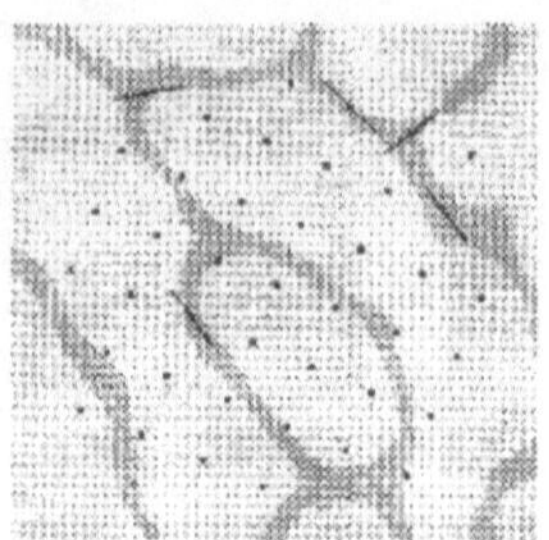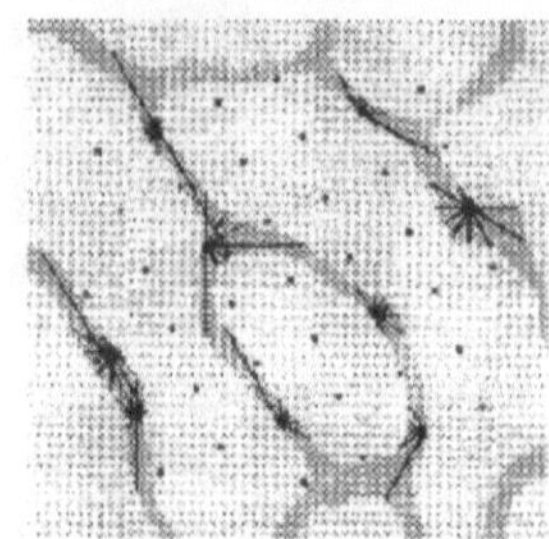

Figure 1.14: Scheme of different methodologies to calculate material orientation (also known as material anisotropy). Mean intercept length (MIL): the number of intersections between a grid of lines and bone is counted for each orientation, producing a polar plot of an ellipse which represents material anisotropy (left). For volume orientation (VO), the orientation of maximum length in bone is calculated at a points grid (middle). Similarly, star length distribution (SLD) applies MIL to a points grid and local orientation distribution is calculated (right). Figure taken from [92].

From that second rank representation, Cowin [105] developed one of the key contributions about morphometry to mechanics relationships in cancellous bone: a generic algebraic relationship between the elasticity tensor of a porous, anisotropic, linear elastic material and its fabric tensor. The relationship derived cannot represent a triclinic material behavior, but at least an orthotropic one, which in the cancellous bone case is a function of its volume fraction and fabric. The relationships reported in [105] were used, combined with fabric and elasticity matrix estimations, to calculate the constants needed in the equations. For example, van Rietbergen et al. [106] determined morpho-mechanic relationships accounting for fabric and bone volume fraction of vertebral whale specimens extracted from a single specimen. The relationships calculated were derived from the work from Cowin [105] and were validated against finite element models developed from high resolution images. A year later, [47] applied the same procedure to human cancellous bone and found high correlations between Cowin's relationships and finite element predictions over a larger range of morphology values.

On the other hand, fractal dimension (D) is used to measure the shape complexity of a structure, that is, how the relationship between the number of characteristics measured at a certain scale changes as we modify the length scale [107]. A fractal is an object with a fractional dimension. For example, if we analyze most planar objects, the number of boxes that cover it if we divide it by 3 would be 3^2. We identify the exponent as the dimension of the object. For fractal geometries, present in nature, that exponent is non-integer. Some authors proposed fractal dimension to define the presence and evolution of cancerous cells [107].

Lopes and Betrouni [108] reviewed methodologies to compute fractal dimension and applications in medicine like brain imaging, mammography or bone analysis. The authors identified fractal characteristics in bone histological sections, like increasing perimeter at higher magnifications, while maintaining its area, or self-similarity. Furthermore, the authors reviewed other works which had found fractal dimension (measured in histological sections) to be able to discriminate between healthy and pathologic cancellous bone.

Among computing methods for fractal dimension, the box-counting method has been extensively used, both in 2 and 3 dimensions [6, 107, 109]. The method consists in dividing the region of interest into boxes of a characteristic length λ and counting the number of boxes needed to fill the whole structure perimeter. Then the procedure is repeated with lower λ values, obtaining a logarithmic relationship, whose slope is the fractal dimension. The method is easy to implement and its extension to 3D is straightforward.

Parkinson and Fazzalari [109] applied fractal principles to evaluate histological sections of trabecular bone and estimated a lower and upper bounds to consider cancellous bone as a fractal (from 25 to 4250 μm). Further, they claimed that sectional fractals, as contrast to single fractal dimension calculated over a whole specimen, could be more easily related to the biology or structure of bone [109].

Another morphometric parameter studied here is connectivity (Conn). Cancellous bone connectivity has attracted attention because it was hypothesized that it has relationships to architectural changes in osteoporosis. Connectivity is a purely 3D characteristic and before the work from Odgaard and Gundersen [110], it was assessed from histological sections. Odgaard and Gundersen [110] proposed a truly 3D procedure based on the Euler characteristic topological invariant. The authors evaluated relationships to other morphometric parameters but they did not found any significant one, so they postulated that connectivity should be considered as an independent parameter.

Later, Kabel et al. [9] evaluated connectivity density itself and in combination with other parameters as a determinant of the mechanical quality of cancellous bone and found that it could only explain very little variance of the stiffness when included in combination with volume fraction. The authors claim that if any relation exists, it would be a negative correlation: stiffness decreases when connectivity density increases [9]. However, Kabel et al. [9] pointed out that connectivity density may have a role to estimate changes in bone properties due to pathologies.

Hildebrand and Rüegsegger [111] proposed a methodology to estimate the mean trabecular thickness (Tb.Th) and separation (Tb.Sp) in 3D images, motivated by the 2D measurements made until that moment, which sometimes included assumptions about the structure type. The procedure proposed in [111] consists in fitting spheres to every point in the bone structure, so local thickness maps are also calculated. The estimation of Tb.Sp is equivalent to Tb.Th but working with the negative of the 3D bone segmented mask.

Some years ago, Doube et al. [112] created an open source application to analyze bone morphometry in 3D, and it is free for anyone to download and use. It facilitates the investigation of bone tissue for free, so authors' altruism must be grateful.

In section 1.5.6, we highlighted the importance of image segmentation on the subsequent morphometric characterization. Following this line, some works in the literature have studied this influence. Hara et al. [113], studied the influence of small threshold variations on the determination of structural and mechanical properties. They pointed out that the influence depends on the volume fraction of the specimen analyzed and the structural parameter. The effect was higher for specimens with low volume fraction (<15%) and for parameters like volume fraction and connectivity, due to the disconnection of trabeculae. On the other hand, Parkinson et al. [114] analyzed the morphometric analysis of cancellous bone performed for different users and by Otsu's algorithm. Their results confirm the importance of defining segmentation criteria that minimize the randomness of user's action. However, the use of an automatic threshold selection (Otsu's method) produced higher differences than the randomness of 3 operators.

On the other hand, it is known that the architectural parameters depend on the bone volume analyzed. Yan et al. [115] addressed the problem of estimating the region of interest dimensions to be representative of the whole structure analyzed. They used 6 human cervical vertebrae and performed a morphometric analysis over 5 architectural parameters (BV/TV, BS/BV, Tb.Th, Tb.N and Tb.Sp) and found trends of their evolution by varying the region of interest size, which were different depending on the morphometric parameter. The authors concluded that, for the samples analyzed, a cubic volume of at least 6 mm side is necessary to be representative of the whole vertebra [115]. However, more robust conclusions would need of the analysis of a wider range of healthy or osteoporotic samples.

1.5.8 Numerical modeling of cancellous bone tissue

Numerical modeling of cancellous bone is an important tool to estimate patient-specific mechanical properties, evaluate disease treatment, implant design, give insight into damage and failure mechanisms at different scales or analyze the influence of microarchitecture on the mechanical competence of the tissue. In contrast to experimental testing, numerical modeling permits to perform multiple simulations either destructive or not, consider complex loading and boundary conditions, evaluate parametric influences or analyze local effects, avoiding the problems related to testing biological materials that suffer from degradation over time and obviously can be only tested destructively once.

1.5.8.1 Simplified parametric models

The complex heterogeneous cancellous bone microstructure have motivated investigations about simplified parametric models. Those models aim at reproducing both the elastic and failure behavior of trabecular tissue whose structure is reduced to depend on a few number of parameters. Finding a base model which can be used as a repetitive structure and reproduce part or the whole mechanical behavior has a great research importance because the influence of variations on the parameters used to construct the model can be isolated from other heterogeneous microstructural characteristics.

The first cancellous bone numerical models described its structure as a periodic repetitive pattern based on simplifications of observations of histological and SEM images [17, 93], see Fig. 1.15. Gibson [17] observed four different structures of cancellous bone as combination of plates and rods configurations and proposed four simplified models: cubic or hexagonal and rod-like or plate-like, respectively. Furthermore, he claimed that the study of the mechanical behavior of cancellous bone can be derived from the mechanisms the wall cell deforms, which actually depend also on its relative density and material properties. The proposed models worked fairly well for different densities and configurations compared to stiffness and strength measurements reported in the literature [17]. Also in 1985, Beaupre and Hayes [93] created an idealized three-dimensional model based on a cubic unit cell containing a spherical centered void to calculate an equivalent homogeneous material that behaved as the simplified model.

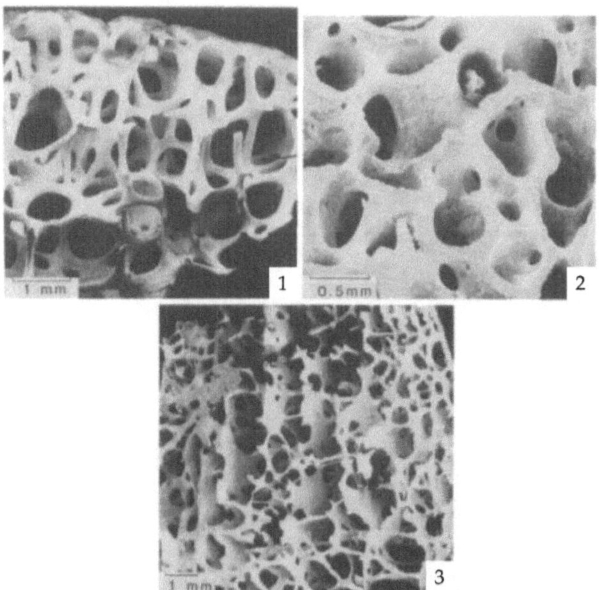

Figure 1.15: Scanning electron micrography of different cancellous bone structure configurations from [17]: Low density cancellous bone with asymmetric rod-like structure 1), high density with asymmetric plate-like structure 2) and plate-like columnar structure 3).

More recently, Kim and Al-Hassani [116] proposed an idealization of vertebral cancellous bone based on observations of microscope images [117], that consisted of an analytical model based on a hexagonal columnar structure with doubly tapered struts (Fig. 1.16 a)). They used the simplified hexagonal model to study the influence of age and gender, based on relationships obtained by Mosekilde [117], on the effective modulus and the collapse stress and compared their results with the obtained using a uniform (non-tapered) model, highlighting the importance of tapered struts on increasing the mechanical competence of the models. However, their comparison lacks of experiments to compare with. On the other hand, Dagan et al. [18] developed a building block of a single trabecula which can be scaled for trabecular thickness and length (Fig. 1.16 b shows a representation of an extension of the building block). The model correlated well with apparent moduli results from osteoporotic bone of human proximal femur.

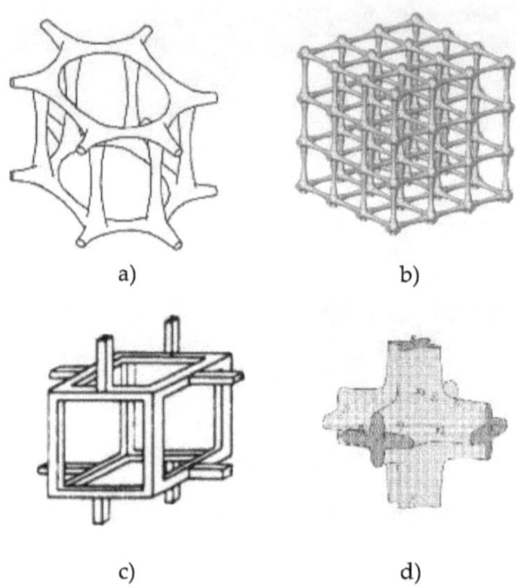

Figure 1.16: Simplified cancellous bone models proposed by other authors in the literature: a) hexagonal based with tapered struts from [116], b) cubic lattice from [18], c) unit cell of idealized periodic model for rod-like cancellous bone from [17] and d) unit cell for a repeatable structure from [118].

Other works [119, 120], used the building block from Dagan et al. [18] to develop their investigations. In [119] the parametric FE model from [18] was modified to include information about the trabecular thickness, separation and BMD from quantitative computed tomography scans. The model was then applied to estimate the stiffness of spine cancellous bone samples extracted from C7 vertebrae of large dogs. Furthermore, they calculated multi variable regressions depending on trabecular thickness, separation and BMD. Then, the authors extended their model to calculate also sample strength by adding an analytical linear relationship obtained by others [120]. The validation of stiffness and strength predictions was performed against uniaxial compression tests on 36 canine and 3 human specimens whose FE input parameters were measured by optical digital microscopy. The accuracy on strength prediction was lower than for the stiffness which can possibly be attributed to the simple analytical expression used for strength estimation. Other authors, like Kowalczyk [118] developed parametric FE models based on cubic or prismatic unit cells (Fig. 1.16 d) to evaluate the complete stiffness matrix of the subsequent orthotropic structures by varying the input morphometric parameters and compared their results with reported values of the literature for real cancellous bone.

To sum up, the first models attempted to describe cancellous bone as a periodic structure based on microscope or SEM observations and incorporating parameters measured on those images. Those studies about simplified parametric models of cancellous bone helped to gain knowledge about the different mechanisms of deformation on cancellous bone structures and were the starting point to develop more precise models.

1.5.8.2   Image-based models

The advances on imaging systems like micro-CT allowed the visualization of cancellous heterogeneous and non-periodic microstructure in conjunction with the estimation of its tissue density [12]. van Rietbergen et al. [48] developed a finite element study explicitly accounting for cancellous bone microstructure based on high-resolution micro-CT images. A new strategy was introduced to directly convert voxels to finite elements, which enabled the estimation of bone elastic properties for different loading cases. In their study, homogeneous material properties were considered, which was stated as a limitation in that moment [48]. Further, they studied the influence of voxel resolution and described that it is more important that the models match the sample's volume fraction rather than the actual voxel size, in the range between 20 to 120 μm. This strategy has motivated numerous studies to develop finite element models based on bone imaging.

However, micro-CT involves high radiation dose in order to achieve high contrast and image resolution, while in vivo imaging systems like HR-pQCT or MDCT permit to work at lower resolutions, between 80 to 168 μm[121, 122]. Therefore, some investigations were focused on the ability of in vivo imaging systems to properly describe cancellous bone microstructure and the performance of the subsequent finite element models to reproduce its mechanical behavior in comparison to micro-CT derived models, which were considered as the reference model [86, 122, 123, 124].

Usually, the highest image resolution available is used for FEM, but sometimes, limitations arise regarding computational costs for large specimens.

Bevill and Keaveny [86] analyzed element sizes ranging from 20 to 120 μm and specimens from different locations and bone volume fractions. The error in yield stress prediction, for different resolutions, depends on the bone volume fraction: coarsened masks with low bone volume fraction have greater relative errors than for higher volume fraction samples [86, 124]. For low density specimens, the element size was more relevant, reporting apparent modulus reduction of up to 41 %, while for higher volume fraction a 10 % reduction was reported [124]. However, in terms of model resolution, 80 μm (clinical resolution) had similar power to detect bone quality than high resolution models of 20 μm [86].

Ulrich et al. [122] studied a wider range of image resolution (between 28 μm to 168 μm resolution) and went a step further by analyzing the influence of meshing techniques on the elastic modulus and von Mises stress estimation. Direct conversion to finite elements was proved against compensated hexahedron and tetrahedron meshes. Compensated hexahedron maintained the BV/TV estimated in the reference model by thickening the trabeculae, as opposite to direct voxel conversion, which showed loss of connectivity due to image coarsening. The meshing technique affects according to the microstructure analyzed: samples of greater trabecular thickness showed minor influence (3 %), which increased up to 40 % for samples of lower BV/TV. In general, lower elastic and von Mises stresses were estimated in the coarse meshes compared to the reference model, which differed up to 40 % in elastic modulus and 46 % in terms of stresses [122].

The prediction of failure load was analyzed by Bauer et al. [123] for artificially coarsened models using Pistoia criterion [125], a linear criterion accounting for high strained volumes. The authors highlighted that not only is important the failure load prediction but also the micro-strain distribution. Maintaining the lattice connectivity showed to be more important than keeping the bone volume fraction alone, which has an increasing value as the resolution is lowered for the same segmentation threshold [123]. In the transition from micro-CT to MDCT (in vivo) resolutions, both imaging techniques combined with Pistoia criterion predicted well both the failure load and local strain distributions [123].

Other approaches to model cancellous bone based on images consider its structure as a combination of plates and rods [126], Fig. 1.17. It implies the difficulty of individual trabeculae segmentation, to explicitly define the plates and rods that compose the structure. Nevertheless, the plates and rods model accurately predict elastic and strength properties compared to voxel-based models and requires 83-fold less memory regarding model size and 324-fold lower computational resources in the nonlinear simulations [126].

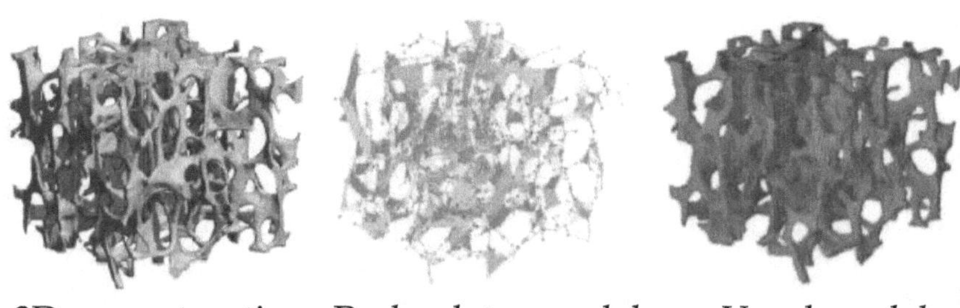

Figure 1.17: Representation of a 3D reconstruction of a cancellous bone specimen (left), subsequent model of plates and rods considering shell and beam elements, respectively (centre) and voxel-based finite element model (right), adapted from [126].

1.5.8.3 Material properties definition

Tissue material properties are usually inferred from several methodologies. Some authors use the attenuation coefficient values and relationships to density and elastic properties [42, 71, 127, 128, 129]. Among experimental approaches, we may distinguish between from nanoindentation measurements [40] or inverse analysis calculation, using experimental results combined with three-dimensional imaging and finite element modeling [10, 24, 46, 47]. Finally, some works assume them following values reported in the literature [128].

In case of images of lower resolution, like in CT or MDCT cases, density-based continuum models are commonly used. These models define the material inside each finite element by averaging its properties depending on the gray level intensity, which is related to tissue density [123, 127]. The elastic modulus to be assigned to each element is defined using a power law that depends on the anatomic site and the apparent density, determined experimentally [130, 131].

Obviously, continuous models do not explicitly account for cancellous bone microstructure but can be used as an initial approximation of its mechanical behavior or as a low computational resources prediction. For example, Bauer et al. [123] used the continuous models to predict cancellous bone failure but low correlations were found between their models and experimental data, possibly due to the failure model considered. An interesting work of Pahr and Zysset [127] dealt with a comparison of continuum finite element models CT based with micro-CT based models, considered as a gold standard. They found that CT based continuum models including patient-specific cortex and density-fabric-based orthotropic cancellous bone material properties provided equivalent predictions as micro-FE models, needing lower computational resources.

In case of high resolution finite element models, equivalent effective isotropic elastic properties are often considered, calculated by inverse analysis from experimental data [47]. This calibration explained up to 95 % of Young's modulus variation compared to experimental testing [47]. Other authors have studied the use of inhomogeneous material properties in micro-finite element models [42, 71, 128, 129]. For example, Bérot et al. [42] considered a randomly distribution of elastic modulus and reported differences lower than 2% on the strain remodeling threshold estimation compared to a homogeneous tissue mechanical properties hypothesis.

Bourne and van der Meulen [128] went a step further and considered inhomogeneities from micro-CT attenuation coefficient on computational models to predict apparent mechanical properties. The authors compared different inhomogeneous specimen-specific properties assignation to homogeneous or generic cancellous bone properties reported in the literature. Their results showed that an homogeneous literature-based elastic modulus tends to overestimate the apparent properties. Moreover, the consideration of an inhomogeneous distribution was more significant for specimens with greater tissue modulus variability, which tended to vanish for more homogeneous specimens [128].

On the other hand, Gross et al. [71] showed that considering mineral heterogeneity has little influence on the estimation of the apparent properties of human cancellous bone, reporting a 2 % overestimation for the homogeneous model. They used synchrotron radiation microcomputed tomography (SR-μ CT) in contrast to standard micro-CT because, in the latter, beam hardening may reduce the accuracy of the estimation of the variation of mineral content and presents inferior signal-to-noise ratio. This reduction was reported explicitly in a study of Kaynia et al. [129], which was a result from lower attenuation coefficients for micro-CT compared to SR-μ CT scanning. A 26 % modulus underestimation was found for micro-CT based [129].

Another option to define the material properties is from nanoindentation [40]. Chevalier et al. [40] compared the effect on the apparent modulus estimation of material property assignation to FE models from nanoindentation and the ones back calculated from experiments. The authors found a 24 % apparent modulus overestimation using nanoindentation. Chevalier et al. [40] hypothesized that the differences were result from side-artifacts during testing that reduced the tissue Young's modulus estimation. In fact, the apparent modulus underestimation was consistent with works analyzing experimental artifacts [53].

1.5.8.4 Elastic properties estimation through homogenization

The determination of the elastic constants that define the behavior of cancellous bone at the apparent level is important to evaluate bone integrity and its relationship to specimen-specific microarchitecture. Moreover, numerical simulations avoid issues related to experimental testing. An orthotropic or transversely isotropic apparent behavior has been reported for cancellous bone on-axis [10, 47].

To calculate cancellous bone elastic constants, van Rietbergen et al. [49] presented a methodology to directly estimate them based on the work from Hollister and Kikuchi [132] that consisted in the application of six unitary strain cases, three pure axial and three pure shear, on the micro-CT reconstruction of two specimens. The procedure does not imply any a priori assumption about the elastic symmetries of the samples and avoid the artifact that sometimes are present in experimental testing. The homogenized elastic properties estimation depends on the boundary conditions applied [133, 134]. The effective (or real) elastic properties are the ones calculating following three main requirements: the structure needs to be periodic, the volume analyzed contains a very large set of microscale elements and periodic boundary conditions have to be applied [134]. Therefore, the application of six unitary strain cases to cancellous bone leads to apparent properties estimation, because it does not fulfill the periodicity requirement necessary to calculate the effective properties. Those apparent properties constitute an upper bound of the effective elastic properties [133].

This procedure was then named as kinematic uniform boundary conditions, and has been applied to calculate the homogeneous properties from different species and locations [47, 49, 106] and to estimate their relationships to bone volume fraction [106]. Besides, it served to calculate the coefficients of the explicit expressions obtained by Cowin [105] between elasticity matrix and fabric tensor. Those coefficients were supposed to be determined experimentally and the procedure proposed avoid the implications regarding experimental artifacts [106]. However, the coefficients between fabric tensor and elasticity should be calculated for other anatomic sites or specimen sets to assess their variability [106].

It has been reported that model size and boundary conditions have a strong influence on the elastic properties prediction [133, 134]. Cancellous bone is a non-periodic structure so its effective elastic properties may not be calculated directly, but does its apparent ones. Pahr and Zysset [134] analyzed the effect of different boundary conditions on the elasticity matrix estimation: uniform displacement (kinematic boundary conditions, KUBCs), uniform traction or uniform displacement-traction (orthogonal mixed uniform boundary conditions, PMUBCs) in contrast to periodic boundary conditions (PBC). PBC permit to calculate effective elastic properties but, in case of a non-periodic structure like cancellous bone, a previous step of mirroring the structure is necessary to be able to apply them [134]. The authors showed that PMUBCs give the same properties than as PBCs, while KUBCs provide an upper bound of the effective elastic properties [133, 134].

More recently, Daszkiewicz et al. [133] proposed to use an embedded configuration to assess the effective elastic properties. This embedded configuration involves the measurement of the elastic properties at a certain distance of the cortex where the boundary conditions are applied, which is defined as *in situ* value. Moreover, the authors studied the effect of the sample size, finding a convergent tendency for increasing volume [133].

1.5.8.5 Failure modeling

The mechanical behavior of bone axial loading until fracture may be divided in three parts: an elastic domain (linear phase where the deformation is reversible), a elastic-continuum damage mechanics domain (diffuse microcracks appear irreversibly) and a fracture mechanics domain (fracture surfaces are developed) [25].

From some decades ago, the numerical resources available have increased but not as much as what clinical practice demands for fracture risk assessment based on micro-FE modeling. Explicitly including cancellous bone microstructure requires of millions of finite elements for a specimen of about 1 cm^3. Therefore, a compromise between accuracy and computational cost is needed for the application of failure models. In the literature, several authors have proposed non-linear micro-finite element models to simulate pre- and post-yielding behavior [24, 44, 48, 75, 135, 136, 137, 138, 139, 140]. However, most of the models proposed to investigate the onset of failure without considering its propagation or the models are complex and require parameters hardly measurable. Furthermore, an experimental validation of the damage models has been little investigated.

Failure models are useful to estimate properties which are difficult to measure experimentally. For example, yielding and fracture strains have been estimated through numerical approaches [72, 73, 141]. Using an effective tissue modulus and considering asymmetric failure strains predicts cancellous bone failure and can be used to back calculate tissue failure properties combining simulations and experiments [72]. Furthermore, it has been used to assess the local strain threshold which is responsible for bone remodeling initiation on osteoporotic cancellous bone [42]. A value of 0.18 % was identified, which is far below the yielding values, but it is within the range of in vivo strains (500-3000 μ strains) [42].

On the other hand, post-yielding has been investigated in the literature from different approaches. For example, Schwiedrzik et al. [135] proposed a continuum cohesive-frictional plasticity model based on Drucker-Prager yield criterion. They validated the model against experimental results with great accuracy in terms of correlations to the experimental stiffness and yield point. On the other hand, García et al. [137] extended 2D to 3D a version of an elastic plastic damage constitutive law for both cortical and cancellous bone, describing its elastic, pure plastic and damaged plastic evolution modes. Further, the model also distinguishes tensile from compressive damage stresses, but their complex model lacks of an experimental validation. Other authors like O'Connor et al. [136], simplified the trabecular network using idealized strut models and applied an asymmetric Mises plasticity formulation.

The Extended Finite Element Method appears, among fracture mechanics approaches, with some potential to model fracture propagation because it needs the crack to be explicitly defined, so it may be used coupled with other techniques to address fracture initiation. However, few works addressed this problem on cancellous bone [139, 140] because a more complex formulation is demanded: a degree of freedom enrichment is required at crack faces and crack tip nodes. Moreover, a 3D version of XFEM presents several geometric difficulties.

An interesting option to simulate failure with a simple model is framed in continuum damage mechanics approaches. The initiation and propagation of cracks is simulated from a smeared crack approach within those models [44, 138, 142, 143, 144]. Nagaraja [75] explains that isotropic damage laws are suitable to reproduce cancellous bone non-linear behavior. Following that argument, Hambli [44] proposed and experimentally validated an isotropic damage law to simulate damage at the microscale in the trabecular lattice. In his model, complete fracture is modeled using an element deletion technique. An interesting investigation by Harrison et al. [141] considered an asymmetric damage approach combined to complete fracture, through element deletion, which further incorporated a cohesive parameter that permits to calibrate brittle-ductile behavior. The approach allows for the estimation of yielding and failure strains and accurately model post-yielding behavior [141].

Levrero-Florencio and Pankaj [145] considered a non-linear homogenization approach to better model damage evolution at the macroscale, incorporation of an isotropic with coupled plasticity and damage constitutive tissue level law and imposing kinematic uniform boundary conditions to calculate the stiffness matrix associated to the specimen. Moreover, three parametric damage coefficients were considered for each orthotropic direction [145]. The model proposed permits to consider strength asymmetry without defining it explicitly and predicts that most damaged elements are on-axis [145], which is in agreement with results from the literature [146].

The approach used in [44] was also applied to reproduce bending failure on a single trabeculae, which gives insight into failure mechanisms: areas subjected to tensile stresses induce damage accumulation and local rupture leading to modulus degradation, while compression areas enhance fracture toughness because microcracks are subjected to closure [24]. A more complex constitutive exponential law was used to model axial and bending failure in single trabeculae, whose results were validated experimentally [73]. Both osteoporotic and healthy donors were analyzed and low variability was found in the yield strain (10-20 %) in contrast to ultimate strain (30-40 %) [73].

However, those complex models require a high number of parameters which are difficult to measure and often need of higher computational resources for the simulations.

1.5.9 Cancellous bone surrogate: rigid polyurethane foams

Rigid polyurethane foams have been used as a cancellous bone surrogate to evaluate orthopedic devices, cement augmentation investigation or mechanical characterization [147, 148, 149]. As they do not suffer from biological degradation or dehydration, and due to its lower costs compared to real bone specimens [150], they have become a reliable alternative to cancellous bone-like structure investigations.

One of the first published studies about polyurethane foams characterization was developed by Menges and Knipschild in 1975 [151], and performed a mechanical characterization of closed-cell rigid polyurethane (PUR) foams based on the conception of a simplified beam structure. From the observation of the behavior of these foams under different loading conditions, they derived analytical expressions relating the strengths of the material, and its elastic modulus with its density. Their mechanical tests supported their theory. Gibson et al. went a step further in the study of the mechanics of cellular materials, first in the two-dimensional case [152] and later it was extended to the three-dimensional one [153]. Their aim was to characterize the homogeneous response in deformation of foams. The investigation was carried out considering simplified cellular models and defining each of the deformation modes involved: bending, elastic buckling and plastic collapse of the struts. Those simplified models for open and closed cell foams were also employed to model cancellous bone simplified structures, as it is also a cellular material [17]. However, by that time Gibson realized that cancellous bone architecture was more complex and proposed other simplified models according to SEM images inspection. In [153], a set of analytical expressions for the mechanical behavior of foams are developed in terms of their geometrical features (strut length and thickness) and then correlated to a relative density parameter. The result is a simplified theoretical law of the foam material in terms of density that agrees with experimental data. A work by Goods et al. [154] corroborated these findings and postulated that this simplified 3D cell model is useful for the prediction of some mechanical properties. More recently, Marsavina et al. [155] modeled uniaxial compression on closed-cell polyurethane foam using the micromechanic model of [153] and obtained accurate results when comparing them with their experimental data. In fact, the three stages of the compressive response of the foam (initially linear elastic, softening stress after yield and plastic plateau) were captured.

Because of the increasing relevance of polyurethane foams in the biomechanical field as a cancellous bone surrogate, several works have been conducted during the last years to characterize this kind of structures [150, 156, 157, 158]. In [159], an extensive review of experimental methodologies to assess metal foam mechanical properties is performed, which can be extended to other foamed structures. Several studies deal with commercial foams [148, 150, 157, 158, 160, 161, 162] while others produce their own foams resembling cancellous bone [147, 156]. Szivek et al. [156] performed uniaxial compression tests over four mixtures preparations of porous polyurethane foams. The mechanical properties obtained from the tests fell all within the range of those of human trabecular bone. The reported compressive strengths ranged from 2.54 to 5.83 MPa, depending on the isocyanate-to-resin ratio. Patel et al. [158] calculated the compressive properties of open cell PUR foams aiming at mimicking osteoporotic human cancellous bone ones, which was achieved only in terms of fracture stress. Further, Thompson et al. [163] studied also the shear properties experimentally and pointed out that to mimic cancellous bone behavior, anisotropy must be also considered.

Calvert et al. [157] tested closed-cell PUR foams (manufactured by General Plastics), widely employed in orthopedic purposes, under the conditions of the ASTM F1839-08 standard [164] for compression testing. Different density samples were chosen for the experimental study and the dependency of the foam elastic modulus on relative density was quantified and showed a good agreement with the law postulated by Gibson et al. [153]. Closed-cell foams exhibit similar static mechanical properties than cancellous bone, but their deformation mechanism is different (stretching in closed-cells vs bending in open-cells) which has influence on fatigue [165]. Fatigue behavior of open-cell PUR was assessed by Johnson et al. [150] in the form of open cell foams and synthetic vertebrae construction, where a plastic cortex was added to the open cell foam. They registered localized fracture in fatigue, which coincides with its monotonic failure. The compression fatigue S-N curves were similar to cancellous bone ones. They also pointed out that the static compressive modulus measured was significantly lower than the values reported by the manufacturer.

Whenever an experimental test is carried out, attention has to be paid to the size of the test specimens as a conditioner of the stress-strain response, as stated by Chiang et al. [166]. They employed a multi-speckle technique (similar to DIC technique) to observe the differences in the strain field between macro and micro-size PUR samples when submitted to tensile loading. While deformation was almost uniform along the largest samples, the micro-size ones revealed heterogeneous patterns. The results of their multi-speckle technique also lack of uniaxial failure initiation at each scale studied, which would have provided information about failure mechanisms. They claim that stiffness is also affected by specimen dimensions (a larger specimen has higher stiffness) but do not assess any relationship to account for the size effect. In this line, Strêk [159] stated that, for tension/compression tests in metal foams, the minimum required sample width/thickness should be seven times the cell size to avoid low specimen size effect.

Indentation on low density polyurethane foams was investigated by Wilsea et al. [167], who further compared their results to fully dense material indentation. They found that indentation hardness of low density foams was very similar to its compression yield strength ($\sigma_{y,c}$) and differs from fully dense material case, where the indentation hardness was 3-fold $\sigma_{y,c}$. Their explanation about this effect comes from the fact that the axial compression for low density foams ($\nu = [0.03 - 0.05]$) produces little lateral expansion, which leads to yielding when the maximum principal stress reaches $\sigma_{y,c}$.

Other studies have addressed fracture properties in PUR foams experimentally [168, 169, 170, 171, 172, 173] by the three-point bending testing of notched specimens. Some of these include numerical modelling of the crack evolution [171, 172], or use the Digital Image Correlation (DIC) technique [166, 171, 173, 174]. The numerical models developed by Marsavina et al. [172] considered homogeneous material and XFEM to model crack propagation under mixed mode testing conditions. The authors highlight the importance of experimental validation (or calibration) of the numerical model, which in their case depends on several parameters.

Among image-based experimental characterization, Jin et al. [173] applied DIC to closed-cell PUR foams and compared the heterogeneous strain estimations to finite element models results, which were similar in a qualitative way. However, little work has been carried out in the literature regarding the finite element analysis of the damage and fracture of unnotched specimens under uniaxial loading conditions.

In foamed structures, microarchitecture has a major influence on the elastic and fracture properties. The advances on imaging systems have motivated studies accounting for an accurate morphological description. Gómez et al.

[162] analyzed the morphometry of two grades of open cell PUR foams by SEM and micro-CT and stated that 0.09 and 0.12 g/cm^3 foams have similar microstructural characteristics than osteoporotic human cancellous bone. Other previous works in the literature have developed finite element models of PUR foams from the segmentation of computed tomography (CT) images [147, 150, 160, 161]. Some of them have applied micro-CT during specimen testing, which provides information about the deformation state at each load increment, which can be used to validate finite element models [147, 160]. Special care has to be taken when modeling is based on high resolution images, because both the characteristic structure parameters and the mechanical properties of the foam may be altered by the micro-CT setting parameters, resolution and the segmentation method applied [160, 175]. Youssef et al. [161] developed finite element models of rigid polyurethane foams of high volume fraction, which were scanned during its testing. The foamed material analyzed did not exactly resembled to cancellous bone, because its microstructure had spherical voids and higher volume fraction. The novelty of the study was the introduction of plasticity, which was observed experimentally at the micro level.

Cement augmentation or infiltration is often tested on synthetic cancellous bone [160]. Zhao et al. [160] modeled foam cement interface using finite elements based on micro-CT images acquired during the compression of a low density open cell foam. They studied frictionless and tied interface contact boundary conditions and validated their models using the micro-CT images in the loaded case. However, their study is only focused on the undamaged case modeling, but the authors propose as future work to include a plasticity and element deletion models to evaluate failure.

Some of the works in the literature dealing with commercial open cell polyurethane foams take into account or refer their results to the average properties provided by the manufacturer [150, 162]. Jonhson and Keller [150] pointed out significant differences between their elastic metrics and the values reported in the literature, which confirm the importance of accurate definition of testing conditions to make the results comparable. Furthermore, the anisotropic characteristics of open cell polyurethane foams should be addressed to better modeling its mechanical behavior, and the heterogeneous architecture of the specimens may have an important role on its mechanical response, as it happens in cancellous bone. Because open cell polyurethane foams are often used to evaluate implant stability and local variations of samples microstructure are relevant on the pull-out strength predictions, finite element models based on high resolution images may help to get insight into failure mechanisms of this kind of structures. A thorough investigation of the influence of foam microarchitecture on its elastic and fracture behavior will be relevant for implant design and failure mechanisms studies at the microscale and will be given in Chapter 4 of this book.

1.5.10 Evaluation of fixation techniques for spine

First of all, the review of evaluation of spine fixation techniques and the subsequent development of chapter 5 was motivated by the four months research stay at the Technique University of Eindhoven (TU/e) under the supervision of Prof. Bert van Rietbergen. We followed one of the research lines that Prof. van Rietbergen is currently studying, framed in a project about different procedures to treat scoliosis, specially for early onset scoliosis (EOS).

Pedicle screw is widely accepted as a standard for stabilization in trauma, deformity correction or fusion procedures [176]. Bilateral pedicle screw fixation permits individual vertebra manipulation, resulting in better derotation of vertebrae compared to hook constructs [177]. In Fig. 1.18, bilateral pedicle screw fixation is depicted, which consists of the insertion of implants on both pedicles towards the vertebral body. The implants are then connected to rods positioned along the spine, which serve as guide in deformity correction. However, fixation with pedicle screws produces higher rates of fusion compared to other techniques, leading to greater failure risk [178]. Stripping on insertion, pullout, migration and loosening failure modes may occur as clinical disorders [179]. Some authors have proposed alternative methods to treat deformity correction, like polymeric sublaminar cables, that would be less invasive [180]. Alternative fixation techniques have special interest for cases like early onset scoliosis severe disorder, where the use of pedicle screws may produce spine growth alteration or restrictive pulmonary disease, due to its higher invasive procedure and the need of periodic surgical interventions [181]. For those cases sublaminar tape fixation permits its use in growth-guidance constructs, avoiding some of the surgical interventions and allowing spinal growth [182, 181]. Nonetheless, pedicle screw remains as the most used procedure.

The development and evaluation of orthopedic implants is based on a combination of surgical experience, engineering expertise and experimental biomechanical testing. Numerical modeling can be an important assistive tool in this process and gives insight into the mechanical processes underlying orthopedic interventions [183]. Imaging systems, like micro-CT, permit to scan non-destructively and provide numerical models which take into account specimen microstructure, insert different implants at different locations and evaluate them from simulation results. Further, the development of image-based finite element models is far less expensive and more versatile than experimental studies. Also, they can be used to simulate multiple situations and loading cases which are difficult to reproduce experimentally.

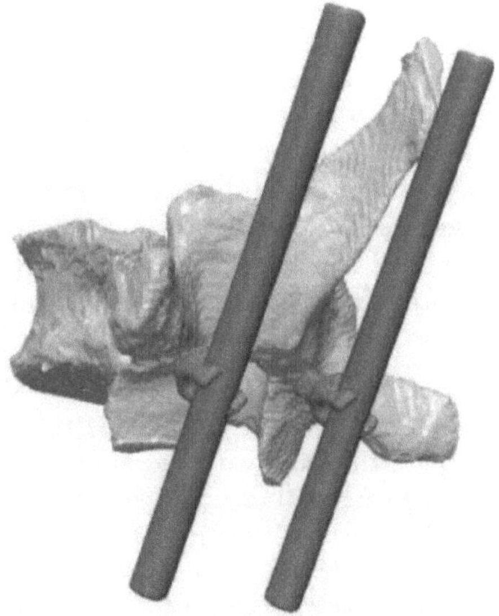

Figure 1.18: Bilateral pedicle screw fixation scheme: implants inserted at each pedicle and connected to rods along the spine, which serve as a guide. The model depicts a thoracic human vertebra with two pedicle implants inserted virtually, scanned by micro-CT and downscaled to a 0.56 mm voxel resolution.

Implant anchorage is claimed to depend on the osseointegration (bone-implant bonding) and peri-implant trabecular bone, being the latter the most important regarding loading capacity [184]. Therefore, it is considered that implant fixation relies primarily on the quality of the bone adjacent to the implant and the geometry of the implant [148, 184, 185, 186, 187]. For example, in [186] the authors investigate implant fixation concerning human cadaveric tibiae, and they claim that the screw pull-out force is affected not only by the quality of the cancellous bone around the screw but also by the proximity to the overlying cortical shell (with particularly significant effects for shell thicknesses over 1.5 mm). On the other hand, Gabet et al. [184] combined experimental pull-out tests with micro-computed tomography to study the importance of the bone architecture around the screw. Failure mainly occurred between 0.5 to 1 mm around the implant, which consisted of buckling of the weakest trabeculae followed by complete failure of peri-implant bone. They claim that the highest correlation to the pull-out stiffness and strength are mean trabecular thickness (Tb.Th) and bone volume fraction (BV/TV) and propose them as target to enhance implant anchorage.

A recent study by Mueller et al. [148] explored implant fixation failure in human femoral heads using a step-wise testing-imaging system. They hypothesized that prior implant fixation failure, significant peri-implant bone failure occurred, which was visualized using their testing-imaging system for large specimens (the supplementary data in [148] shows clearly the effect). From their observations, they analyzed correlations between ultimate force and bone peri-implant morphometry and found a significant relationship with bone volume fraction. However, the bone volume analyzed in the correlation was arbitrary.

Some standards (such as ASTM) have accepted the pull-out test as the standard method to simulate the axial withdrawal of a screw [164, 188]. The displacement ranges assumed for pull-out test vary widely from 0.005 to 1.0 mm for common orthopedic screws [149, 187, 189, 190]. However, some experimental studies report a range of displacement values between 1.0 to 3.0 mm [191, 192]. From our point of view, this scattering within the displacement values depends on how the displacement is measured. High displacement values would be related to global measurements (for example: direct crosshead displacement or maybe not avoiding the compliance of the testing machine) while small values would be related to local measurements (for example: optical techniques, displacement gages or extensometers attached to the specimen), where fixtures displacement would be avoided in the measurement. Therefore, for an accurate bone-screw relative displacement measurement, local metrics would be preferred over global ones. In [184], the authors provide micro-CT images of the bone-implant construct before and after the pull-out test and the images reveal displacements less than 0.2 mm.

There are many studies in the literature that examine the pull-out strength on either real or synthetic bone specimens, both experimentally [176, 177, 193] or numerically [179, 187, 189, 194]. Some of them focus on the influence of using implants of different features [195] or on parametric studies to assess the influence of the insertion angle, insertion depth or density on the pull-out strength [196, 197]. Some authors [191, 192, 195], have analyzed the holding power of a screw inserted in synthetic low density cancellous bone, experimentally and through homogeneous continuum finite element models, which highlights the importance of such synthetic materials on implant design and evaluation.

The recent work of Steiner et al. [198], reviews computational approaches to analyze the primary implant stability in trabecular bone either with simplified or image-based finite element models. Within the simplified models, Brown et al. [179] proposed a 2D axisymmetric finite element model to identify parameters to enhance the pull-out strength and proposed cement augmentation to improve osseointegration. Ruffoni et al. [199] considers a cubic volume of interest (VOI) of 17 mm side in form of a beam lattice model, to explore the role of the peri-implant bone architecture on the mechanics of the bone-implant system.

Some works have addressed parametric analysis of implants with bone continuum finite element models [149, 189]. In [149] a parametric study is presented about the characteristic dimensions of a screw on its holding power, considering a homogeneous continuum cancellous bone model. Zhang et al. [190] analyzed how different bone material properties affected using a continuum model developed in [189]. Their results show that the pull-out strength was proportional to bone material shear strength.

Among realistic finite element models in the literature, Wirth et al. [200] studied the mechanical competence of the bone-screw system combining micro-CT and finite element analysis on ten sheep vertebral bodies with orthopedic screws inserted. They found a correlation between bone volume and pull-out strength and used a high strained criterion [125] to determine failure. The same authors analyzed implant stability and its variations about the cancellous microstructure and found that peri-implant bone density was the best single morphometric parameter to predict implant stability [201]. Piper and Brown [187] explored the influence of cancellous bone microstructure on the pull-out strength, using numerical models micro-CT based whose differences resulted from changing thresholding segmentation parameters on the same original bone model. A recent work by Steiner et al. [202] proposes to quantify implant stability using micro-FE and considering cancellous bone damage due to screw insertion [203] to achieve more accurate predictions. They claim that without that consideration, the predictions of the stiffness were overestimated by over 330%.

Regarding modeling screw-bone contact, different approaches may be found. Some of them used a simplified bone-screw geometry, considering surface-to-surface friction contact [189, 190, 192, 195]. Piper and Brown [187] considered asymmetric pure penalty friction contact while other approaches dealt with perfectly bounded contact in the bone-screw interface [149, 199, 200, 201, 202].

The high computational cost associated both to image-based numerical modeling and solving non-linear contact failure problems, motivates the development of either simple failure criteria for numerical modeling or analytical expressions, based on experimental observations that allow their application to clinical practice. However, one should be aware of the simplifications made both in modeling and failure criteria if the objective is to study local effects at the bone-implant interface.

Chapter 2

Cancellous bone: morphometric characterization

2.1 Introduction

The increasing percentage of aged population in our society makes the prediction of bone failure clinically relevant, with high economic and social costs associated [3]. Cancellous bone constitutes the primary insertion location of orthopedic implants and it is known to have major importance on bone mechanical state and fracture behavior, controlled by density and microstructure [10, 14]. Bone diseases which produce mechanical competence loss, like osteoporosis, are known to be related to cortical cortex thinning and cancellous bone degradation [1, 3]. Therefore, the improvement of fracture risk assessment needs of an accurate estimation of cancellous bone elastic and failure properties, which even after some decades of major worldwide research interest has not been totally solved and it is still being investigated nowadays. Mechanical properties are commonly assessed either experimentally, through numerical simulations or measuring microstructural features that are related to bone's mechanical competence. Bone mineral density (BMD) is the actual gold standard method for bone's mechanical state diagnosis. However, an indication of BMD is not enough for a complete cancellous bone deterioration characterization and fracture risk assessment, because not only the amount of bone loss is important but also is it the nature and degree of the atrophy [6]. In other words, the amount of cancellous bone (determined by BMD and/or BV/TV measurement) explains some degree of variation of its mechanical properties, but cannot fully characterize it [8, 10, 11, 14, 47, 92].

In this chapter, cancellous bone morphometry is characterized through the analysis of images acquired using micro-computed tomography (micro-CT). First, we present the porcine vertebral cancellous bone specimens used in this book, together with their preparation and storage protocol. Then, the micro-CT acquisition and the density calibration phantoms are described, and the procedure to segment the subsequent images is given. The morphometric parameters calculated and their assessment method are defined. After that, the morphometry results are presented and discussed. Finally, the sensitivity to variations of the segmentation threshold, corresponding to the action of different users, is studied on both the morphometry derived from the segmentation and the elastic properties calculated from image-based finite element models. The results presented in this chapter will be used to explore relationships between morphometry and mechanical properties in Chapter 3.

2.2 Description of specimens: vertebral cancellous bone

In this chapter, the experimental work is performed on porcine vertebral cancellous bone specimens. The vertebral column serve as protection of the spinal cord and gives structural stability to the skeleton. For the sake of completeness we first compare human and pig skeletons, Fig. 2.1. Both human and porcine spines may be divided into cervical, thoracic, lumbar and sacral vertebrae. Some mammals have also caudal vertebrae, corresponding to tail bones (coccyx in humans). The cervical vertebrae are located in the neck, the thoracic are attached to the ribs, the lumbar are between the ribs and the pelvis, while the sacral and the caudal are in the pelvis area.

Fig. 2.2 shows a 3D reconstruction of two human thoracic vertebrae (T11 (left) and T3 (right)) where their different parts can be distinguished, scanned by micro-CT at the Technique University of Eindhoven (TU/e). In general, vertebrae can be divided between its body (or centrum) and its arch. Vertebral body is mainly composed of cancellous bone and a cortex of cortical bone. Within the vertebral arch, other structures can be distinguished: spinous process, transverse process, articular process, pedicles and facets. The components of the vertebral arch have a thick layer of cortical bone and are the location of muscles and tendons anchor, while the pedicles are the union between the vertebral body and arch and are commonly the placement spot for implants to treat trauma, deformity correction or fusion [176]. Furthermore, bone spurs are marked in Fig. 2.2, which are abnormal bone growth that occurs in osteoarthritic spinal joints due to misalignments or damage in the discs and soft tissues.

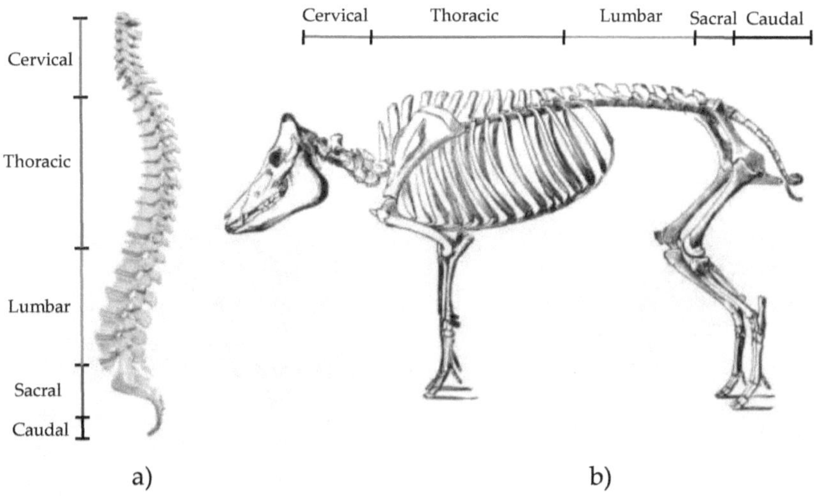

Figure 2.1: Scheme of a) human spine and b) pig skeleton where morphological similarities can be found. Figures a) and b) are free of copyright, b) image attribution is Andrew Clifford [204]

Many works in the literature use animal bones to develop their investigations due to their similarities to human bones, the limited supply of human cadavers, their higher cost and ethical concerns present on the use of human specimens. Further, implants and surgical procedures are often tested pre-clinically on animal spines. It is said that the porcine spine is the most representative model for the human spine [205, 206]. Several investigations dealing with animal models have compared human and porcine spines from anatomical or mechanical perspectives [205, 206, 207, 208, 209].

Busscher et al. [205] compared the complete spine of 6 human and 6 pigs and measured anatomical dimensions on CT images. Their results confirm great similarities between human and porcine spines [205]. Other authors have compared human data from the literature to biomechanical measurements by testing single joint segments under pure flexural moment conditions in the three main anatomical planes of porcine spines to assess the range of motion of each segment and its flexion/extension response [208]. They warn that porcine spine is not suitable for modeling all regions of the human spinal column.

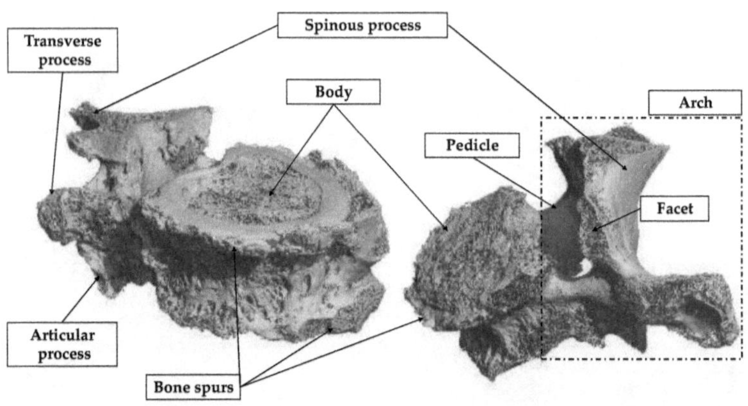

Figure 2.2: 3D reconstruction of two thoracic human vertebrae suffering osteoarthritis. The different parts of a vertebra are highlighted.

Moreover, Aerssens et al. [209] performed an interspecies comparison about composition, density and mechanical characteristics between 7 vertebrates that are commonly used in bone research (human, dog, pig, cow, sheep, chicken and rat). In their study they distinguish between cortical bone from femurs and cancellous bone from lumbar vertebrae. Cancellous bone cylinders were tested under compression conditions and the results show that human and porcine samples have similar fracture stress, which were the lowest compared to the rest of species. In addition, little composition variation was found among species and the ash concentration of pigs, dogs and sheep was similar to the human one. However, the relation between fracture stress and mineral density form separate entities in the interspecies comparison [209].

2.2.1 Preparation of specimens

Cancellous bone specimens were prepared at Instituto de Biomecánica de Valencia (IBV) from skeletally mature pigs recently euthanised. Specifically, a total of 41 specimens constitute the complete data set for this book. The specimens belonged to thoracic and lumbar vertebrae and were cut out of the vertebral body with a precision saw (Accutom-2, Struers, Copenhagen, Denmark) whose blade was appropriate to cut 70-400 HV hardness materials. Cutting parameters varied depending upon the original sample morphology and were the maximum saw blade shaft speed and the minimum saw blade feed. Several clamp adapters were used to ensure sample faces parallelism, which has a major importance for unconfined compression testing [22]. In ad-dition, a combination of ultrasonic bath and water jet was used to eliminate bone marrow from the specimens.

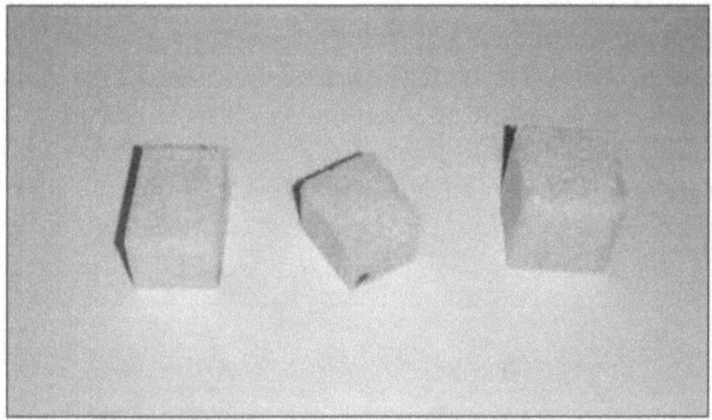

Figure 2.3: Three of the cancellous bone specimens analyzed in this book.

After the extraction, specimens had parallelepiped-shape with at least 10 mm side (Fig. 2.3) and the samples were stored in saline serum at a temperature of -25°C until their scanning and testing [39]. The bone growth plates were avoided in the specimen preparation. The main trabecular orientation of each specimen was also identified after machining and was defined as the principal compression test direction. Three different sets of cancellous bone were defined, as a function of the use of calibration phantoms and the purpose of analysis: set A (8 specimens) and B (28) were scanned without calibration phantoms, while set C (5 specimens) was scanned together with phantoms.

However, 3 specimens from set A suffered from experimental artifacts related to stress concentrations due to non-parallel faces leading to crushing at the edges (Sec. 3.2), and were discarded from the study. Regarding the purpose of analysis, the morphometry of the whole data set was calculated. Set A and C were used to further model its compression fracture, while set B was used to explore morpho-mechano relationships derived from elastic properties homogenization.

2.3 High resolution scanning: Micro-Computed Tomography (μCT, micro-CT)

Two different μCT services were used to scan the specimens because the latter included the possibility of using density calibration phantoms. Specimens from sets A and B were scanned by μCT (V|Tome|X s 240, GE Sensing and Inspection Technologies, shown in Fig. 2.4) using the CENIEH (Burgos, Spain) micro-CT service, with an isotropic voxel resolution of 22 μm (voltage 110 kV, intensity 280 μA, integration time 200 ms, Cu filter). On the other hand, set C was scanned using the μCT service at Estación de Bioloxía Mariña de A Graña (Universidad de Santiago de Compostela, Ferrol, Spain), whose scanner is a Skyscan1172 (Bruker, Kontig, Belgium), with an isotropic voxel resolution of 13.58 μm (voltage 100 kV, intensity 100 μA, Al/Cu filter).

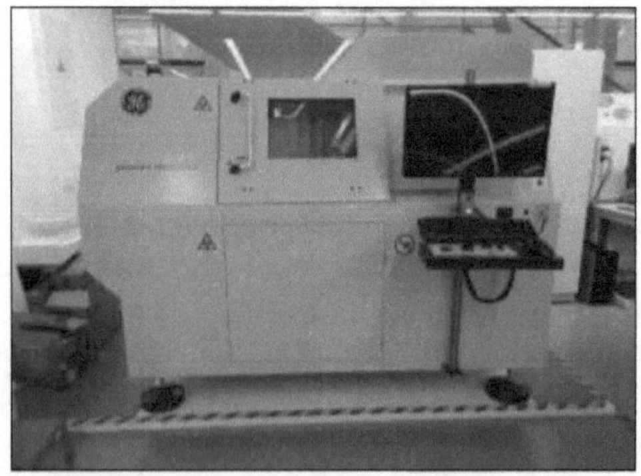

Figure 2.4: V|Tome|X s 240 μCT scanner used for high resolution images acquisition for sets A and B (CENIEH, Burgos, Spain).

Micro-CT acquisition results in a 3D matrix where each voxel has the value of the attenuation coefficient corresponding to the material scanned, directly related to material density. Manual thresholding segmentation method consists in determining a gray level value or range were bone is found, which would be equivalent to choosing a range of densities. However, the attenuation coefficient depends on acquisition parameters (tube current, voltage or integration time) [210], so, calibration phantoms, which are materials with a priori known density, need to be scanned using the same acquisition configuration, enabling the determination of a relationship to estimate density.

The phantoms that are used the most to assess BMD are hydroxyapatite (HA) phantoms and dipotassium phosphate (K_2HPO_4) solutions. HA is known to be the mineral component of bone tissue, whereas K_2HPO_4 is used because of its similar characteristics to HA in terms of effective atomic number or density [210, 211]. Equivalent density measurements through calibration phantoms have been proved to correlate to ash density, but an offset correction subtraction factor of 0.2 g/cm^3 may be necessary [210].

2.3.1 HA phantom

Two hydroxyapatite (HA, $Ca_5(PO_4)_3OH$) phantoms of 250 and 750 mg HA/cm^3 (Bruker, Kontig, Belgium) were used as solid phantoms, depicted in Fig. 2.5.

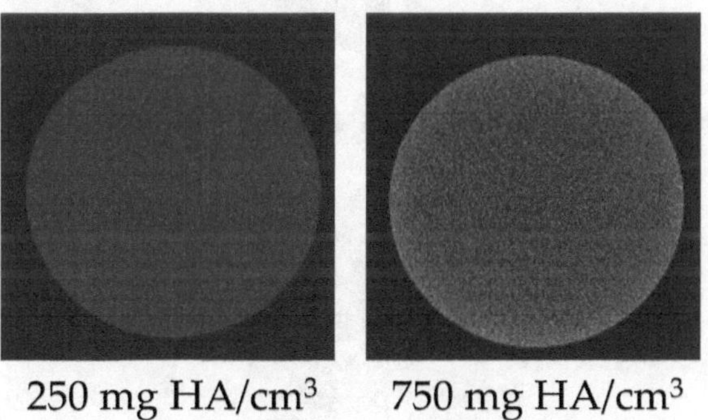

Figure 2.5: Micro-CT images of HA phantoms used to define the density calibration relationship.

The phantoms were scanned at a 13.58 μm isotropic resolution using the micro-CT service of Estación de Bioloxía Mariña de A Graña from Santiago de Compostela University (USC) (Ferrol, Spain) using the equipment and setting aforementioned. A calibration relationship was calculated between density and gray scale values (GS), Eq. 2.1, depicted in Fig. 2.7.

$$\rho = 1.364\ GS + 1056 \tag{2.1}$$

2.3.2 K_2HPO_4 phantom calibration

In 1970, Witt and Cameron [211] developed a stable bone equivalent material composed of K_2HPO_4 in water, which was reproducible in other laboratories and with a mass attenuation coefficient very similar to that of compact bone. They performed an inter-comparison study between six laboratories, which confirmed the idea that a K_2HPO_4 phantom was easily reproducible. Regarding the plastic containers of the solutions, they claimed that even not exactly simulating bone in soft tissue, they can still serve as standard and to calibrate scans [211]. The stability of K_2HPO_4 solutions over time did not show significant differences for a three months study [210].

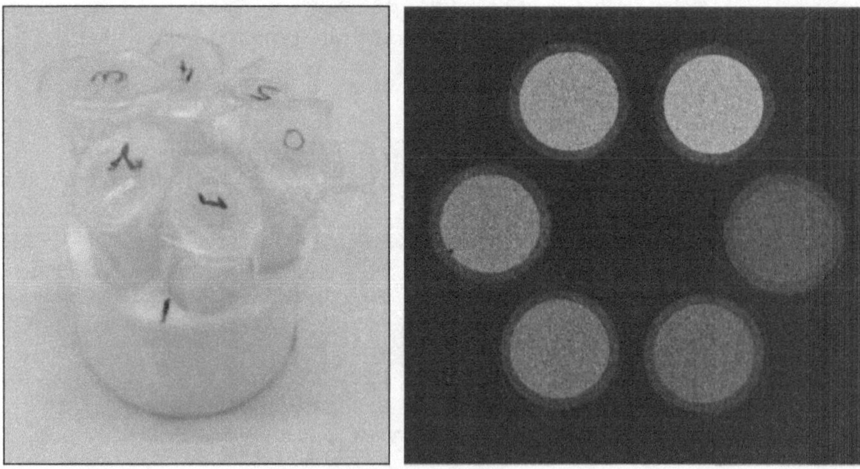

Figure 2.6: K_2HPO_4 phantom in its container (left) and micro-CT image of the same phantom, where the different gray scale values represent different solution concentrations (right).

The K_2HPO_4 phantoms of different solute concentrations used in this book were prepared at Instituto de Biomecánica de València, presented in table 2.1 together with their equivalent densities. Each solution was preserved inside a plastic Eppendorf tube and mounted in a cylindric container, as shown in Fig. 2.6. The liquid phantom was scanned by micro-computed tomography (Skyscan 1172, Bruker, Ferrol, Spain) with an isotropic voxel resolution of 13.58 μm and the same settings than cancellous bone samples from set C. The representation of density values as function of GS values for both the liquid and solid phantoms is presented in Fig. 2.7.

Table 2.1: Dipotassium phosphate (K_2HPO_4) phantom concentrations in terms of mass per volume [g/mL], equivalent densities [mg HA/cm^3] and corresponding mean and standard deviation gray scale values from segmentation.

	Concentration [g/mL]	Density [mg HA/cm^3]	Gray value [-]
Phantom #0	0	58.2	-731.58 ± 88.14
Phantom #1	0.1050	154.1	-661.21 ± 90.03
Phantom #2	0.1934	225.5	-608.89 ± 91.63
Phantom #3	0.2990	297.8	-555.84 ± 95.73
Phantom #4	0.5016	423.8	-463.51 ± 93.84
Phantom #5	0.7270	523.4	-390.49 ± 103.34

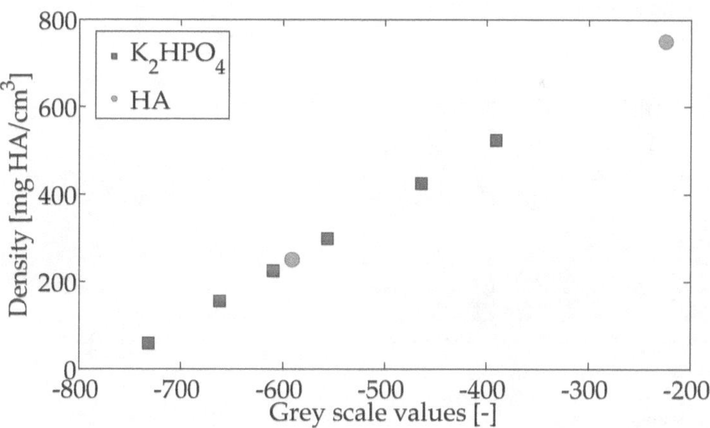

Figure 2.7: K_2HPO_4 and HA phantoms density as function of the gray scale value.

2.4 Image segmentation

2.4.1 Introduction

Segmentation is a key part of image-based finite element modeling. Its accuracy depends both on image quality and on the procedure followed to distinguish between image components. It also has major importance for the estimation of morphometry, which is calculated from the 3D voxel segmented mask.

2.4.2 Segmentation procedure

The segmentation procedure followed in this work for cancellous bone μCT images is divided into three steps: first, a Gauss filter is applied to smooth image contours. Then, a manual threshold is chosen, defining the interval where we can distinguish bone tissue. Finally, a connectivity analysis is conducted on the resulting 3D mask aiming to detect the existence of groups of voxels non-connected to the main trabecular structure. Those non-connected voxels are deleted from the mask in order to avoid problems during the FE simulations. Fig. 2.8 shows the segmentation procedure for bone images in this **book**. In red, a non-connected group of pixels is rounded which was deleted from the segmented mask. In the initial micro-CT image, air, bone marrow and bone can be distinguished with different gray levels.

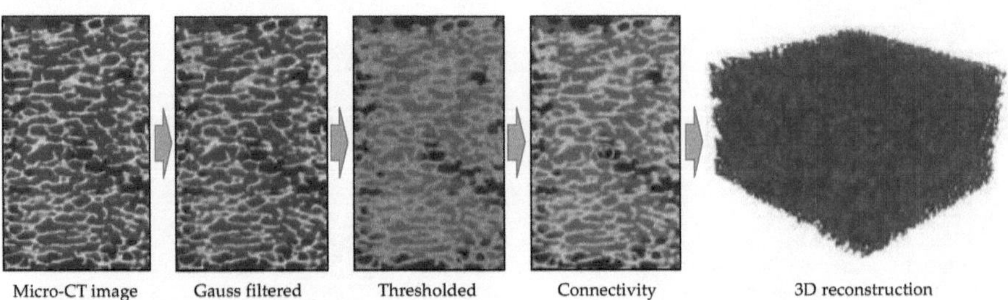

Figure 2.8: Segmentation procedure followed to segment cancellous bone tissue: a Gauss filter is applied to the initial image, then it is thresholded manually and a connectivity analysis is performed, which allows to eliminate groups of voxels (rounded in red) non-connected to the main structure.

The above mentioned procedure (manual or automatic) is considered as a standard to segment cancellous bone μCT images in the literature [12, 13, 41, 95]. From the 3D segmented masks, a 3D reconstruction is useful to visualize cancellous bone microstructure (Fig. 2.9). The segmented mask also serves as input to assess morphological features of each specimen, which has been proved to influence the mechanical performance of cancellous bone specimens [8, 10].

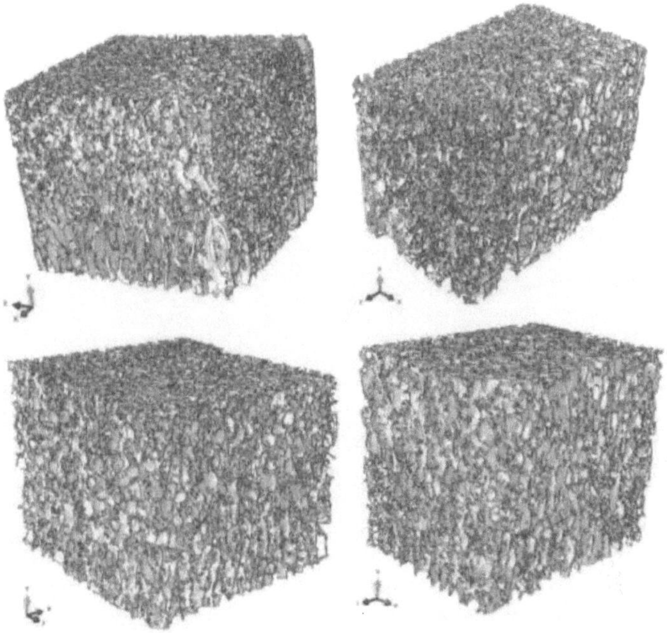

Figure 2.9: 3D reconstruction of four cancellous bone vertebral samples from their segmented masks.

Manual thresholding depends on the user's criterion, so if we compare masks processed by two users, differences may be found, which may have an influence on the estimation of the microstructural parameters. In section 2.5.12 we aim at investigating the effect of variations on the segmentation threshold (sensitivity) due to the action of different users on the morphometry and the elastic properties estimated using image-based models.

2.5 Morphometric characterization at the microscale

2.5.1 Introduction

In this section, the morphometric parameters estimated in this book are presented. The methodology to calculate each parameter is also described and some parameters are applied to reference problems in order to assess their performance. The parameters were calculated using Matlab (MATLAB 2014a, The MathWorks Inc., USA) (BV/TV, Tb.N, D_{2D}, D_{3D}, $DA_{MIL,2D}$, $DA_{MIL,3D}$), BoneJ, which is a free, open source tool for bone image analysis [112], (Tb.Th, Tb.Sp and Conn.D) or from the surface mesh (BS/BV, BS/TV).

2.5.2 Bone volume fraction (BV/TV)

Bone volume fraction (BV/TV) represents the ratio inside the volume of interest (VOI) between the voxels which represent bone tissue and the total number of voxels (Eq. 2.2), calculated through segmented 3D mask analysis. Often, BV/TV is expressed in [%].

$$\text{BV/TV} = \frac{\text{number of bone tissue voxels}}{\text{number of total voxels}} \tag{2.2}$$

2.5.3 Bone surface to total volume ratio (BS/TV)

BS/TV is the relationship between cancellous bone surface and the apparent total volume, expressed in mm^{-1}. We estimate bone surface from the surface mesh, where A_i represents the surface mesh area discretized and N is the total number of surfaces, while total volume (TV) is measured using a caliper, Eq. 2.3.

$$\text{BS/TV} = \frac{\sum_{i=1}^{N} A_i}{\text{TV}} \tag{2.3}$$

2.5.4 Bone surface to volume ratio (BS/BV)

BS/BV is the ratio between the exterior bone surface and its volume. Bone surface calculation is analogous to BS/TV, while bone volume is estimated by bone mask voxel counting. BS/BV may be expressed by Eq. 2.4 (mm^{-1}).

$$BS/BV = \frac{\sum_{i=1}^{N} A_i}{\text{number of bone voxels}} \qquad (2.4)$$

2.5.5 Mean trabecular thickness (Tb.Th)

Tb.Th represents the mean value of the trabeculae thickness of the 3D image model, usually given in mm. In other words, it defines the mean value of the distance between the bone mask contour and its skeleton (Fig. 2.10).

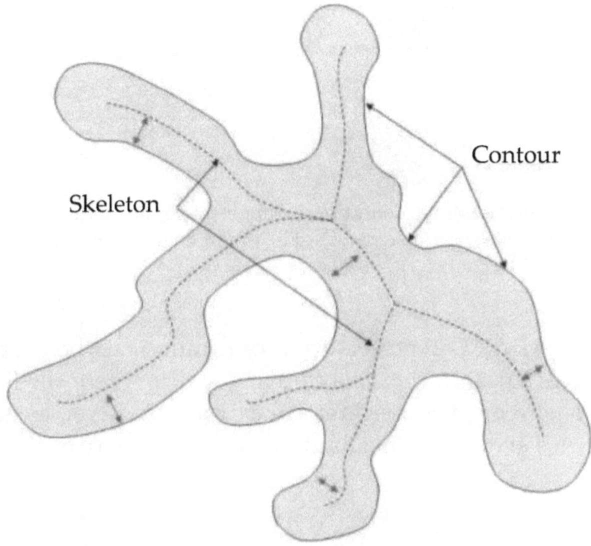

Figure 2.10: Scheme of the definition of Tb.Th parameter in a trabecular-like image from [6].

The method used to calculate the mean trabecular thickness fits spheres of maximum radii in the trabecular structure [111] and permits to calculate Tb.Th without a priori assumptions about the type of structure analyzed. It is a fully 3D method, in contrast to other methods in the literature that tend to overestimate Tb.Th [6].

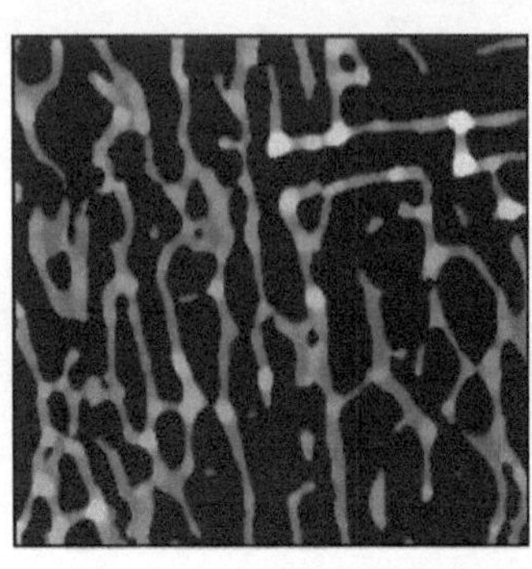

Figure 2.11: Local thickness representation through maximum radii spheres fitting in 2D (left) and in 3D for a whole specimen (right). The brighter the color, the larger the thickness.

Fig. 2.11 shows a 3D representation of a cancellous bone specimen with maximum spheres fitted in the structure and a slice where the local thickness spheres are visualized. The brighter colors refer to larger local thicknesses, which for the case shown are localized in the central part of the specimen.

2.5.6 Mean trabecular separation (Tb.Sp)

The mean trabecular separation (Tb.Sp) defines the mean value of marrow voids in a cancellous bone specimen. The calculation procedure is analogous to the one for Tb.Th but applied to the negative of the 3D segmented mask, that is, changing 1's per 0's and vice versa. A 3D representation and a 2D slice of the local trabecular separation is depicted in Fig. 2.12, obtained using BoneJ [112].

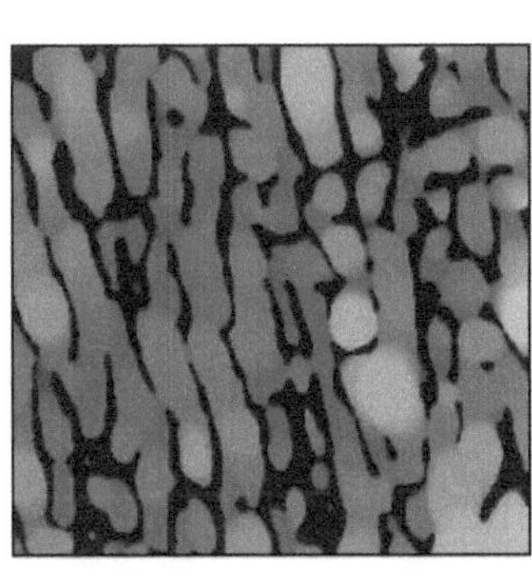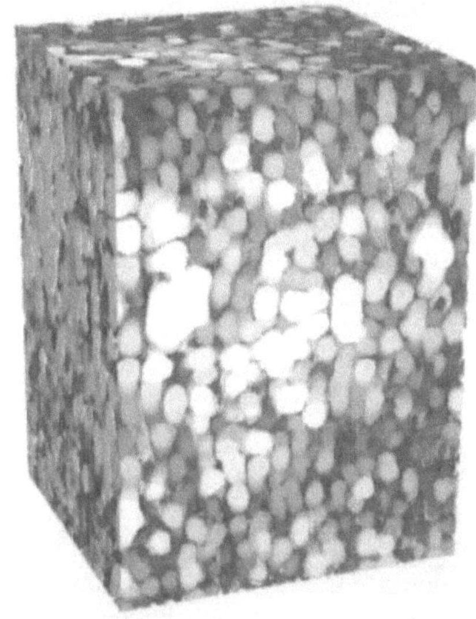

Figure 2.12: Local trabecular separation calculated in the negative of the segmented mask in 2 dimensions (left) and voids representation for a whole specimen in 3D (right).

2.5.7 Trabecular number (Tb.N)

Tb.N relates the bone tissue present in the VOI and the mean trabecular thickness, also named mean trabecular plate density [9]. Its calculation is given by Eq. 2.5 for a plate-like model [102] and is expressed in (mm^{-1}). Assuming a plate-like model is reasonable for the porcine vertebral cancellous bone specimens analyzed, because mostly plates were observed in the reconstructed models.

$$\text{Tb.N} = \frac{\text{BV/TV}}{\text{Tb.Th}} \tag{2.5}$$

2.5.8 Fractal dimension in 2D (D_{2D}) and 3D (D_{3D})

Fractal dimension is commonly used to measure the complexity of a heterogeneous structure like cancellous bone. In other words, fractal dimension is an exponent that gives an idea of how the space is filled while varying the length scale of analysis. Fractal geometries are present in nature and cancellous bone has some fractal characteristics, like increasing perimeter for increasing analysis resolution or self-similarity [108]. There is not an unique fractal dimension, but in some cases they match [212].

Fractal dimension is able to discern between healthy and osteoporotic patients, with higher D values for the healthy case [213]. The reduction of cancellous bone connections produce fractal dimension to decrease, so fractal analysis may be sensitive to cancellous bone connectivity [213, 214].

Commonly, for cancellous bone analysis, the box-counting fractal dimension is calculated. If we consider an object of euclidean dimension D, for example a square of side size 1, and divide it by a factor $1/\lambda$ at each direction, $N = \lambda^D$ boxes would be needed to cover the original object perimeter, and its dimension (euclidean or topological) would be defined as Eq. 2.6.

$$D_{eucl} = \frac{\log N(\lambda)}{\log 1/\lambda} \tag{2.6}$$

If we apply the same argumentation to a fractal object, varying the characteristic length of analysis, λ, the data will fit the following expression, Eq. 2.7.

$$\log N = -D \log \lambda + k \tag{2.7}$$

where D is the fractal dimension, N is the number of boxes needed to cover the perimeter, λ is the characteristic length of analysis and k is a constant of proportionality. Fig. 2.13 depicts an scheme for fractal dimension calculation which, in 2 dimensions can be explained as follows. The field of analysis is divided according to the characteristic length λ and the number of boxes of λ size needed to cover the whole perimeter is counted. The process is repeated for lower λ values, obtaining a logarithmic relationship, whose slope is the fractal dimension D.

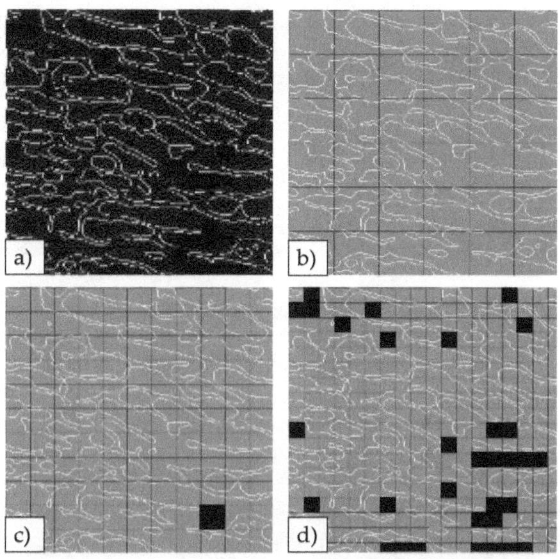

Figure 2.13: a) Cancellous bone contour detection from the segmented mask. b) Overlapping a grid of a characteristic length of 53 pixels all boxes contain bone contour, while for c) a grid of 29 pixels characteristic length, only one box does not contain contour, d) increasing to 32 for a decreasing characteristic length of 18 pixels.

This box-counting method was implemented in Matlab (MATLAB 2014a, The MathWorks Inc., USA) both for 2D and 3D and applied to the perimeter of the segmented mask. In 2D, the 3D structure was analyzed along its 3 main directions, obtaining three measurements of D_{2D}, whose values range between 1 and 2. Two of them, visualizing the main trabecular orientation, and the other one for the transversal plane, as shown in Fig. 2.14. We define $D_{2D\text{-}1}$ and $D_{2D\text{-}2}$ as the fractal dimension calculated over planes a) and b) from Fig. 2.14, while $D_{2D\text{-}3}$ corresponds to the transversal plane c) in Fig. 2.14.

The extension to 3 dimensions of the box-counting method is analogous to 2D, changing squares by cubes. The perimeter of the 3D mask is calculated and the number of cubes containing bone contour is accounted for each characteristic length λ. Then, the data is fitted according to Eq. 2.7, whose value ranges between 2 and 3.

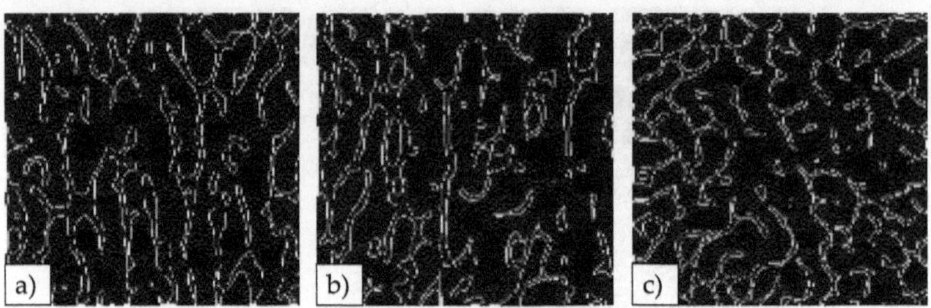

Figure 2.14: Representation of the three planes along D_{2D} is calculated: in a) and b) the preferred trabecular orientation is clearly distinguished, while c) is the transversal plane.

2.5.8.1 Application to reference problems

In order to validate the implementation of the 2D and 3D versions to calculate fractal dimension, we applied them to two reference problems with known solution: D_{2D} was proved against Sierpinski's triangle (Fig. 2.15) while D_{3D} was validated against the Menger Sponge (Fig. 2.16).

Sierpinski's triangle has a fractal dimension of $log(3)/log(2) = 1.585$ and our implementation gives a value of 1.588, with an error of 0.2 %, represented in Fig. 2.15.

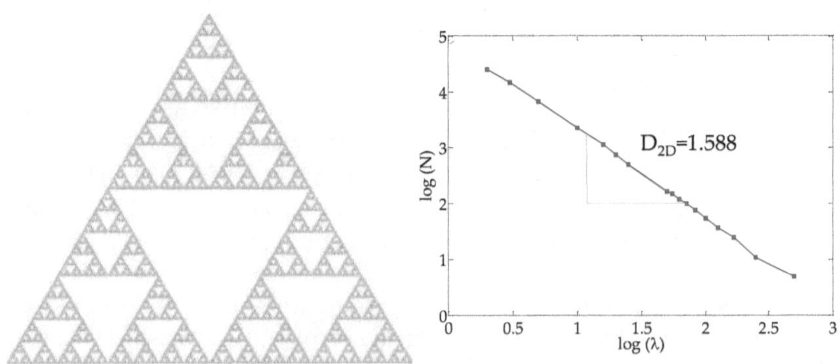

Figure 2.15: Representation of Sierpinski's triangle for D_{2D} validation. The figure has license for free use [215] and it is attributed to Beojan Stanislaus (left). Fractal dimension assessment of a Sierpinski's triangle through box-counting method (right).

In case of Menger sponge fractal, it has a known fractal dimension of $log(20)/log(3) = 2.727$ and our implementation gives a 2.763 fractal dimension values, with an error of 1%.

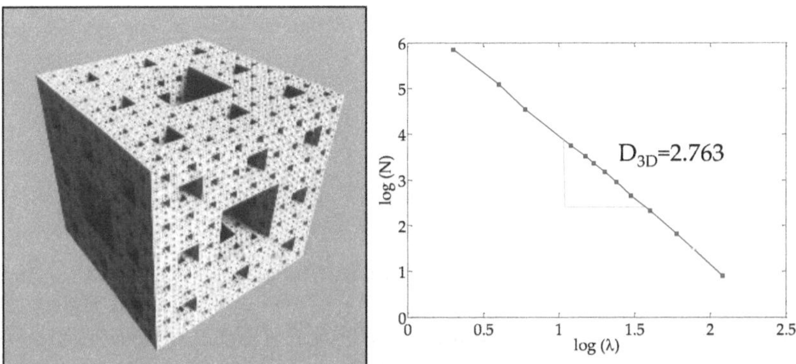

Figure 2.16: Menger sponge representation to validate D$_{3D}$ estimation. Figure attribution: Daniel Schwen, free use license [216] (left) and validation of the 3D implementation of the box-counting method against menger sponge fractal (right).

2.5.9 Fabric tensor to estimate the degree of anisotropy (DA)

The fabric tensor describes the material anisotropy degree of orthotropic materials like cancellous bone [92, 104]. Harrigan and Mann [104] proved that the representation of the mean intercept length (MIL), calculated over a histological section of cancellous bone resulted in an ellipse, whose main axis was aligned to the main trabecular orientation, expressed by Eq. 2.8 or as a tensor (Eq. 2.9).

$$ax^2 + bxy + cy^2 = k \tag{2.8}$$

$$[M] = \begin{bmatrix} a & b/2 \\ b/2 & c \end{bmatrix} \tag{2.9}$$

The application of the mean intercept length to a 3D cancellous bone mask produces an ellipsoid oriented according to the preferred trabecular direction, which may be expressed like Eq. 2.10 or in a tensorial form (Eq. 2.11). The tensorial description permits to determine preferred orientations from principal axis analysis or to include anisotropic material properties. The relationship between the long and short axis of the ellipse, and between the longest and shortest axis of the ellipsoid may be defined as the degree of anisotropy (DA).

$$Ax_1^2 + Bx_2^2 + Cx_3^2 + 2Dx_1x_2 + 2Ex_1x_3 + 2Fx_2x_3 = 1 \qquad (2.10)$$

$$[M] = \begin{bmatrix} A & D & E \\ D & B & F \\ E & F & C \end{bmatrix} \qquad (2.11)$$

The degree of anisotropy is important in cancellous bone analysis [9, 217]. Some authors relate it to the mechanical state, combined with the apparent density or volume fraction, while others have proved its relationship to the elastic stiffness matrix, from the work of Cowin [105].

2.5.9.1 Degree of anisotropy based on mean intercept length method in 2D (DA_{MIL2D})

The mean intercept length is a parameter that measures the mean distance between phases for a particular analysis direction. The method is applied to the segmented mask, that is, a binarized image, so the segmentation process may have a significant influence on its estimation. The implementation of the mean intercept length in 2D (MIL2D) may be described as follows: a set of parallel proof lines of total length h, defined by its angle θ from a reference axis and separated a distance d, are traced, and the number of intersections $C(\theta)$ between them and the phases interface are counted, see Fig. 2.17. Then the mean intercept length for that angle θ is calculated as defined in Eq. 2.12:

$$\text{MIL}(\theta) = \frac{h}{C(\theta)} \qquad (2.12)$$

If the phase is oriented along the probe lines, few intercepts are counted and MIL gets a higher value than for the non-oriented case, where more interceptions appear and MIL value is lower. The process is repeated for θ values in the range [0° - 180°] and the resulting MIL values may be plotted as a rose diagram (Fig. 2.18 right). The data is fitted to an ellipse through the application of the least squares method and the relationship between its long and short axis is defined as the anisotropy degree (DA).

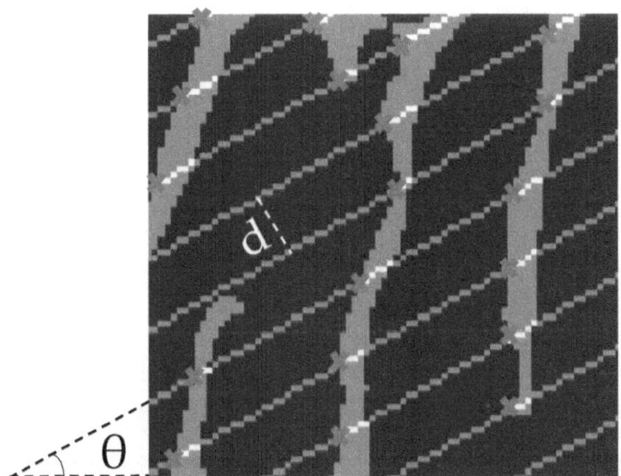

Figure 2.17: Scheme of mean intercept length method: A set of parallel lines characterized by an angle θ and separated a distance d are traced and the number of intersections between phases are counted. MIL is then calculated using Eq. 2.12.

Fig. 2.18 shows an example of the application of MIL method to a cancellous bone micro-CT segmented image. A preferred orientation, perpendicular to the horizontal direction is clearly distinguished, which is captured in the polar plot of the mean intercept length. The relationship between the ellipse axis is defined as the degree of anisotropy based on the mean intercept length (DA_{MIL2D}). The accuracy of the method depends on the angle discretization and the separation between prove lines.

The mean intercept length method has limitations that should be mentioned. In general, it can only be applied to materials whose anisotropy and orientation is determined by their boundaries [218]. For example, it should not be applied to analyze the microstructural anisotropy of a circle lattice like the one depicted in Fig. 2.19, since its anisotropy is determined by the distribution of circles and not by their boundaries.

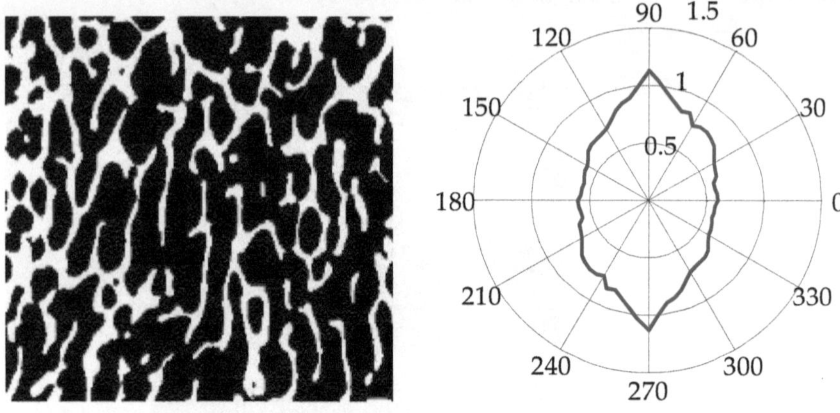

Figure 2.18: Example of application of MIL to an image of cancellous bone. Segmented mask of cancellous bone tissue, where the preferred orientation is clearly distinguished (left) and rose diagram representation of MIL, which is capable to detect the preferred orientation at a 90° orientation (right).

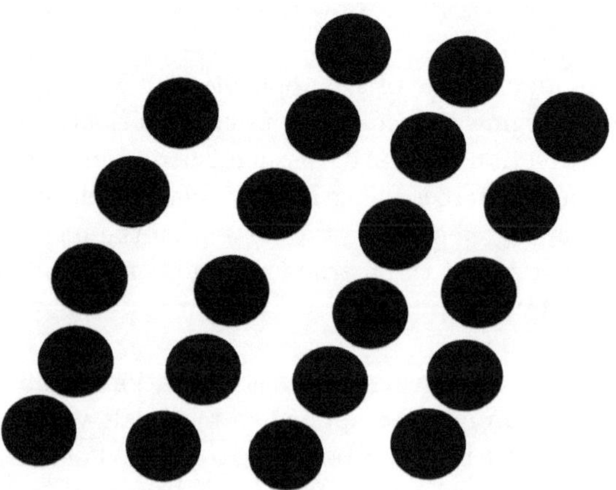

Figure 2.19: Representation of a lattice composed by circles. MIL is not capable to assess its anisotropy because it is not determined by its boundaries but its spacial distribution.

2.5.9.2 Degree of anisotropy based on mean intercept length method in 3D (DA$_{\text{MIL3D}}$)

The extension of the implementation to 3D consisted of including an additional angle (ϕ). Therefore, we define the set of lines for a particular orientation described by their azimuth (θ) and elevation (ϕ), which will vary according to Eq. 2.13 to cover the whole volume of analysis.

$$0 \leq \theta < 360° \quad 0 \leq \phi < 90° \tag{2.13}$$

A linear uniform distribution of azimuth and elevation angles is not desirable because, if plotted in a sphere, points would tend to concentrate near the poles. It can be explained by the area differential definition in spheric coordinates, Eq. 2.14.

$$\text{dA} = r^2\cos\phi \ \text{d}\phi\text{d}\theta \tag{2.14}$$

In order to uniformly distribute the prove angles, a cube projection method is considered. First, the cube faces are meshed uniformly and then, the values of azimuth and elevation of that points are calculated. Fig. 2.20 shows an example of a cube discretization to be projected to an uniformly discretized sphere. The traced line, characterized by θ and ϕ is replicated over the volume of interest and the procedure to calculate MIL is analogous to 2D.

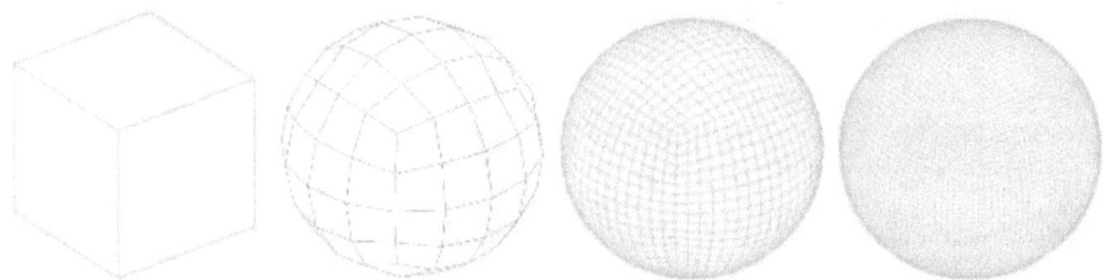

Figure 2.20: Different levels of discretization for a uniform distribution of probe lines for MIL calculation.

MIL results are then fitted to an ellipsoid of Eq. 2.10 by the least squared method and the anisotropy degree is calculated as the ratio between the longest and the shortest axis of the ellipsoid.

This methodology was applied to three examples: a grid of perpendicular planes, a rhomboid and a trabecular bone sample (Fig. 2.21). For each example, the method is capable to detect the presence of main material orientation. Perpendicular grid planes case predicts two main equivalent transversal directions and a main orientation (Fig. 2.21 left). The anisotropy degree associated has a 4.42 value. On the other hand, the rhomboid case also predicts the existence of three main orthogonal directions, with a DA value of 3.75 (Fig. 2.21 middle). Finally, the application of MIL to a trabecular bone sample estimates a DA value of 1.76 and the orientation of the resulting ellipsoid matches the one of the segmented mask, determined by visual inspection (Fig. 2.21 right).

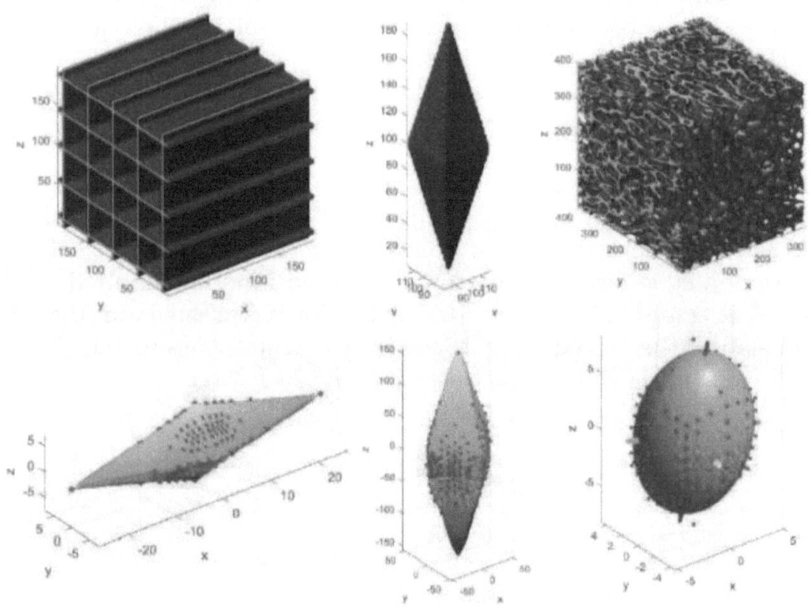

Figure 2.21: Examples of application of the 3D version of MIL to determine anisotropy degree. At the top of the figure we represent the segmented masks for each example: perpendicular grid planes (left), rhomboid (centre) and trabecular bone sample (right). At the bottom of the figure a representation of MIL points distribution is shown (left and centre) and the subsequent fitted ellipsoid (right).

2.5.10 Connectivity density (Conn.D)

The connectivity density (Conn.D) of cancellous bone is believed to play a role in stiffness and strength changes due to pathologies like osteoporosis [110]. The determination of Conn.D values was performed using BoneJ application [112], which is based on the works from Odgaard and Gundersen [110] and Toriwaki and Yonekura [219]. The connectivity value is determined using the Euler-Poincaré equation (Eq. 2.15), that depends on the topological invariant Euler characteristic number (χ):

$$\chi = \beta_0 - \beta_1 - \beta_2 \tag{2.15}$$

where β_0 is the number of parts in the structure, β_1 is the connectivity (Conn) and β_2 is the number of voids surrounded by bone. In case of cancellous bone, it is expected to have just one connected structure ($\beta_0=1$), with no closed cavities because it is an open cell structure ($\beta_2=0$). The connectivity density is calculated normalizing Eq. 2.15 to the volume (V), Eq. 2.16:

$$\text{Conn.D} = \frac{1 - \chi}{V} \tag{2.16}$$

The calculation of the Euler number in a 3D digitized image may be described as in Eq. 2.17 [219].

$$\chi = n_0 - n_1 + n_2 - n_3 \tag{2.17}$$

where n_0 represents the number of vertex in the object, n_1 is the number of edges, n_2 is the number of faces and n_3 corresponds to the number of voxels. Obviously, those numbers depend on the connectivity neighborhood definition (Fig. 2.22), which conditions whether each entity of a voxel defines the same entity of the 3D object or a connection between voxels and does not contribute to the Euler number (χ).

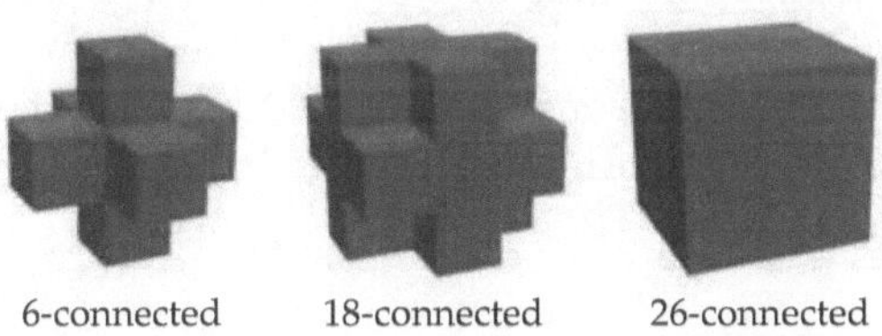

Figure 2.22: 3D connectivity definitions for a digitized image.

2.5.11 Morphometry results of cancellous bone specimens

In this section, the morphometric description of the datasets analyzed is presented. As mentioned, we divide the datasets as follows: set A corresponds to 5 samples scanned without calibration phantoms and tested destructively under quasi-static compression conditions (Table 2.2), set B is composed of 28 samples scanned without phantoms and simulated to estimate apparent elastic mechanical properties through homogenization (Table 2.3) and set C is composed of 5 samples scanned together with calibration phantoms and tested under the same conditions than set A (Table 2.4). The specimens of each set belonged to different animals and lumbar or thoracic vertebrae. The data estimation for sets A, B and C has been also represented as violin plots in Figures 2.23, 2.24 and 2.25. Each violin plot represents the data distribution as its probability density for each value.

We have estimated bone volume fraction (BV/TV), bone surface to total volume ratio (BS/TV), bone surface to volume ratio (BS/BV), mean trabecular thickness (Tb.Th), mean trabecular separation (Tb.Sp), trabecular number (Tb.N), fractal dimension (D_{2D}, D_{3D}), anisotropy degree (DA_{MIL2D}, DA_{MIL3D}) and connectivity density (Conn.D). As mentioned above, both D_{2D} and DA_{MIL2D} were applied to the samples along their three main directions, two of them containing the main trabecular orientation, while the other comprises their transversal plane.

The first we can notice in Tables 2.2, 2.3 and 2.4 is that some parameters do not vary much. The reason may be the origin of the specimens since all came from healthy mature pigs.

In case of BV/TV, a mean value of 22.5 % is obtained for set A, 21 % for set B and around 20 % for set C, so regarding mean values, the three sets analyzed are very similar. Looking at individual values, the highest bone volume fraction (28 %) and the lowest value (14 %) are found on two specimens belonging to set B. The values measured for BV/TV lay in the range of both osteoporotic (5-23 %) and normal cancellous bone (10-50%), which overlap according to Nazarian et al. [103].

The relationship between bone surface area and specimen apparent volume (BS/TV) presents less scattering than BS/BV. The wider variation of BS/BV parameter makes it more suitable to be used to detect changes on bone microstructure. Specifically, a mean BS/BV value of 22.68 mm^{-1} (range of 19.2 - 25.43 mm^{-1}) was calculated for set A, 23.25 mm^{-1} (ranging 17.72 - 31.79 mm^{-1}) for set B and a significantly higher mean value of 31.96 mm^{-1} (ranging 27.20 - 34.95 mm^{-1}) was obtained for set C.

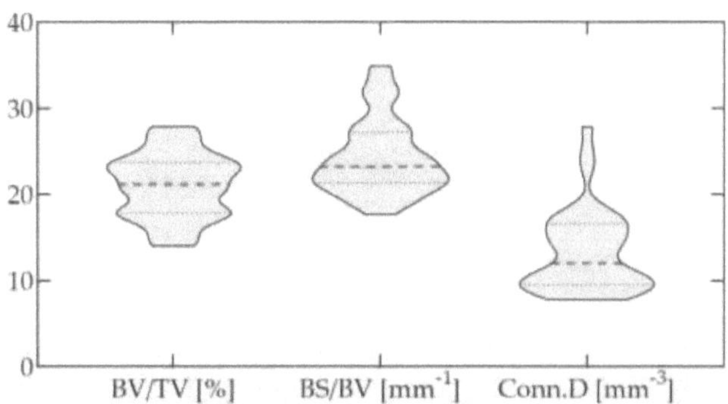

Figure 2.23: Violin plot representation of the bone volume fraction (BV/TV), bone surface to volume ratio (BS/BV) and connectivity density (Conn.D) values. The plot was generated considering sets A, B and C. The median (red dash line) and interquartile ranges (dash lines) are shown.

The mean trabecular thickness (Tb.Th) shows negligible variations between sets. The minimum Tb.Th value (0.1 mm) is found for Specimen B#27, which corresponds to the one of the lowest BV/TV, while the highest Tb.Th (0.16 mm) is found for the specimen of the highest BV/TV. In this sense, Tb.Th parameter is not capable to discern variations of BV/TV, because all the samples range in a narrow set of Tb.Th values. Tb.Th estimations are in the range of values reported for normal cancellous bone from different locations [8, 220].

On the other hand, the mean trabecular separation (Tb.Sp) presents similar scattering between sample sets (standard deviation of 0.07 - 0.08 mm). In terms of mean values, sets A and C have the same mean Tb.Sp, which is significantly higher in case of set C (mean value of 0.62 mm in contrast to 0.52 mm). The higher Tb.Sp values for set C may be related to the slightly lower mean BV/TV of the set. Analyzing individual values, 0.39 mm is the lowest Tb.Sp value, while the maximum one is 0.69 mm.

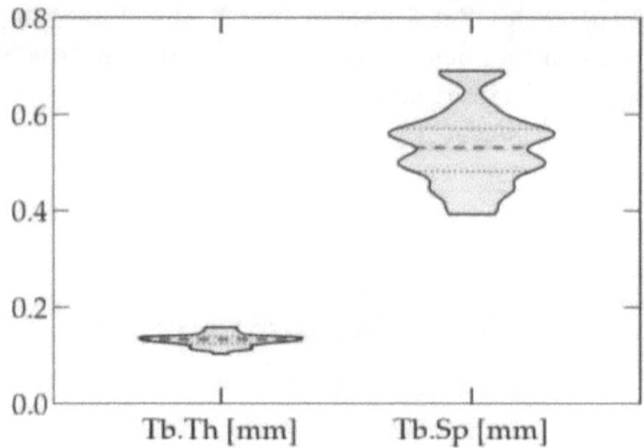

Figure 2.24: Violin plot representation of the mean trabecular thickness (Tb.Th) and mean trabecular separation (Tb.Sp) values. The plot was generated considering sets A, B and C. The median (red dash line) and interquartile ranges (dash lines) are shown.

Trabecular number (Tb.N) relates to the amount of cancellous bone (BV/TV) and the mean value of its trabecular thickness (Tb.Th). As discussed above, a narrow range of values was obtained for Tb.Th and, as a consequence, the variation of Tb.N value in this study varies in the range of $[1.2 - 1.99]$ mm^{-1}, distributed around a mean value of 1.56 mm^{-1}. Our results are in the range of normal cancellous bone (1.25 mm^{-1} in [220] and 1.36 mm^{-1} in [221]) from different locations (1.26 mm^{-1} for lumbar spine, 1.39 mm^{-1} for iliac crest, 1.42 mm^{-1} for femoral head and 1.45 mm^{-1} for calcaneus samples in [8]) and are lower than the Tb.N values reported in [222] (7.78 mm^{-1}).

We assessed fractal dimension in 2D along the three main 3D image axis, Fig. 2.14. As can be noticed in Tables 2.2, 2.3 and 2.4, the application of fractal dimension to planes containing the main trabecular orientation (D_{2D-1}, D_{2D-2}) gives similar values (between 1.50 and 1.72), while transversal plane fractal analysis (D_{2D-3}) results in a slightly different fractal dimension value, around a 3 % higher, for the three sets analyzed.In addition, 3D fractal dimension was calculated, giving lower values for set C (mean value of 2.63) compared to sets A and B (2.72 and 2.75). Values of D_{3D} range from 2.57 to 2.81.

The application of the 2D version of MIL parameter to the three main planes, which define the 3D image, led to interesting results. First, a clear preferred orientation direction is detected by MIL parameter ($DA_{MIL2D-1}$, $DA_{MIL2D-2}$), with anisotropy degree values of around 1.65 for the whole dataset. Besides, the values for planes containing the preferred trabecular orientation give almost the same DA prediction. In contrast, the transversal direction ($DA_{MIL2D-3}$) is described as nearly isotropic according to MIL parameter (mean $DA_{MIL2D-3}$ value of around 1.05, 1 defines isotropy). Moreover, the extension to 3D of the MIL provides very similar results than the 2D application to the main orientation planes, which supports the idea that the specimens were machined identifying the main orientation, which is close to match global specimen directions.

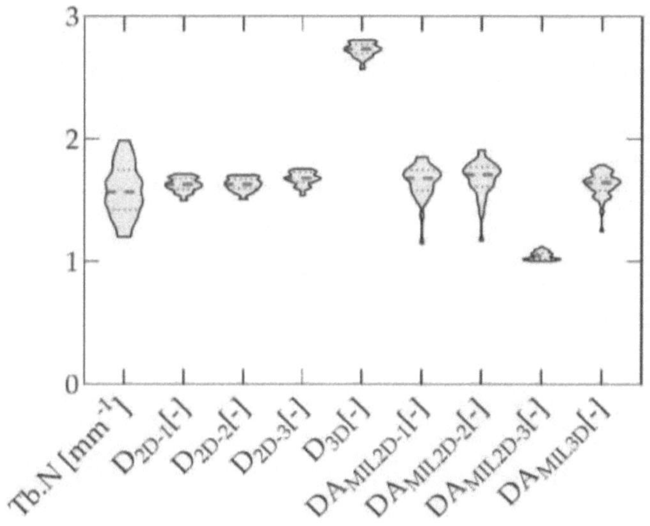

Figure 2.25: Violin plot representation of the trabecular number (Tb.N), fractal dimension (D) and anisotropy degree (DA) values. The plot was generated considering sets A, B and C. The median (red dash line) and interquartile ranges (dash lines) are shown.

Finally, connectivity density (Conn.D) estimations present values ranging from 7.8 to 25 mm^{-3}. The values obtained are in the upper range of the

reported by Kabel et al. [9] and Uchiyama et al. [222] and are an order
of magnitude higher than the values reported by Hambli [44]. Other works
report negative values that may be taken carefully because they may be result
of noisy images analysis or the presence of multi particles within bone structure [221]. The results do not show a clear relationship to other morphometric
parameters, which is consistent with other results reported in the literature
[9, 110]. A weak dependence on BV/TV and Tb.N is reported, but the authors
themselves question the relationship and postulate Conn.D as an independent
parameter [110].

Table 2.2: Morphometric analysis of specimens of set A under study, mean values and standard deviation for each parameter are also presented. BV/TV=bone volume fraction, BS/TV=bone surface per total volume, BS/BV=bone surface per bone volume, Tb.Th=mean trabecular thickness, Tb.Sp=mean trabecular separation, Tb.N=trabecular number, D_{2D}=fractal dimension 2D (calculated along three main directions: 1 and 2 correspond to planes containing the preferred trabecular orientation, while 3 correspond to the transverse plane), D_{3D}=fractal dimension 3D, DA_{MIL2D}=bone degree of anisotropy in 2D (calculated along the three main directions, defined like for fractal dimension 2D), DA_{MIL3D}=bone degree of anisotropy in 3D, Conn.D=connectivity density of the trabecular structure.

Specimen	BV/TV [%]	BS/TV [mm^{-1}]	BS/BV [mm^{-1}]	Tb.Th [mm]	Tb.Sp [mm]	Tb.N [mm^{-1}]	D_{2D-1} [-]	D_{2D-2} [-]	D_{2D-3} [-]	D_{3D} [-]	$DA_{MIL2D-1}$ [-]	$DA_{MIL2D-2}$ [-]	$DA_{MIL2D-3}$ [-]	DA_{MIL3D} [-]	Conn.D [mm^{-3}]
A#1	27.07	4.66	19.2	0.16	0.56	1.67	1.64	1.66	1.69	2.72	1.84	1.78	1.02	1.74	7.83
A#2	20.47	5.34	23.9	0.14	0.56	1.47	1.62	1.63	1.68	2.69	1.55	1.61	1.05	1.53	11.8
A#3	17.63	4.48	25.43	0.13	0.59	1.34	1.63	1.6	1.65	2.68	1.7	1.77	1.02	1.68	13.38
A#4	22.6	5.31	23.49	0.14	0.41	1.59	1.71	1.66	1.69	2.74	1.53	1.44	1.1	1.52	24.94
A#5	24.73	5.29	21.39	0.14	0.5	1.79	1.69	1.69	1.73	2.77	1.75	1.79	1.02	1.68	13.57
Mean	22.5	5.02	22.68	0.14	0.52	1.57	1.66	1.65	1.69	2.72	1.67	1.68	1.04	1.63	14.3
SD	3.66	0.41	2.42	0.01	0.07	0.17	0.04	0.03	0.03	0.04	0.13	0.15	0.03	0.1	6.38

Table 2.3: Morphometry results of set B. We report individual results and mean and standard deviation values. All the parameters were estimated on cubic volumes of 7 mm side.

Sample	BV/TV [%]	BS/BV [mm^{-1}]	Tb.Th [mm]	Tb.Sp [mm]	Tb.N [mm^{-1}]	$D_{2D\text{-}1}$ [-]	$D_{2D\text{-}2}$ [-]	$D_{2D\text{-}3}$ [-]	D_{3D} [-]	$DA_{MIL2D\text{-}1}$ [-]	$DA_{MIL2D\text{-}2}$ [-]	$DA_{MIL2D\text{-}3}$ [-]	DA_{MIL3D} [-]	Conn.D [mm^{-3}]
B#1	27.91	17.72	0.16	0.5	1.76	1.68	1.67	1.73	2.78	1.78	1.68	1.01	1.67	8.2
B#2	21.3	20.05	0.15	0.57	1.46	1.62	1.62	1.66	2.72	1.58	1.55	1.09	1.54	8.52
B#3	20.08	21.55	0.14	0.57	1.47	1.61	1.62	1.67	2.73	1.62	1.73	1.07	1.64	9.57
B#4	24.78	19.08	0.15	0.52	1.64	1.65	1.66	1.71	2.76	1.48	1.61	1.08	1.53	10.3
B#5	21.01	21.31	0.14	0.55	1.52	1.62	1.63	1.68	2.73	1.72	1.75	1.01	1.66	9.57
B#6	23.72	19.12	0.15	0.54	1.55	1.65	1.64	1.68	2.74	1.49	1.5	1.06	1.47	8.76
B#7	18.18	27.88	0.11	0.49	1.62	1.64	1.64	1.7	2.75	1.67	1.73	1.07	1.66	17.5
B#8	26.31	21.29	0.13	0.44	1.96	1.7	1.71	1.76	2.8	1.68	1.75	1.03	1.66	14.38
B#9	22.15	21.19	0.14	0.56	1.61	1.64	1.65	1.69	2.75	1.56	1.62	1.06	1.52	11.38
B#10	17.84	24.39	0.12	0.56	1.43	1.6	1.6	1.66	2.71	1.76	1.83	1.01	1.75	10.67
B#11	25.6	21.52	0.13	0.44	1.91	1.69	1.7	1.75	2.8	1.72	1.91	1.12	1.79	14.9
B#12	22.38	21.55	0.13	0.51	1.67	1.65	1.65	1.71	2.76	1.84	1.82	1	1.75	9.85
B#13	21.51	19.64	0.15	0.56	1.46	1.61	1.61	1.68	2.73	1.77	1.9	1.05	1.75	8.4
B#14	27.48	20.61	0.14	0.44	1.99	1.72	1.7	1.76	2.81	1.75	1.61	1.1	1.67	14.85
B#15	20.78	24.6	0.13	0.48	1.66	1.66	1.66	1.72	2.76	1.68	1.71	1.02	1.63	16.61
B#16	23.79	23.01	0.13	0.45	1.83	1.69	1.69	1.74	2.79	1.7	1.71	1.01	1.65	16.57
B#17	22.83	24.25	0.12	0.46	1.87	1.68	1.69	1.74	2.79	1.62	1.74	1.1	1.62	16.88
B#18	23.33	23.99	0.13	0.39	1.74	1.72	1.71	1.73	2.8	1.15	1.17	1.09	1.25	27.9
B#19	23.22	22.83	0.14	0.4	1.66	1.69	1.69	1.74	2.8	1.53	1.49	1.1	1.55	23.05
B#20	23.93	22.69	0.13	0.48	1.86	1.69	1.69	1.74	2.79	1.68	1.74	1.04	1.65	14.81
B#21	17.86	26.8	0.12	0.51	1.53	1.63	1.63	1.68	2.74	1.75	1.77	1.01	1.71	16.09
B#22	15.07	25.31	0.13	0.69	1.2	1.55	1.56	1.61	2.67	1.69	1.73	1	1.62	10.04
B#23	16.44	22.77	0.13	0.69	1.24	1.56	1.57	1.61	2.67	1.58	1.67	1.02	1.6	8.84
B#24	14.05	27.42	0.12	0.61	1.2	1.56	1.55	1.61	2.67	1.73	1.67	1.07	1.64	10.46
B#25	18.66	21.94	0.14	0.63	1.38	1.59	1.6	1.65	2.7	1.62	1.69	1.03	1.6	8.64
B#26	17.43	27.61	0.11	0.5	1.52	1.62	1.63	1.69	2.74	1.7	1.81	1.07	1.74	17.4
B#27	14.05	31.79	0.1	0.51	1.35	1.59	1.59	1.65	2.7	1.8	1.74	1.05	1.71	18.56
B#28	15.57	29.21	0.11	0.49	1.4	1.6	1.6	1.67	2.72	1.86	1.81	1.04	1.75	17.53
Mean	20.97	23.25	0.13	0.52	1.59	1.64	1.64	1.69	2.75	1.66	1.69	1.05	1.64	13.58
SD	3.96	3.37	0.01	0.08	0.22	0.05	0.05	0.04	0.04	0.14	0.15	0.04	0.11	4.91

Table 2.4: Morphometry results of set C. We report individual results and mean and standard deviation values.

Sample	BV/TV $[\%]$	BS/TV $[mm^{-1}]$	BS/BV $[mm^{-1}]$	Tb.Th $[mm]$	Tb.Sp $[mm]$	Tb.N $[mm^{-1}]$	D_{2D-1} $[-]$	D_{2D-2} $[-]$	D_{2D-3} $[-]$	D_{3D} $[-]$	$DA_{MIL2D-1}$ $[-]$	$DA_{MIL2D-2}$ $[-]$	$DA_{MIL2D-3}$ $[-]$	DA_{MIL3D} $[-]$	Conn.D $[mm^{-3}]$
C#1	18.01	5.74	31.89	0.14	0.69	1.32	1.51	1.51	1.56	2.60	1.74	1.64	1.05	1.68	9.22
C#2	23.44	7.43	31.72	0.13	0.54	1.80	1.59	1.58	1.63	2.70	1.60	1.56	1.07	1.59	12.36
C#3	19.99	5.44	27.20	0.12	0.57	1.67	1.56	1.58	1.61	2.66	1.38	1.39	1.03	1.41	15.12
C#4	17.25	6.03	34.95	0.13	0.68	1.33	1.50	1.51	1.54	2.57	1.60	1.63	1.02	1.59	10.47
C#5	19.66	6.69	34.02	0.13	0.60	1.51	1.56	1.56	1.60	2.64	1.66	1.66	1.02	1.61	10.38
Mean	19.67	6.27	31.96	0.13	0.62	1.53	1.54	1.55	1.59	2.63	1.60	1.58	1.04	1.57	11.51
SD	2.39	0.80	3.00	0.01	0.07	0.21	0.04	0.04	0.04	0.05	0.13	0.11	0.02	0.10	2.31

2.5.12   Influence of cancellous bone images segmentation on morphometric and elastic response determination

In this section, we aim at investigating the effects of the selection of the segmentation threshold on the morphometry and the estimation of the elastic response through image-based FE modeling. We analyze the influence of varying the user's threshold choice by a ±15% for three samples of different bone volume fraction: Specimen B#1, B#15 and B#27.

A detail of the segmented masks resulting from a ±15% threshold variation for a cancellous bone mask is depicted in Fig. 2.26, where noteworthy dissimilarities can be noted. Similar influence is expected for other cancellous bone samples.

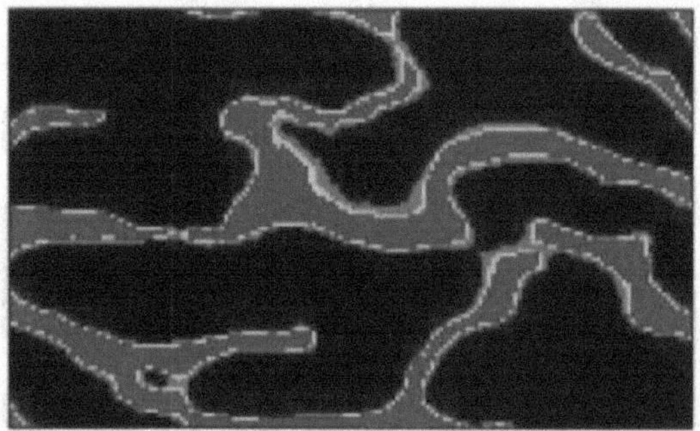

Figure 2.26: Segmented masks detail for a ± 15% segmentation threshold variation from the user's choice. Slight differences between masks can be noticed (in blue: +15% threshold variation, in yellow: original threshold, in red: -15% threshold variation).

For each threshold, the resulting mask is analyzed in terms of its morphometry and a FE model is generated maintaining the element type (C3D4 coded in Abaqus) and element size. For each specimen, a compression along its main orientation direction is simulated and the apparent stiffness is calculated, considering a tissue Young's modulus of 1 GPa to only account for changes due to the microarchitecture.

Fig. 2.27 shows the effect of a ± 15 % threshold variation on the 3D reconstruction for Specimens B#1, B#15 and B#27. It can be noted that threshold variation affects differently depending on the BV/TV of the specimen. Specimen B#1 had a BV/TV of 28 % and the threshold variation produces a change in the range of 19 to 36 % and a plate-like structure is observed in general, with increasing thicknesses for a lower segmentation threshold. Specimen B#15 shows a similar variation in terms of structure type, with an original BV/TV of around 20 %, which turned to between 11.5 to 30 % and, for 15 % threshold variation makes the microstructure more rod-like. In case of Specimen B#27, with an original volume fraction of around 15 %, changing the segmentation threshold strongly affected the trabecular structure connectivity. A 15 % threshold variation produces the disruption of the trabecular structure, resembling an osteoporotic cancellous bone specimen, see Fig. 2.27.

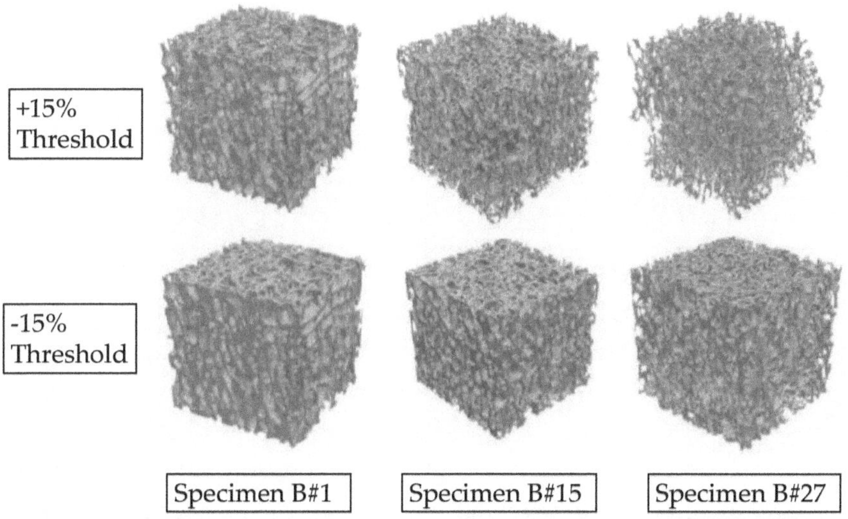

Figure 2.27: Reconstruction of the effect of a ± 15 % variation of the segmentation threshold on three vertebral cancellous bone specimens. Each specimen had a different original volume fraction, summarized in Table 2.3, which allows to study a wider range of BV/TV.

Table 2.5 summarizes the influence of threshold variation on the morphometry of the samples analyzed, while Table 2.6 shows the variation of the apparent modulus. It can be noted that, for the morphometry, different evolutions arise depending on the specimen initial bone volume fraction.

Fig. 2.28 depicts the effect of BV/TV on the apparent modulus, which follows a power law. We considered a Young's modulus of 1 GPa for all the models to only study the influence of the microstructure. This effect is analogous to the reported for cancellous bone in the literature [10, 14, 40].

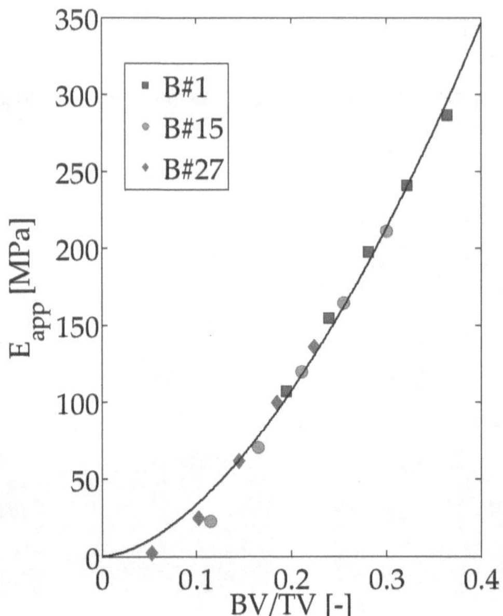

Figure 2.28: Sensitivity analysis of the influence of varying the user's segmentation threshold ± 15% on the apparent modulus estimated through finite element modeling with respect to bone volume fraction. The data is fitted to a power law whose expression is $E_{app} = 1619 \, BV/TV^{1.683}$ ($R^2 = 0.9907$).

Some parameters are more sensitive to segmentation threshold variation. For example, the apparent modulus (E_{app}) is influenced linearly by the thresholding, but its magnitude changes as a function of the BV/TV of the specimen, see Fig. 2.29 top right. In case of specimen B#27, with the lowest BV/TV, a ± 15 % variation produces up to 120 % modulus change, which decreases to 45 % for specimen B#1, with the highest BV/TV.

Analogous behavior is observed for BV/TV but with a lower amplitude (Fig. 2.29 top left): up to 63 % BV/TV reduction for specimen B#27 for a

Table 2.5: Influence of segmentation threshold variation (Δ Thr) on the morphometry of three samples of different original bone volume fraction.

Sample	Δ Thr	BV/TV [%]	BS/TV [mm^{-1}]	BS/BV [mm^{-1}]	Tb.Th [mm]	Tb.Sp [mm]	Tb.N [mm^{-1}]	$D_{2D\text{-}1}$ [-]	$D_{2D\text{-}2}$ [-]	$D_{2D\text{-}3}$ [-]	D_{3D} [-]	$DA_{MIL2D\text{-}1}$ [-]	$DA_{MIL2D\text{-}2}$ [-]	$DA_{MIL2D\text{-}3}$ [-]	DA_{MIL3D} [-]	Conn.D [mm^{-3}]
B#1	+15%	19.45	5.07	26.05	0.13	0.55	1.46	1.62	1.62	1.68	2.73	1.74	1.68	1.02	1.73	11.27
	+7.5%	23.94	5.29	22.09	0.15	0.53	1.62	1.66	1.65	1.71	2.76	1.75	1.67	1.00	1.71	9.36
	0%	28.09	5.36	19.07	0.16	0.38	1.73	1.68	1.67	1.73	2.78	1.75	1.66	1.02	1.69	8.2
	-7.5%	32.18	5.36	16.66	0.18	0.49	1.79	1.69	1.68	1.74	2.79	1.73	1.65	1.03	1.69	7.4
	-15%	36.44	5.32	14.61	0.2	0.48	1.83	1.7	1.69	1.75	2.8	1.71	1.63	1.04	1.64	6.7
B#15	+15%	11.43	4.3	37.59	0.1	0.55	1.09	1.54	1.54	1.6	2.67	1.61	1.7	1.05	1.64	16.26
	+7.5%	16.46	5.14	31.24	0.12	0.51	1.4	1.61	1.62	1.67	2.73	1.64	1.69	1.03	1.64	18.33
	0%	21.08	5.55	26.31	0.13	0.49	1.62	1.66	1.66	1.72	2.76	1.66	1.68	1.01	1.62	16.61
	-7.5%	25.49	5.72	22.44	0.15	0.48	1.75	1.69	1.69	1.74	2.79	1.66	1.66	1.00	1.61	14.27
	-15%	30.01	5.79	19.3	0.16	0.46	1.85	1.71	1.7	1.76	2.81	1.65	1.64	1.01	1.59	12.64
B#27	+15%	5.27	2.57	48.79	0.09	0.74	0.6	1.33	1.33	1.41	2.51	1.74	1.74	1.00	1.69	7.3
	+7.5%	10.19	4.1	40.25	0.1	0.55	1.04	1.52	1.52	1.59	2.65	1.72	1.72	1.02	1.69	15.63
	0%	14.47	4.86	33.6	0.11	0.52	1.32	1.59	1.59	1.65	2.71	1.75	1.71	1.05	1.69	18.56
	-7.5%	18.47	5.26	28.48	0.12	0.5	1.51	1.64	1.63	1.69	2.74	1.77	1.69	1.06	1.69	17.38
	-15%	22.36	5.45	24.39	0.14	0.49	1.64	1.67	1.66	1.72	2.77	1.76	1.66	1.07	1.67	15.66

Table 2.6: Influence of segmentation threshold variation (Δ Thr) on the apparent modulus (E_{app}) estimated through image-based finite element models of three samples of different original bone volume fraction.

Sample	Δ Threshold	E_{app} [MPa] [1*]
B#1	+15%	107.2
	+7.5%	154.6
	0%	197.7
	-7.5%	240.7
	-15%	286.8
B#15	+15%	22.9
	+7.5%	70.4
	0%	120.1
	-7.5%	164.5
	-15%	211.4
B#27	+15%	1.9
	+7.5%	24.6
	0%	61.9
	-7.5%	99.7
	-15%	136.0

1* E=1 GPa for all the samples.

15 % increment of the threshold, which decreases to 46 % for specimen B#15 and to 31 % for B#1.

In case of BS/BV (Fig. 2.29 bottom left), the influence of the initial bone volume fraction is less significant than for other parameters analyzed, with only between a 4 to 9 % difference between samples. The influence for each sample is linear with an associated variation of 50 % for a 15 % increasing threshold for specimen B#27.

The ratio between the bone surface area to the total volume shows less influence for the highest BV/TV, which increases as the BV/TV decreases, see Fig. 2.29 bottom right. The relationships observed are non-linear and of greater importance for a 15 % threshold variation (up to 22.5 % for B#15 and 47 % for B#27). Decreasing the segmentation threshold affects less to BS/TV parameter, up to 12 % for specimen B#27.

Fig. 2.30 shows the effect of varying the segmentation on the mean trabecular thickness (Tb.Th), mean trabecular separation (Tb.Sp), trabecular

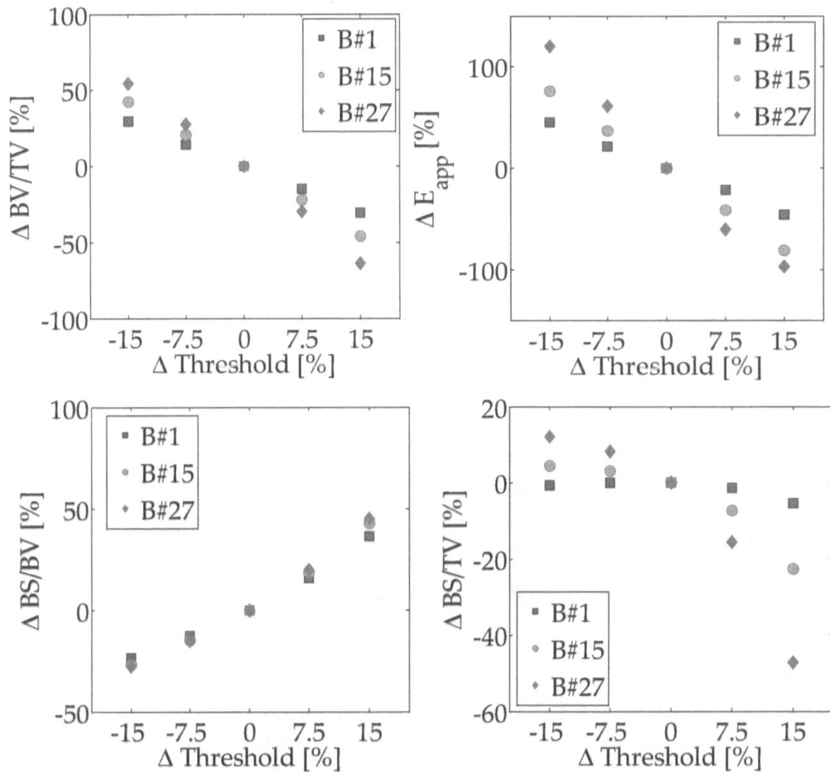

Figure 2.29: Influence in percentage of a ± 15% threshold variation on the estimation of the bone volume fraction (BV/TV), bone surface to volume ratio (BS/BV), bone surface to total volume (BS/TV) and apparent modulus (E_{app}).

number (Tb.N) and connectivity density (Conn.D). For Tb.Th, the effect of samples of different BV/TV is negligible, while the influence of applying various thresholds is linear. A threshold increase of 15 % results in a Tb.Th reduced around a 20 %. Underestimating the threshold a 15 % shows a similar but higher effect of around 23 %.

Connectivity is also affected differently according to the BV/TV, see Fig. 2.30 bottom right. The connectivity density (Conn.D) increases for increas-

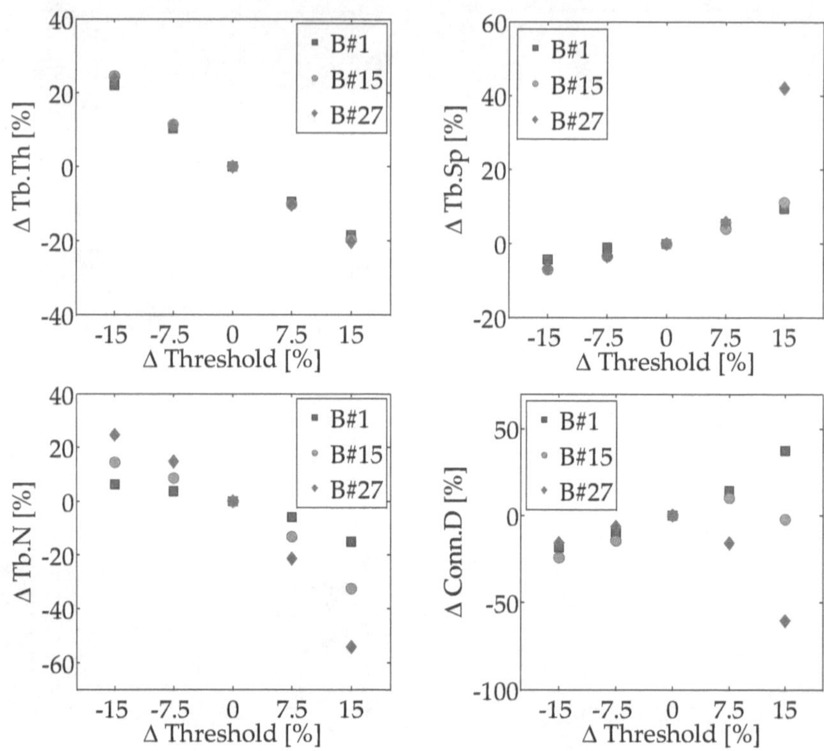

Figure 2.30: Influence in percentage of a ± 15% threshold variation on the estimation of the mean trabecular thickness (Tb.Th), mean trabecular separation (Tb.Sp), trabecular number (Tb.N) and connectivity density (Conn.D).

ing threshold for sample B#1, which has the highest BV/TV and presents a plate-like structure after the threshold variation, that affects between -18 and 37 %. As the BV/TV of the sample is reduced, a disruption on the trabecular lattice is produced. For example, for specimen B#15, the connectivity increases until a 7.5 % threshold increment. Beyond this point the connectivity is reduced. This effect is also seen in the lowest BV/TV sample. In that case, the connectivity is strongly reduced: up to 60 % for a 15 % threshold.

As the threshold increases, so does the mean trabecular separation, because

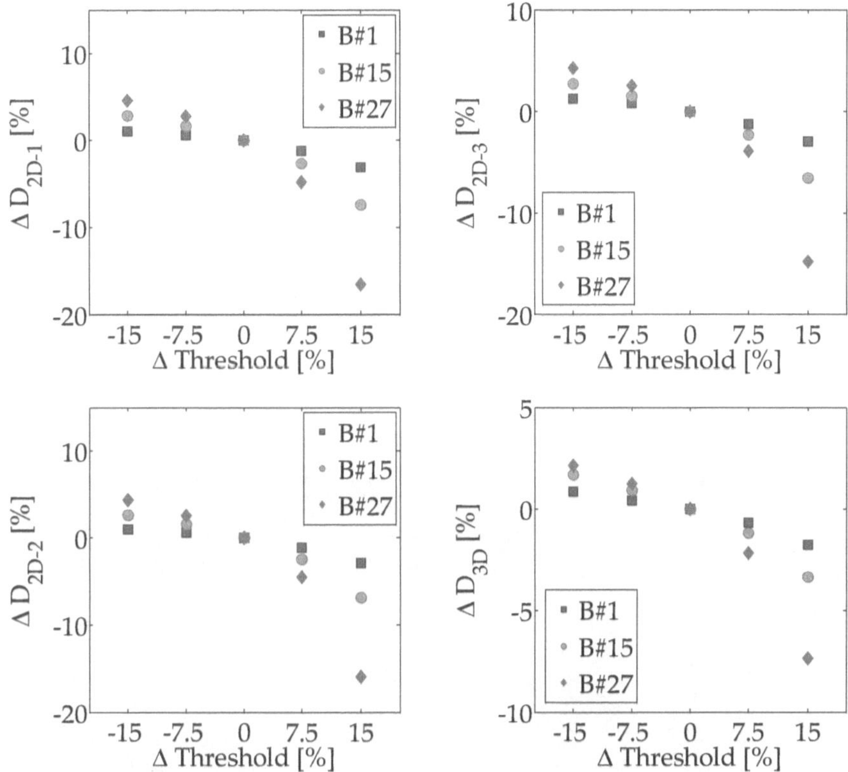

Figure 2.31: Influence in percentage of a ± 15% threshold variation on the estimation of the fractal dimension in 2D ($D_{2D\text{-}(1,2,3)}$), along the three main directions (1 and 2 refer to planes containing the preferred trabecular orientation, while 3 to the transversal plane) and in 3 dimensions (D_{3D}).

less bone is taken into account. For samples B#1 and B#15, a linear effect is observed (see Fig. 2.30 top right) with an influence between -7 and 11 %. In case of B#27, the increment of the segmentation threshold produces a disruption of the trabecular lattice, as depicted in Fig. 2.27, which leads to an increasing value of Tb.Sp up to 42 %. For a 7.5 % variation, the connectivity has already been disrupted but at a lower degree, and Tb.Sp value does not show such an important increment.

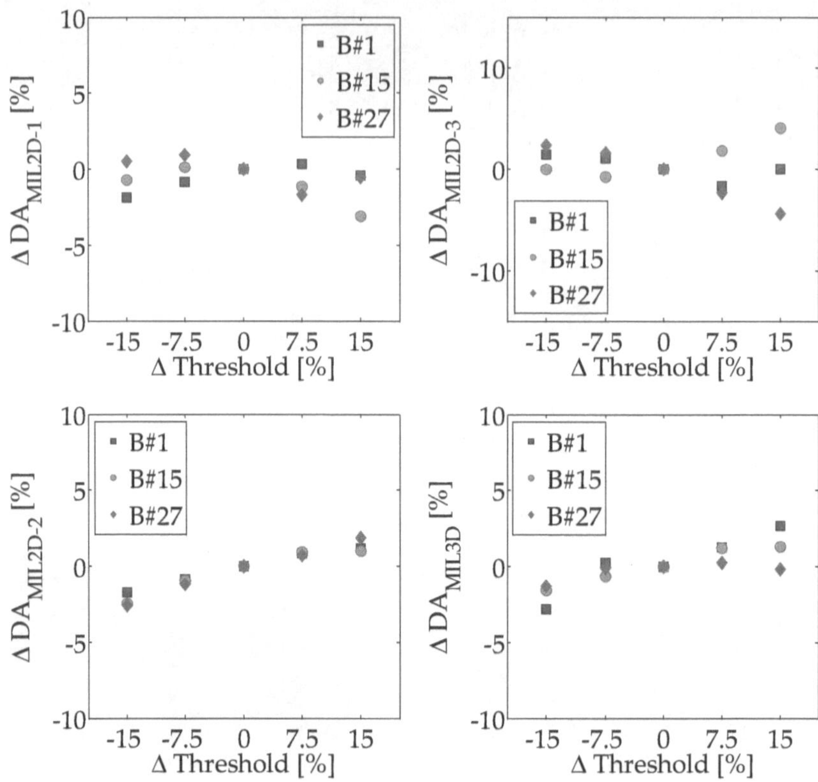

Figure 2.32: Influence in percentage of a $\pm$ 15% threshold variation on the estimation of the anisotropy degree, estimated through the mean intercept length, in 2D ($DA_{MIL2D-(1,2,3)}$), along the three main directions (1 and 2 refer to planes containing the preferred trabecular orientation, while 3 to the transversal plane) and in 3 dimensions (DA_{MIL3D}).

Trabecular number shows decreasing values for increasing segmentation threshold, which is consistent according to the definition that we used, which relates BV/TV and Tb.Th. Again, the lower the BV/TV, the higher the influence, with a -54 % variation for a 15 % threshold case.

Fractal dimension in 2 and 3 dimensions are affected similarly in percentage, see Fig. 2.31. If we analyze the data from Table 2.5, the calculation of the fractal dimension in 2D over the preferred orientation planes (1 and 2)

matches and the values are around a 4 % lower than for the transversal plane
(3). As the BV/TV of the sample increases, so does the fractal dimension,
but with a lower degree. Analyzing the evolution of fractal dimension (D) for
threshold variation, it shows a non-linear behavior where the amplitude of the
effect increases for a decreasing BV/TV. In 2 dimensions, a 15 % threshold
variation results in a 16 % decreasing fractal dimension (D) value for the lowest BV/TV, a 7 % for the middle case and only a 3 % decreasing value for
the highest BV/TV sample. Modifying a -15 % the segmentation threshold
affects less to the fractal dimension, with a maximum value for B#27 of 4.5
%.

The morphometric parameters that are less sensitive to variations on thresholding are the degree of anisotropy, measured from the mean intercept length,
both in 2D and 3D, see Fig. 2.32 and Table 2.5. The application of the MIL
method to the transversal plane of the samples revealed no preferred orientations, with values of the anisotropy degree (DA_{MIL}) close to 1 and a maximum
percentage variation of 4 %. On the other hand, the results from the analysis of the preferred orientation planes (directions 1 and 2) show a degree of
anisotropy of around 1.7 for the samples studied. This parameters presents
low sensitivity to threshold variations, less than 3 %. In case of the 3D version of MIL method, the results are very similar than the 2D versions for the
preferred orientation, with values around 1.7 and a low influence of the segmentation. Therefore, the application of MIL 2D to the preferred orientation
planes and MIL 3D produce analogous results.

Our results about the influence of the segmentation on the morphometry
are in line with others reported in the literature [113, 114]. For example, Hara
et al. [113] investigated threshold variation in a smaller range ($\pm 1\%$) and obtained analogous trends for the same range of BV/TV. They also analyzed the
effect of low volume fraction, where threshold variation may disconnect trabecular structures. In that case, the influence of threshold variation was higher
than for specimens of higher volume fraction as supported by our results.
They also pointed out the importance of threshold selection when studying
connectivity, with variations up to 7% for a 0.5% threshold variation.

Parkinson et al. [114] analyzed the effect of segmentation variation when
performed by different users and Otsu's algorithm [98]. Variations up to 7%
of the selected threshold were reported, so our threshold variation $\pm$ 15% is a
bit higher compared to typical user random errors reported in [114].

On the other hand, our results about the apparent modulus are in line with the ones reported in [40]. Chevalier et al. [40] analyzed the influence of a $\pm$ 10% threshold variation on the estimation of the apparent modulus, calculated from voxel-based finite element models. The authors analyzed 6 human femoral cancellous bone samples of different volume fraction. Their results show a dependence of the apparent modulus estimation on the volume fraction of the sample: low density samples present greater variations than high density samples. Within each sample, a linear influence is found related to threshold variation, in line with our observations. However, the representation of the whole dataset together shows that the linear influence seen for each sample turns to a power law for a wide range of BV/TV, as reported in the literature.

2.6 Conclusions

In this chapter, we have presented the cancellous bone specimens that constitute the dataset analyzed, together with their extraction and storage procedure. Then, the imaging system used to scan the samples and the phantoms used to assess bone density were shown. Two different calibration phantoms were used: liquid (K_2HPO_4) and HA-based phantoms. The micro-CT images were segmented using a global thresholding method. The morphometric parameters that we used to characterize cancellous bone microstructure from the segmented masks were presented, and their calculation method was defined.

A parametric analysis of the segmentation threshold was performed, studying its influence on both the morphometry and the apparent stiffness estimated through finite element modeling. Three vertebral cancellous bone samples of different bone volume fraction were selected from the data set, representative of samples of high, medium and low BV/TV, which allowed us to study a wider range of variation of the results.

The variation of the segmentation threshold in a $\pm$ 15 % produced changes in the microstructure as a function of the BV/TV of the sample. In case of the sample of lowest BV/TV, the increment of the segmentation threshold produced a disruption of the microarchitecture, with a loss of connectivity, and the change from a plate-like to a rod-like structure. Therefore, the segmentation threshold has a greater importance for the analysis of samples of lower BV/TV, which is the case of the osteoporotic ones, because it may cause the loss of connectivity and wrong estimations of morphometry and elastic modulus.

A power law relationship between the apparent modulus and bone volume fraction was obtained from the study, which agreed other relationships reported in the literature. This power law relationship could be obtained thanks to the segmentation influence analysis, because the data sets used in this book corresponded to mature healthy porcine vertebral cancellous bone samples, so less data scattering was present.

Some morphometric parameters were little influenced by segmentation threshold variation, such as the anisotropy degree in 2 and 3 dimensions, with a maximum effect of 4 % for a 15 % threshold increment.

The apparent modulus is highly sensitive to the segmentation threshold.

We report variations between 45 and 120 % for the limits that we considered for threshold variation. A linear influence was observed, like in the case of BV/TV and Tb.Th. For the latter parameters, an associated maximum range of parameter variation of -64 to 55 % and -20 to 24 % was found, respectively.

A non-linear influence of varying the threshold was observed for BS/BV, BS/TV, Tb.Sp, Tb.N, Conn.D and fractal dimension, which was higher for the sample of lower BV/TV. Both versions, 2D and 3D, of fractal dimension presented very similar behavior. On the other hand, the connectivity density (Conn.D) was affected differently according to the volume fraction: increasing the segmentation threshold increased the connectivity density up to a point, which defined the beginning of the disruption of the trabecular connections.

The results we reported in this chapter are in line with other from the literature, but we went a step further analyzing both morphometry and elastic properties together and accounting for various bone volume fractions, which permit to study the effect on healthy and osteoporotic cancellous bone. Besides, we considered a unique tissue modulus for all the samples in order to give insight into effects purely due to changes in the microarchitecture.

Chapter 3

Cancellous bone: experimental and numerical mechanical characterization

3.1 Introduction

In this chapter, we aim at calculating cancellous bone mechanical properties at the macro- and microscales. In both cases we determine elastic, yield and failure properties. At the macroscale, we use quasi-static compression testing and numerical homogenization to measure the global elastic response of parallelepiped-shaped specimens on their three main directions. Then, the objective is to find relationships between those homogeneous elastic properties and the underlying microstructure, to give insight into how microstructural changes affect the elastic response of cancellous bone. Single and multiple parameter analysis are performed to assess the morphometric variables that control the explanation of elastic properties variation.

On the other hand, tissue material properties are determined at the microscale. To achieve this goal, we apply different approaches: a combination of compression testing, micro-CT and finite element modeling, a phantom-based approach and the application of digital image correlation to images taken during testing. We use the first of them to estimate both elastic and failure properties, the second one to calculate Young's modulus at the tissue level, while the third one is used to estimate yield and failure strains. A comparison between the approaches is also reported.

We calculate properties that define the quality and integrity of cancellous bone at the apparent and micro levels and their relationship to cancellous architecture. The regressions obtained permit to estimate those mechanical properties that describe the state of a specimen. This avoids testing and numerical modeling. The first is time consuming, imply the possibility of specimen degradation and may include experimental artifacts, while numerical modeling involves high time and computational costs.

The tissue material properties estimated in this chapter may be used in other numerical models to study yielding and post-yielding behavior and to investigate observations reported in the literature. Specifically, we use them to analyze failure properties variability calculated through numerical approaches, against the hypothesis that cancellous bone yield strain is relatively constant over a range of apparent densities and failure strain presents a wider range of variation. Moreover, we analyze a single strain parameter (equivalent strain, $\varepsilon_{\mathrm{eq}}$) as an accurate descriptor of cancellous bone compression failure both through DIC and FE analysis.

3.2 Experimental characterization

In this section, the results of the estimation of cancellous bone mechanical properties are presented divided into elastic and failure properties. The calculation method is defined for each case. Within elastic properties we estimate the apparent stiffness (E_{app}), tissue level elastic modulus (E) and homogeneous stiffness matrix (C) for each specimen. Regarding failure properties, the yield and complete failure properties are calculated at the macroscale (σ_{y}, ε_{y}, σ_{f}, ε_{f}) and microscale ($\varepsilon_{\mathrm{y,c}}$, $\varepsilon_{\mathrm{f,c}}$). For these purposes, we used the following methods: compression testing, combination of compression tests and FEM, phantom-based estimation and elastic homogenization.

3.2.1 Compression tests

Quasi-static compression tests were carried out along the main trabecular orientation in order to estimate the apparent Young's modulus (E_{app}), yield stress (σ_{y}), yield strain (ε_{y}), failure stress (σ_{f}) and failure strain (ε_{f}) of 13 cancellous bone specimens. The testing protocol is detailed in the following. First, the specimens were thawed at 4°C the night previous to testing, maintained moist in 0.9% saline solution and wrapped in a gauze. Specimen dimensions were determined using a dial caliper, identifying the anisotropy direction and defining it as the testing direction. Compression tests were conducted using an electromechanical testing machine (MTS Criterion C42, MTS Systems, USA, Fig. 3.1), with aluminum compression platens (MTS ref.: FYA502A) and measuring the displacement between them using a displacement gauge (MTS ref.:632.06H-20).

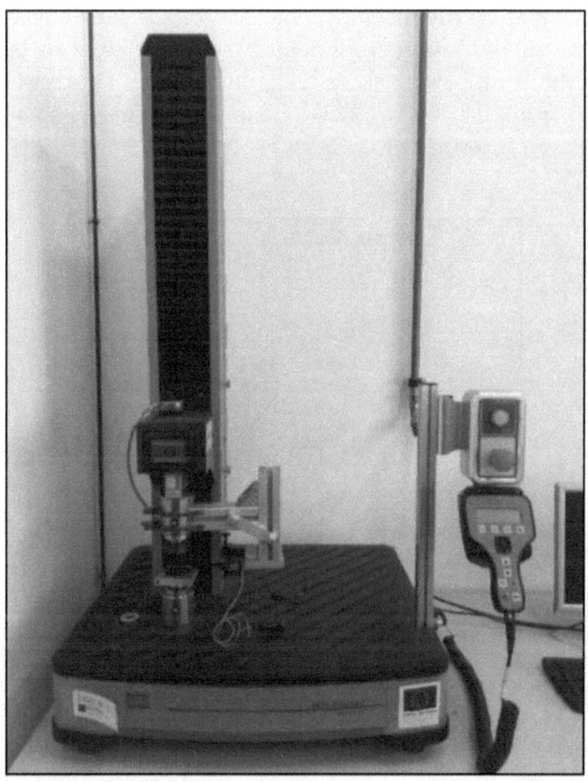

Figure 3.1: Electromechanical testing machine used for experimental testing: MTS Criterion c42.

Due to the small specimens dimensions, positioning the displacement gauge between compression platens could cause damage to it. In order to avoid any damage during testing, a metal surface was added to the lower compression platen where the displacement gauge contact point was positioned. The testing rig is shown in Fig. 3.2. A 10 N pre-load was defined. Then, load was applied after 5 preconditioning cycles [52] with a displacement rate of 1 mm/min between 0.1% to 0.5% strain levels, to avoid damage within specimens [57]. After a few preconditioning cycles, apparent modulus estimation tended to stabilize [52, 57]. Experimental artifacts from different sources were minimized following recommendations given in [30]. However, different levels of damage at the specimen-compression platen interface was observed in some cases, due to the cut of the trabeculae at the machined surfaces of the specimen [23, 56]. Three specimens that suffered from experimental artifacts due to their non-complete parallelism of the compression faces [22], which acted as stress concentrators, were discarded from the study. This phenomenon caused specimen crushing at specimen-platen interface (Fig. 3.3).

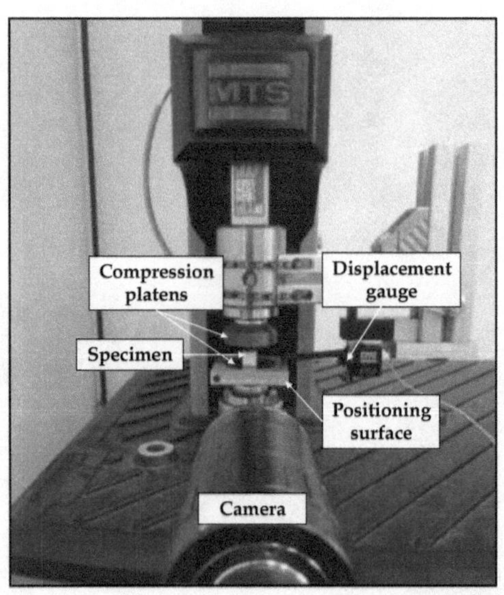

Figure 3.2: Experimental setup for the compression tests and digital image correlation (DIC) system.

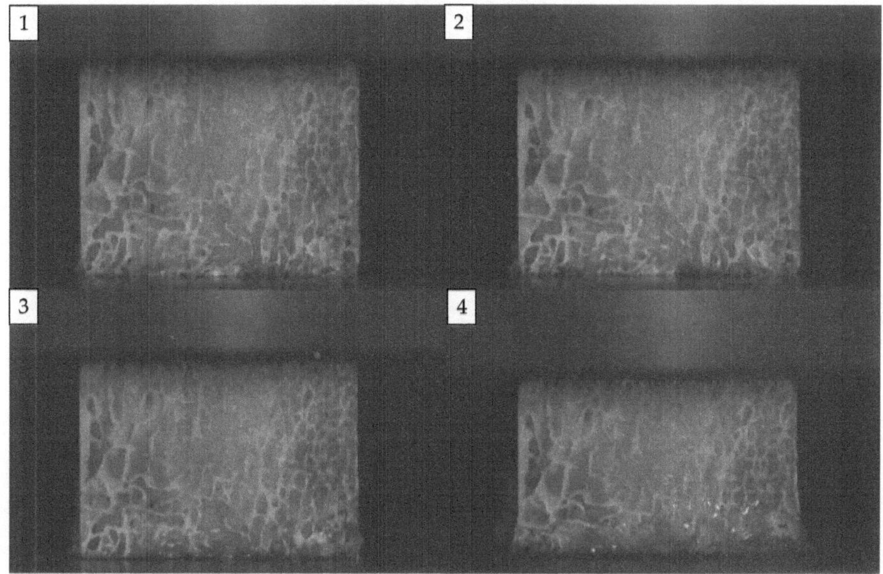

Figure 3.3: Experimental artifacts observed on the three specimens discarded from the study. The specimens suffered from crushing at the bottom compression platen interface due to the non-parallelism of specimen faces. This specimen presents a thin layer of a closed and mineralized bone growth plate (left side).

The force-displacement response was employed to compute the stress-strain relationships of the specimens, which is displayed in Fig. 3.4 for set A, see section 2.2.1 for sets definition. The apparent Young's modulus (E_{compr}) was determined as a linear fit in the last cycle from the stress-strain response. The failure stress (σ_f) was defined as the peak value of the stress following the elastic response and the failure strain (ε_f) was defined as the strain at σ_f. We also estimated the yield stress (σ_y) and strain (ε_y) following the 0.2 % offset method. It consists in drawing a line of the initial slope of the linear response with an offset of 0.2 % in strain. The yield parameters are obtained at the intersection between the drawn line and the experimental response.

As described in the literature, cancellous bone compression response may be divided into the following parts, which can be distinguished in Fig. 3.4: first, a linear elastic phase where the tissue deforms reversibly (the preconditioning cycles are applied in this domain). Then, from the yield point, a loss of linearity with material softening occurs until the maximum load is reached. Later, failure spreads on the specimen developing diffuse damage, microcracks and complete trabecular fractures. Once the trabecular structure stacks after collapsing, the load increases again in the final part of the response. Table 3.1 summarizes set A results of apparent compression stiffness (E_{compr}), stress at failure (σ_{f}), strain at failure (ε_{f}), yield stress (σ_{y}) and yield strain (ε_{y}) measured through experimental compression tests. In addition, Table 3.2 presents also the apparent modulus values for specimens from set C for the transversal plane ($E_{\text{trans-1}}$, $E_{\text{trans-2}}$).

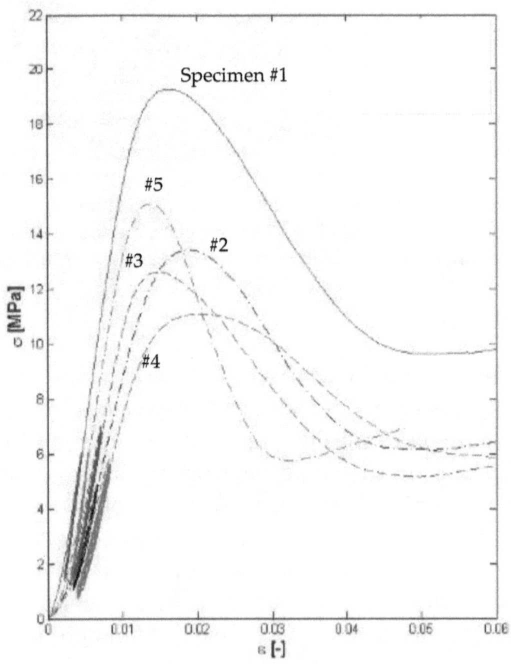

Figure 3.4: Stress-strain curve registered in compression testing for specimens belonging to set A. Ten preconditioning cycles are also displayed.

In our results, the apparent compression stiffness ranges from around 0.9 to 1.9 GPa for the main orientation direction (Tables 3.1 and 3.2). The apparent modulus in the transversal directions is about a third of the preferred orientation value, ranging between 229 to 487 MPa, and both transversal directions are quite similar, thus they may define a plane of isotropy. The apparent modulus is known to depend on the bone volume fraction, so comparisons need to be referred to it. Our results of apparent elastic modulus are in the range of values for similar BV/TV of specimens extracted from different anatomical locations (Table 1.1).

Table 3.1: Mechanical parameters measured in experimental quasi-static compression tests for set A.

Sample	E_{compr}[MPa]	σ_y[MPa]	ε_y [%]	σ_f[MPa]	ε_f [%]
A#1	1943.8	17.8	1.11	19.3	1.65
A#2	1118.4	11.6	1.31	13.4	1.93
A#3	1481.8	11.9	1.18	12.6	1.49
A#4	1078	9.7	1.3	11.1	2.07
A#5	1915.3	13.6	1.05	15.1	1.38
Mean	1507.5	12.9	1.19	14.3	1.7
SD	416.3	3.06	0.12	3.1	0.29

Table 3.2: Mechanical parameters measured in experimental quasi-static compression tests for set C. Failure parameters are referred to the main trabecular orientation, while elastic values are reported for the three main directions: E_{compr} for the main direction and $E_{\mathrm{trans\text{-}1}}$ and $E_{\mathrm{trans\text{-}2}}$ for the other two transversal directions.

Sample	E_{compr}[MPa]	$E_{\mathrm{trans\text{-}1}}$[MPa]	$E_{\mathrm{trans\text{-}2}}$[MPa]	σ_y[MPa]	ε_y [%]	σ_f[MPa]	ε_f [%]
C#1	879.2	229.1	253.4	10.1	1.55	10.5	1.9
C#2	1416.1	408.1	486.7	14.1	1.30	14.7	1.65
C#3	909.5	464	306.6	8.7	1.27	9.2	1.75
C#4	927.3	306.2	315	8.5	1.24	8.8	1.53
C#5	982.3	322.8	278.6	8.9	1.25	9.2	1.45
Mean	1022.9	346.0	328.1	10.08	1.32	10.5	1.66
SD	199.4	81.9	82.2	2.1	0.11	2.2	0.16

Yield stress (σ_y) values measured through compression in the main direction take a value between 8.5 to 17.8 MPa, while stress at failure (σ_f) values are between 8.8 to 19.3 MPa, Tables 3.1 and 3.2. Failure stresses reported in the literature present a wide scattering (Table 1.3). Our results lie in the range of values reported in the literature and are similar to the ones reported for human femoral neck [45], bovine tibia [26, 87] or vertebral whale [84].

A mean value for yield strain (ε_y) of 1.25 %, with a minimum value of 1.05 % and a maximum value of 1.55 % was estimated, while the mean failure strain (ε_f) is 1.68 %, ranging from 1.38 to 2.07 %, Tables 3.1 and 3.2. Our results for yield and failure strains are in the range of values reported in the literature (Table 1.3).

Linear regressions between elastic and failure properties measured in compression tests were investigated, Table 3.3. The apparent modulus (E_{compr}) correlates well to the yield and failure stresses (R^2 values of around 0.8 for both cases), while both stresses correlate to each other (R^2=0.978). This relationship between modulus and strength has been observed and reported in other works [10, 26, 43, 72, 78, 125] and permits to estimate cancellous bone strength through non-destructive testing. The stiffer cancellous bone is, the proportionally stronger it is.

The high correlation obtained between yield and failure strains may be a result from the calculation method, which was the 0.2 % offset procedure. Modulus and strength parameters do not show correlation to the strain metrics (Table 3.3, R^2 values between 0.193 to 0.299), which supports the idea that yield and failure strains are relatively constant and independent of density and microstructure. This can be explained because yield and failure strains are controlled by local tissue properties and the deformation mechanisms occur at the nanoscale. Therefore, density and microstructure would condition the apparent elastic modulus and strength, while they would not affect failure strain values.

Table 3.3: Correlation of the linear regressions estimated between elastic and failure parameters for specimens from set A and C.

	Correlation coefficient (R^2)				
	E_{compr}	σ_y	ε_y	σ_f	ε_f
E_{compr}	1	0.8	0.296	0.805	0.246
σ_y		1	0.193	0.978	0.176
ε_y			1	0.299	0.986
σ_f		Symm.		1	0.283
ε_f					1

3.2.1.1 Relationships between microstructural parameters from sets A and C and mechanical parameters from quasi-static compression tests

Linear regressions were estimated between parameters defining specimen microstructure and the experimentally measured compression stiffness (E_{app}), yield stress (σ_y), yield strain (ε_y), stress at failure (σ_f) and strain at failure (ε_f). A total of n=10 specimens were used for the regression analysis. Therefore, the regressions estimated need to be confirmed in larger data sets.

The Pearson correlation coefficients (R^2) of the relationships under study are presented in Table 3.4, whereas some of the most significant correlations are depicted in Figs. 3.5, 3.6, 3.7 and 3.8. Moreover, we present the linear regression coefficients calculated for the most significant relationships, Table 3.5. It is important to note that the Pearson correlation coefficients obtained are not enough to consider the regressions as significant and it would be more correct to design them as tendencies. Nonetheless, the relationships in bold in Table 3.4 present a p-value<0.05.

Table 3.4: Pearson correlation coefficients (R^2) of the linear regressions estimated between morphometric and elastic and failure parameters for specimens from set A and C.

	Correlation coefficient (R^2)				
	E_{app}	σ_y	ε_y	σ_f	ε_f
BV/TV	**0.582**	**0.632**	0.273	**0.679**	0
BS/TV	0.128	0.053	0.115	0.09	0.011
BS/BV	0.489	0.387	0.285	**0.507**	0.025
Tb.Th	0.35	**0.517**	0.042	**0.573**	0.033
Tb.Sp	0.145	0.067	0.155	0.12	0.068
Tb.N	0.298	0.257	0.221	0.269	0.016
$D_{2D\text{-}1}$	0.395	0.212	0.296	0.305	0.012
$D_{2D\text{-}2}$	**0.524**	0.333	0.423	0.448	0.001
$D_{2D\text{-}3}$	**0.542**	0.364	0.364	0.483	0.001
D_{3D}	**0.521**	0.354	0.318	0.447	0.001
$DA_{MIL2D\text{-}1}$	0.414	0.407	0.068	0.355	0.162
$DA_{MIL2D\text{-}2}$	0.458	0.322	0.226	0.289	0.399
$DA_{MIL2D\text{-}3}$	0.072	0.011	0.239	0.003	**0.618**
DA_{MIL3D}	0.397	0.38	0.063	0.32	0.191
Conn.D	0.028	0.103	0	0.057	0.219

The combination of experiments and morphometric analysis has revealed some tendencies in the correlations, Table 3.4. Among them, BV/TV correlates to the apparent modulus in either a linear or power law, Fig. 3.5. The investigation of a power law relationship is motivated because other works report that sort of dependence between BV/TV and the apparent modulus. The more bone volume fraction, the higher the apparent elastic modulus. If we look at Fig. 3.5, there is a point at the left side of the regression line that may be due to experimental errors. We have considered it on the study but, if deleted, the power law correlation coefficient (R^2) increases to 0.86, which is very similar than values reported elsewhere [8]. Anyway, the influence of BV/TV parameter is known to be major on the modulus variation. However, some of the variation needs to be predicted for other parameters [8].

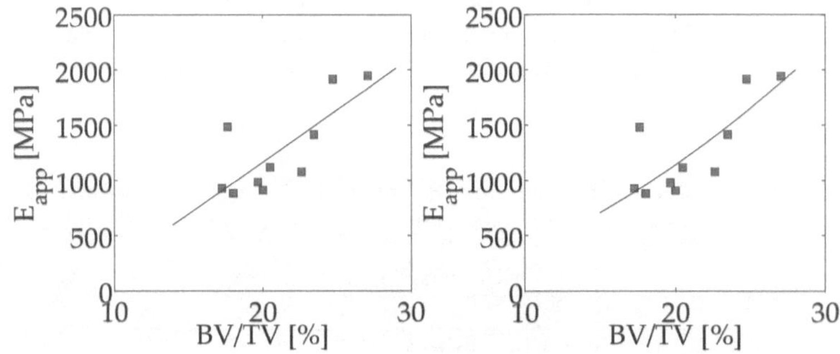

Figure 3.5: Relationships between bone volume fraction (BV/TV) and apparent compression modulus (E_{app}) for specimens from sets A and C. Linear (left) and power (right) relationships are analyzed.

Bone volume fraction also presents a relationship to the yield and failure stresses (Fig. 3.6 left and centre), with R^2 values of 0.63 and 0.68 respectively (Table 3.4). As expected from yield to failure stress relationship, the slope and intercept values for these regressions are comparable (Table 3.5). These influences of BV/TV on modulus and strength have been widely reported in the literature: the amount of bone that constitutes the specimen is relevant for its mechanical behavior and it is known to explain most of the variation of cancellous bone modulus and strength [8, 10, 103, 217].

On the other hand, the ratio between bone surface and bone volume correlates with the stress at failure (R^2=0.5). The higher is BS/BV, the lower strength, Fig. 3.6 right. Similarly, but presenting weaker correlations, BS/BV may also be related to the apparent modulus and yield stress, Table 3.4.

Table 3.5: Linear coefficients of the regressions of higher correlation (highlighted in Table 3.4) estimated between morphometric and mechanical variables, in the form Mech(morph)=slope*morph+intercept.

Mech(morph)	Slope	Intercept
E_{app}(BV/TV)	94.35	-724.3
E_{app}($D_{\text{2D-2}}$)	4722	-6281
E_{app}($D_{\text{2D-3}}$)	4873	-6717
E_{app}(D_{3D})	4747	-11450
σ_y(BV/TV)	0.722	-3.73
σ_y(Tb.Th)	199.4	-15.58
σ_f(BV/TV)	0.8386	-5.29
σ_f(Tb.Th)	234.8	19.55
σ_f(BS/BV)	-0.4303	24.15
ε_f(DA_{MIL3D})	6.544	-5.126

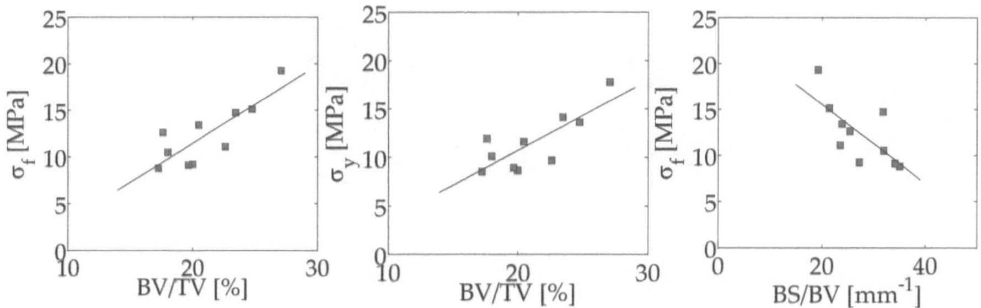

Figure 3.6: Relationship between failure stress and bone volume fraction (left), yield stress and bone volume fraction (centre) and bone surface to bone volume ratio and failure stress (right).

The mean trabecular thickness (Tb.Th) influences both the yield and failure stresses, with R^2 values of 0.52 and 0.57 respectively, Fig. 3.7 left and centre. Besides, a weak but significant correlation (R^2=0.35, p-value<0.05) is found to the apparent modulus. These correlations have been previously reported with analogous correlation coefficients [221]. Furthermore, a combination of BV/TV and Tb.Th was reported to improve the elastic modulus variation explanation [8].

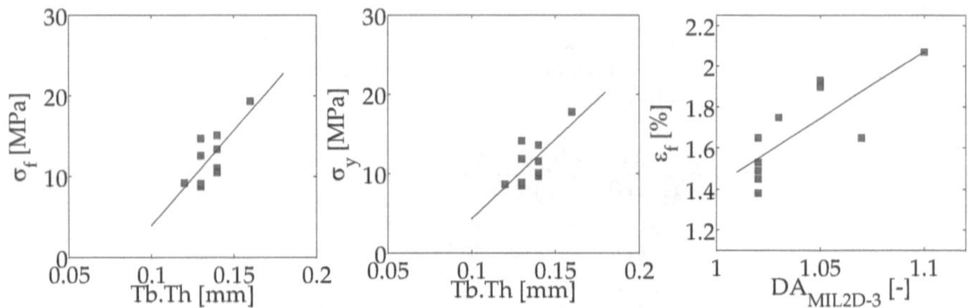

Figure 3.7: Linear regressions estimated between mean trabecular thickness (Tb.Th) and failure stress (left) and yield stress (centre) and between anisotropy degree in 2D along the transversal plane and failure strain (right).

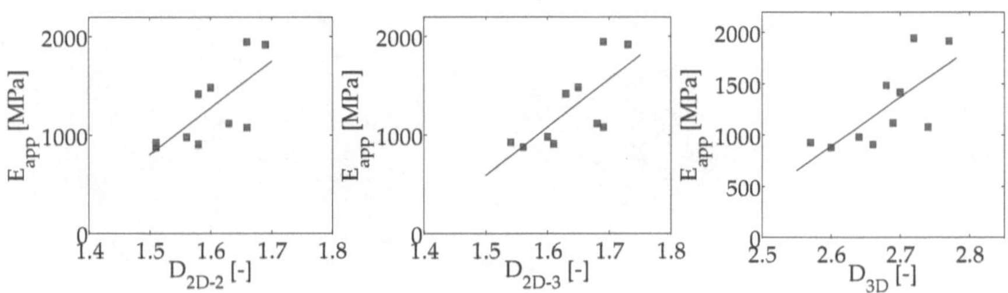

Figure 3.8: Linear regressions between fractal dimension (2D and 3D versions) and apparent modulus (E_{app}).

Fractal dimension, both in 2D and 3D, presents a positive tendency to the apparent modulus (Fig. 3.8). It is interesting that both versions of fractal dimension lead to similar regression results, even for the transversal plane direction (D_{2D-3}). The coefficients of the linear regressions show similar slope values for the 2D and 3D versions, Table 3.5. In case of the intercept, fractal dimension regression for the 2D version differs from the 3D version, which is significantly higher in modulus, Table 3.5. Therefore, our results reveal that a relationship exists between cancellous bone complexity and specimen stiffness. This influence was already observed [214, 221]. As happens in our results, the correlation was significant (p-value<0.05) for all three directions but their R^2 values were lower than the presented in Table 3.4.

Fractal dimension has been proved to distinguish between normal and osteoporotic cancellous bone, with higher D values for healthy bone [223]. Furthermore, it is directly related to bone volume fraction, as it gives an idea of how bone fills the space [213, 224]. A representation of BV/TV and fractal dimension confirms the results reported by others in the literature, Fig. 3.9. Therefore, it makes sense that a positive correlation between fractal dimension and apparent modulus exists because of the relationsip between BV/TV and fractal dimension.

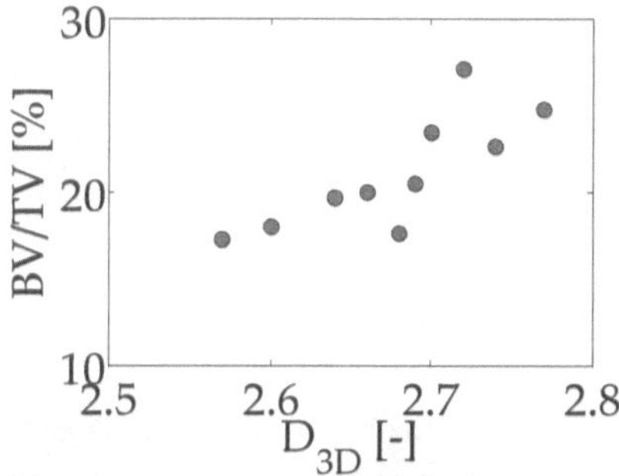

Figure 3.9: Representation of bone volume fraction with respect to fractal dimension in 3D. A positive correlation can be distinguished.

Furthermore, a tendency of weaker correlation coefficient than for apparent modulus, is obtained to failure and yield stresses, Table 3.4. The linear relationship between apparent modulus and failure stress reported in the literature supports our observations [10].

On the other hand, the anisotropy degree presents a weak but significant correlation to the apparent modulus, Table 3.4. Specifically, the 2D version of MIL, applied to the planes containing the preferred trabecular orientation and the 3D version correlate to the apparent modulus, while if applied to the transversal plane, the correlation vanishes. In the literature, some authors claim that including DA values to BV/TV regressions improve the prediction of the apparent elastic modulus [8, 217].

Some morphometric parameters do not show a significant correlation to the mechanical properties evaluated, like BS/TV, Tb.Sp, Tb.N or Conn.D. The lack of relationship between Conn.D and specimen mechanical response confirms the observations reported in the literature [9, 221, 222]. Kabel et al. [9] stated that Conn.D presents a very limited value to assess on the elastic properties of the cancellous bone and they claim that, if any relationship exists, their study suggested that the stiffness decreases when Conn.D increases. In case of Tb.Sp and Tb.N, some works report no significant correlations to the apparent modulus [222], while other report significant relationships [217, 221].

Finally, yield and failure strains do not show correlation (or present weak correlation) to the morphometric parameters, except for the case of anisotropy degree in 2D, calculated along the transversal plane (Fig. 3.7 right). However, we consider that this correlation is not evident because the anisotropy degree values obtained for that plane do not vary much and correspond to a nearly isotropic case, so this relationship needs to be confirmed with larger datasets. In addition, yield and failure strains have been reported to be relatively constant and independent from specimen microstructure [10, 26, 50], which is supported by the lack of correlation between morphometry and strain variables presented in our results (Table 3.4). This lack of correlation can be explained because yield and failure strains depend essentially on local tissue properties and not much on the morphology of the sample. Deformation mechanisms occur from nano scale, where microstructure obviously has no influence.

3.2.2 Tissue Young's modulus estimation through compression tests combined with μCT-based FEM

We used a combination of compression tests and μCT-based finite element modeling to estimate cancellous bone Young's modulus at tissue level. This approach has been applied in numerous works in the literature [42, 44, 46, 47, 50, 72, 75] to estimate tissue elastic properties and is depicted in Fig. 3.10. It is an inverse analysis procedure which consist of two main steps: recording the force-displacement response of each specimen and generating finite element models with detailed microstructure, considering as boundary conditions the experimental ones. Then, a linear simulation is performed and the apparent compressive stiffness is computed and compared to the experimental. The tissue Young's modulus is then calibrated so that the simulations match the test response. A scheme of the elastic properties estimation methodology is depicted in Fig. 3.10.

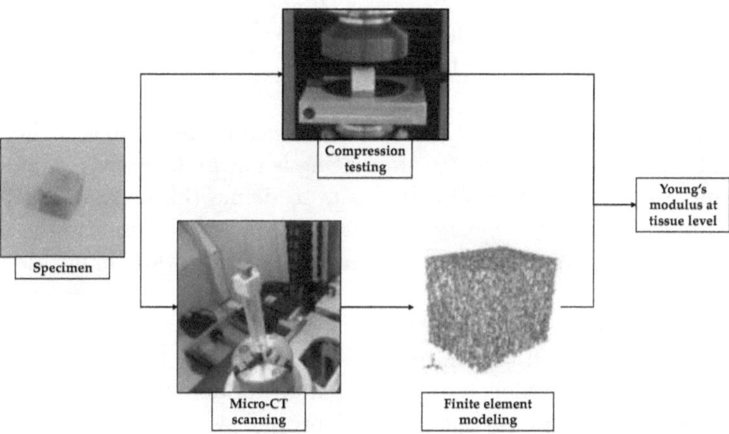

Figure 3.10: Scheme of the procedure followed to estimate tissue-level Young's modulus combining testing and μCT-based FEM.

Table 3.6 presents the tissue Young's modulus estimation for each specimen following the approach explained in this section. A mean value of 11.09 GPa with a standard deviation of 1.69 GPa resulted from our estimations. Low scattering is found in Table 3.6, with a minimum value of 9 GPa and a maximum value of 15.25 GPa. The values reported in the literature for the methodology used here are between 5.6 and 18.8 GPa (Table 1.2), so our results are within the range of values reported for a combination of testing and FE modeling.

Table 3.6: Estimation of the Young's modulus for cancellous bone tissue through a combination of compression tests and μCT-based FEM

Specimen	E [GPa]
A#1	10.84
A#2	10.6
A#3	15.25
A#4	12.15
A#5	12.11
C#1	8.99
C#2	9.54
C#3	10.36
C#4	11.17
C#5	9.87
Mean	11.09
STD	1.69

Some limitations of the method should be mentioned. First, if the level of discretization of the mesh used for simulating is not high enough it may stiffen the results. In our case, we did some tests to define the mesh characteristics and the level of discretization reached was chosen as a compromise between accuracy and computer resources available. On the other hand, cancellous bone tissue is considered homogeneous, which is not accurate for some loading conditions. However, several investigations in the literature have accounted for material heterogeneity in the finite element models [71, 128, 225], reporting a significant but minor influence on the apparent modulus [71, 128]. Therefore, the assumption of homogeneous material properties does not induce considerable error. In that way, Kabel et al. [47] found that an effective isotropic tissue modulus is enough to predict cancellous bone apparent properties.

Other authors claim that this methodology may lead to tissue modulus estimation errors, because the experiments used to calibrated tissue level properties may include experimental artifacts that underestimate E up to a 50 % [40], but following some recommendations it is possible to minimize them [30, 52, 56] and get accurate results [40].

3.2.3 Phantom-based estimation

In this section we aim to estimate the Young's modulus at the tissue level based on density measurement. Section 2.3 presents the use of phantoms of known densities to estimate bone mineral density. Some works in the literature have investigated stiffness-density expressions [130, 131, 226]. A literature review from Helgason et al. [131] highlighted the lack of consensus about a unique stiffness-density relationship, which the authors associate to the different testing protocols used to develop the expressions. However, even for protocols that minimize the presence of experimental artifacts, different stiffness-density relationships were found according to specimen location [130].

Moreover, Schileo et al. [226] reported a detailed protocol to accurately estimate stiffness based on density measurements. In short, two steps are necessary: first, a linear calibration is needed to transform the phantom-based densities ($\rho_{\mu CT}$) to ash density (ρ_{ash}). Schileo et al. [226] calculated similar but different relationships between $\rho_{\mu CT}$ and ρ_{ash} for cancellous and cortical bone, and also proposed a combined expression. We compare the predictions of using the cancellous (Eq. 3.1) and the combined one (Eq. 3.2). Then, a scaling is necessary to calculate the apparent density (ρ_{app}) used in the stiffness-density expressions, Eq. 3.3.

$$\rho_{\mu CT} = -0.05 + 0.98\ \rho_{ash} \tag{3.1}$$

$$\rho_{\mu CT} = -0.09 + 1.14\ \rho_{ash} \tag{3.2}$$

$$\frac{\rho_{app}}{\rho_{ash}} = 0.6 \tag{3.3}$$

All density definitions in mg/mm^3.

Regarding the Young's modulus-density equation, we applied the one proposed in [130] for vertebral cancellous bone (Eq. 3.4), plotted in Fig. 3.11.

$$E_t(GPa) = 4.73\ \rho_{app}^{1.56} \tag{3.4}$$

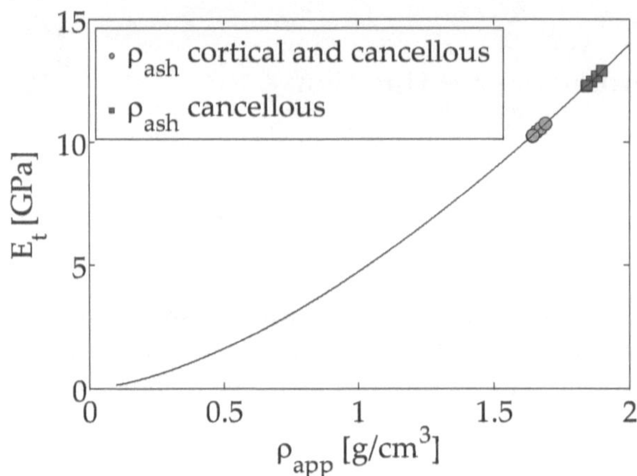

Figure 3.11: Representation of the Young's modulus of the tissue as a function of apparent density (Eq. 3.4) including the specimens predictions using ash density expressions for cortical and cancellous bone (Eq. 3.2) or only cancellous bone (Eq. 3.1).

Specifically, we calculate a mean Young's modulus according to the mean mineral content of each specimen (Table 3.7) which was estimated using calibration phantoms and the gray level-mineral content relationship calculated ($\rho = 1.364\ GS + 1056$).

Table 3.7: Young's modulus estimation through density measurement using calibration phantoms.

Specimen	Mean gray level	Mean density [mg HA/cm^3]
C#1	-8.00	1045.1
C#2	-0.32	1055.6
C#3	-16.78	1033.1
C#4	8.26	1067.3
C#5	-15.31	1035.1

The results for the estimation of the Young's modulus of the tissue based on density calibration phantoms are presented in Table 3.8, where we compare the predictions using Eq. 3.1 and 3.2 to determine ash density. It can be noted that the results using the ash density equation fitted only for trabecular bone provides results about 20 % stiffer than the one fitted for both cortical and trabecular bone. Little scattering is found on the predictions, which points out

Table 3.8: Tissue Young's modulus estimation through density measurement using calibration phantoms. The first column results make reference to ash density estimation using Eq. 3.1 (for trabecular bone), while the second one to Eq. 3.2 (for cortical and cancellous bone).

Specimen	E_t [GPa] Eq. 3.1	E_t [GPa] Eq. 3.2
C#1	12.48	10.42
C#2	12.67	10.57
C#3	12.27	10.25
C#4	12.88	10.74
C#5	12.30	10.28
Mean	12.52	10.45
STD	0.23	0.18

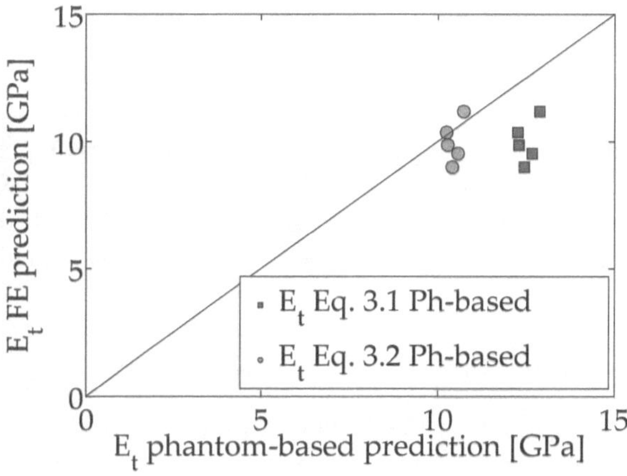

Figure 3.12: Tissue Young's modulus comparison between phantom-based and FE predictions.

that the specimens analyzed were similar in terms of density. Furthermore, a comparison between phantom-based and finite element Young's modulus estimation is shown in Fig. 3.12. FE and phantom-based predictions are very similar, although differences up to 38.5 % are found when using the ash density expression for trabecular bone only (Eq. 3.1), while lower differences are found when using ash density equation using cortical and trabecular bone.

3.2.4 Digital Image Correlation

Digital image correlation (DIC) is an optical displacement measurement technique that emerged on the 80s of the last century [62, 63, 228]. The need of time-consuming post-processing motivated the development of algorithms to track displacements between subsequent images and since then, high accuracy has been achieved [228]. This technique has some advantages compared to other measurement techniques, especially for biological tissues testing, where damage may be induced to the specimen due to measurement system attachment. However, DIC only provides surface displacement metrics, although what happens in the internal sections influences the surface results [51]. The DIC technique presented in this section will be also applied to characterize cancellous bone surrogates displacement fields at failure in Chapter 4.

Digital image correlation method divides the region of interest in squared faces to track their displacement and it requires for an image matching method to determine them. Here, we present the template matching method, that minimizes the difference between the reference (F) and deformed (G) images gray values, the so-called sum of squares deviation (SSD), to determine the average facet motion (Eq. 3.5) [228]. The method assumes no lighting changes between images.

$$\vec{\mathbf{d}}_{opt} = argmin \sum \mid G(\mathbf{x} + \vec{\mathbf{d}}) - F(\mathbf{x}) \mid^2 \tag{3.5}$$

The optimal average facet displacement may be solved using an iterative algorithm by a first-order Taylor series expanding of Eq. 3.5, as function of the current average displacement estimation in x and y directions (d_x, d_y) and motion updates in the iteration (Δ_x, Δ_y).

$$\chi^2(d_x + \Delta_x, d_y + \Delta_y) = \sum \mid G(\mathbf{x} + \vec{\mathbf{d}}) - \frac{\partial G}{\partial x}\Delta_x - \frac{\partial G}{\partial y}\Delta_y - F(\mathbf{x}) \mid^2 \tag{3.6}$$

Then, taking partial derivatives and setting to zero, results in the Lucas-Kanade tracker algorithm, Eq. 3.7, used to iteratively solve the average facet motion.

$$\begin{bmatrix} \Delta_x \\ \Delta_y \end{bmatrix} = \begin{bmatrix} \sum (\frac{\partial G}{\partial x})^2 & \sum \frac{\partial G}{\partial x}\frac{\partial G}{\partial y} \\ \sum \frac{\partial G}{\partial x}\frac{\partial G}{\partial y} & \sum (\frac{\partial G}{\partial y})^2 \end{bmatrix}^{-1} \begin{bmatrix} \sum \frac{\partial G}{\partial x}(F - G) \\ \sum \frac{\partial G}{\partial y}(F - G) \end{bmatrix} \tag{3.7}$$

In order to further deformation estimation, the cost function (SSD) needs to include a subset shape function $\xi(x, p)$ to transform the coordinates after deformation [228] and Eq. 3.5 turns to:

$$\chi^2(\mathbf{p}) = \sum (G(\xi(\mathbf{x} + \mathbf{p}) - F(\mathbf{x}))^2 \tag{3.8}$$

Where the subset shape function to consider an affine transformation may be written as follows, Eq. 3.9.

$$\xi(\mathbf{x}, \mathbf{p}) = \begin{bmatrix} p_0 \\ p_1 \end{bmatrix} + \begin{bmatrix} 1 + p_2 & p_3 \\ p_4 & 1 + p_5 \end{bmatrix} x \tag{3.9}$$

To minimize the cost function and estimate the affine transformation (which includes translation, scaling, rotation, shear mapping among others) of the subset it is necessary to derive Eq. 3.8 with respect to $\mathbf{p}$ parameters, and its iterative update may be computed using Eq. 3.10 [228].

$$\Delta \mathbf{p} = \mathbf{H}^{-1} \mathbf{q} \tag{3.10}$$

Where $\mathbf{H}$ is the Hessian matrix (Eq. 3.11) and $\mathbf{q}$ is defined by Eq. 3.12. The partial derivative is denoted by subscripts, i.e., $G_x = \frac{\partial G}{\partial x}$.

$$\mathbf{H} = \begin{bmatrix} \sum G_x^2 & \sum G_x G_y & \sum G_x^2 x & \sum G_x^2 y & \sum G_x G_y x & \sum G_x G_y y \\ & \sum G_y^2 & \sum G_x G_y x & \sum G_x G_y y & \sum G_y^2 x & \sum G_y^2 y \\ & & \sum G_x^2 x^2 & \sum G_x^2 xy & \sum G_x G_y x^2 & \sum G_x G_y xy \\ & & & \sum G_x^2 y^2 & \sum G_x G_y xy & \sum G_x G_y y^2 \\ & \text{Symm.} & & & \sum G_y^2 x^2 & \sum G_y^2 xy \\ & & & & & \sum G_y^2 y^2 \end{bmatrix} \tag{3.11}$$

$$\mathbf{q} = \begin{bmatrix} \sum G_x (F - G) \\ \sum G_y (F - G) \\ \sum G_x x (F - G) \\ \sum G_x y (F - G) \\ \sum G_y x (F - G) \\ \sum G_y y (F - G) \end{bmatrix} \tag{3.12}$$

However, this methodology assumes no changes in lighting between images, which is far from real experiments. To solve this issue, a photometric function (Φ) is applied to the gray values of G. If the photometric transformation consists of a scaling, it leads to the normalized sum of squared difference criterion (NSSD), Eq. 3.13, while if $\Phi(G) = aG + b$, it leads to the zero-mean normalized sum of squared difference (ZNSSD) [228].

$$\chi^2_{NSSD} = \sum \left(\frac{\sum F_i G_i}{\sum G_i^2} G_i - F_i \right)^2 \tag{3.13}$$

Now, we have defined the matching pattern criterion to account for facet (or subset) deformation, including optimization criteria for a changing lighting case. In order to apply this technique, we used VIC-2D Digital Image Correlation software (v.6.0.2 Correlated Solutions Inc., US), a high resolution fixed focal lens (HF7518V-2, Myutron, Japan) with 12 Mpx resolution and 75 mm focal length, and a spotlight. Fig. 3.13, shows a scheme of the DIC procedure.

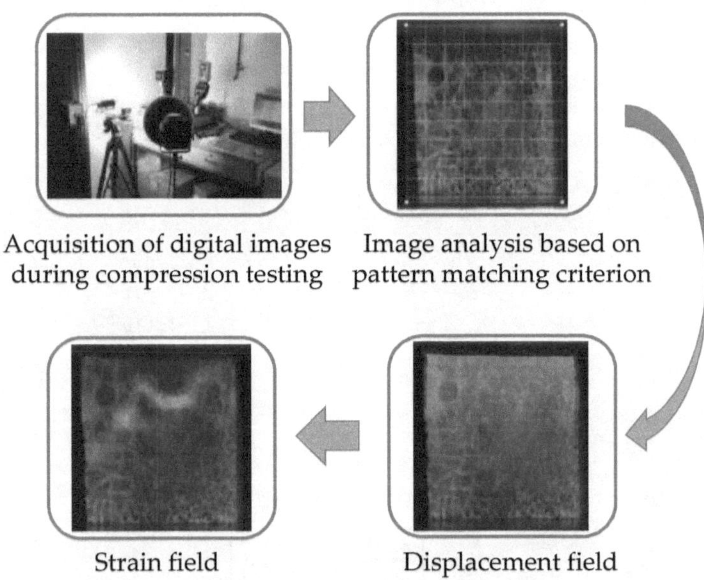

Figure 3.13: Scheme of digital image correlation (DIC) procedure. DIC is applied to the images acquired during testing, which are analyzed based on a pattern matching criterion, resulting in the displacement field estimation. The strain field is computed according to the chosen tensorial description.

Our application of DIC technique to cancellous bone specimens aims at:

- Analyzing the influence of DIC parameters on the estimation of failure properties

- Finding the best descriptor to characterize cancellous bone fracture patterns during quasi-static compression testing

- Estimating failure properties following a criterion based on failure localization and fracture pattern determination accuracy

3.2.4.1 Comparison of displacement measurements between DIC and displacement gauge

To begin with, we present a comparison of DIC performance on displacement measurement with the displacement gauge signal for one of the specimens, Fig. 3.14. As can be seen, both displacements nearly match, but DIC slightly underestimates the measurements (the maximum difference between signals was 0.03 mm). Similar results were obtained for the other samples. The displacement gauge from the testing machine provides an accurate local metric so a maximum difference of 0.03 mm to the DIC signal shows a good DIC displacement measurement performance.

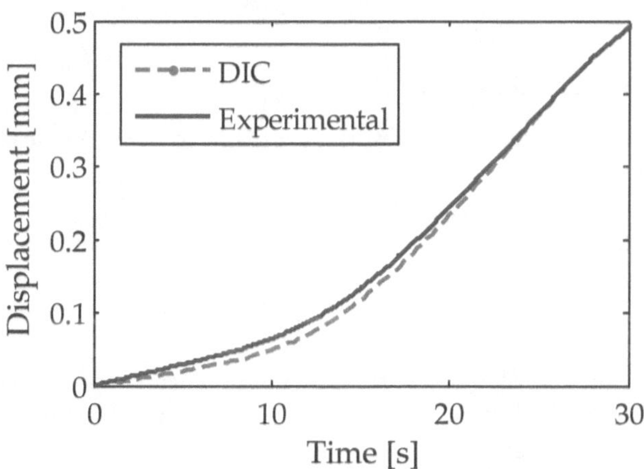

Figure 3.14: Displacement signals measured with MTS displacement gauge and DIC for a cancellous bone specimen.

3.2.4.2 Analysis of DIC parameters influence on failure variables estimation

In relation to the parametric analysis, we study the influence of the following parameters:

- Facet (or subset) size

- Step size

- Speckle vs non-speckle

- Pattern matching criterion

- Incremental vs non-incremental correlation

We performed the analysis of DIC parameters influence on Specimen #C1. For each case, we registered the maximum equivalent strain, defined by Eq. 3.14, for the image corresponding to the yield point and the one of the fracture point. Moreover, the accuracy and localization of the fracture pattern was evaluated for a post-yielding image.

$$\varepsilon_{\mathrm{eq}} = \sqrt{\frac{2}{3}\varepsilon_{ij}\varepsilon_{ij}} \tag{3.14}$$

3.2.4.2.1 Facet/Subset size

This parameter controls the area of the grid that is used to track the displacement between images. It has to ensure that there is sufficient pattern inside the area to perform the correlation [228, 229]. The facet size depends on the application, the use of speckle and, in case of random reticular structures, the void size. Fig. 3.15 shows in yellow a representation of subsets of different sizes for ROI of an open cell polyurethane foam.

The following subset sizes were used in the parametric study: 31, 51, 81, 101, 125 and 151 pixels size. The rest of the parameters were set to the following values: step size of 10 pixels, normalized squared differences pattern matching criterion, incremental correlation and a strain filter size of 9 pixels.

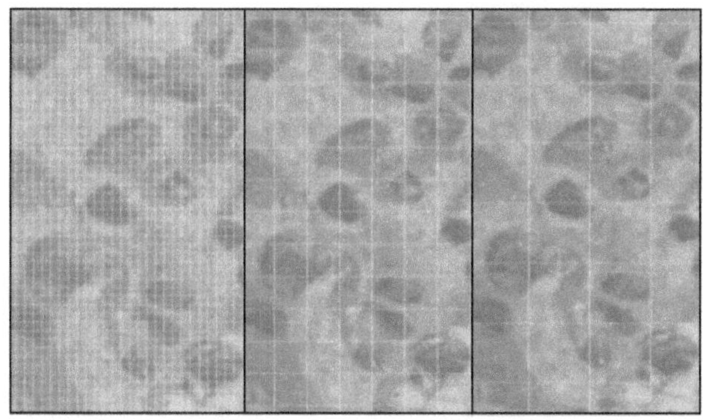

Figure 3.15: Subset size variation example: 21x21 (left), 81x81 (middle) and 151x151 (right) subset pixel size.

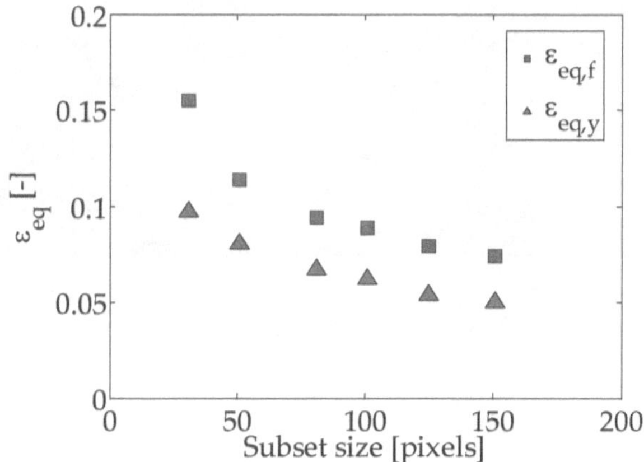

Figure 3.16: Effect of subset size variation on the fracture and yielding strains for Specimen #C1.

The results of failure strain variation with respect to the facet size are presented in Fig. 3.16. It can be observed that both the yield strain and the strain at fracture decrease as the subset size increases and it tends to stabilize. As more material is included in the facet, less localized measurement is made. The difference between failure strains is almost constant (about

0.04), except for the lowest subset size. However, for that case, DIC results present many voids on the solution, which indicates that it could not solve the correspondence problem and the results should be discarded, as is the case for 31 and 51 pixels of facet size in Fig. 3.17. It can be noted that failure localization is described by any of the subset sizes, but it is detected more clearly for larger subset values (125 and 151 pixels of facet), Fig. 3.17.

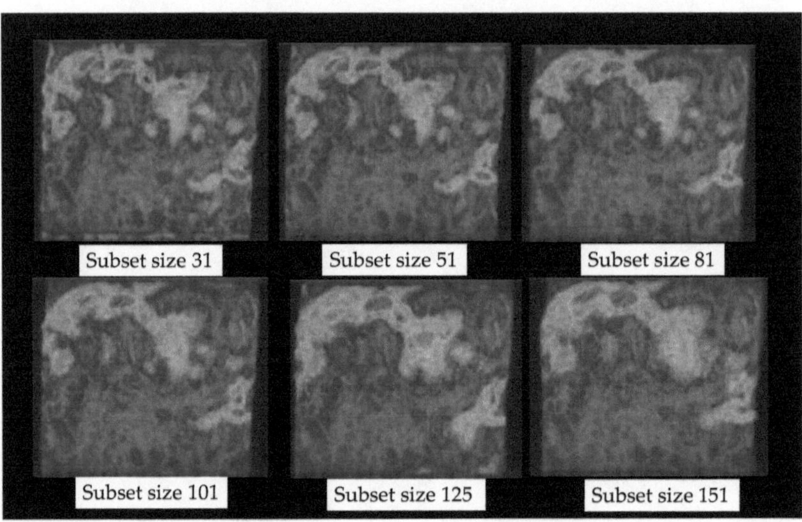

Figure 3.17: Distribution of equivalent strain (ε_{eeq}) for subset size variation for Specimen #A1. Failure localization can be distinguished for any of the facet sizes analyzed.

3.2.4.2.2 Step size

Step size controls the spacing of the points analyzed during correlation and is recommended to be roughly 1/4 of the subset size, although the smaller the step size is, the more accurate displacement estimation [229]. Then, we will vary the step size between 5 and 20 pixels and for two subset sizes, 81 and 125 pixels, Fig. 3.18.

The tendency of step size variation is analogous to step size variation for both subset sizes analyzed: failure strains values decrease for larger step sizes, Fig. 3.18. The variation in the step size also affected the estimation of the failure properties while a 10-pixel size yielded a variation around 15%, a 5-pixel range increased the variation up to a 34%. Failure localization spreads for larger step sizes, Fig. 3.19. A step size of 5 pixels permits an accurate localization, but in a region of the right part of the specimen it vanishes. Therefore, we chose a step size of 10 pixels for failure properties estimation.

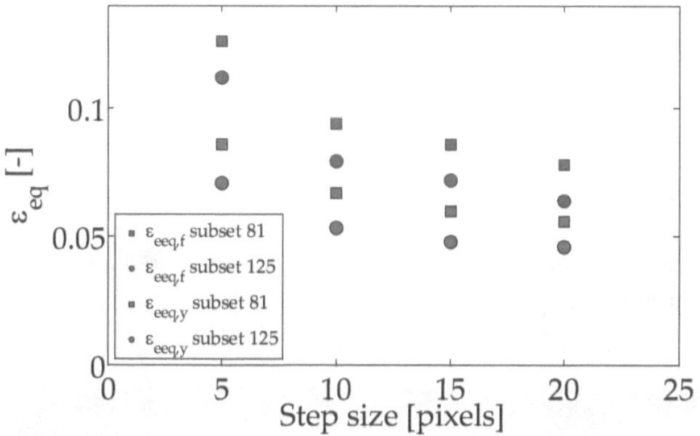

Figure 3.18: Effect of step size variation on the fracture and yielding strains for 81 and 125 pixels subset size.

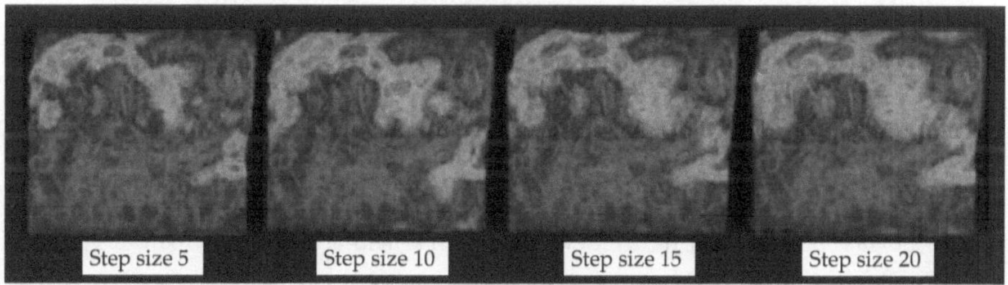

Figure 3.19: Effect of step size variation the equivalent strain distribution for a subset size of 125 pixels.

3.2.4.2.3   Using speckle in a reticular structure

DIC technique usually needs a speckle to calculate displacements, especially for plain surface materials. Luckily, the heterogeneous non-periodical microstructure of the cancellous bone can be used as pattern to be track in DIC. A speckle is a set of points on specimen surface, used for contrasting pattern recognition, which is commonly painted using a spray to ensure randomness. However, it needs to fulfill some requirements [228, 229]:

1. Randomly distributed

2. Non-repetitive

3. High contrast to specimen surface

4. Isotropic (not bias to one orientation)

5. Speckle size depends on both the application and the parameters used for the correlation (see Fig. 3.20)

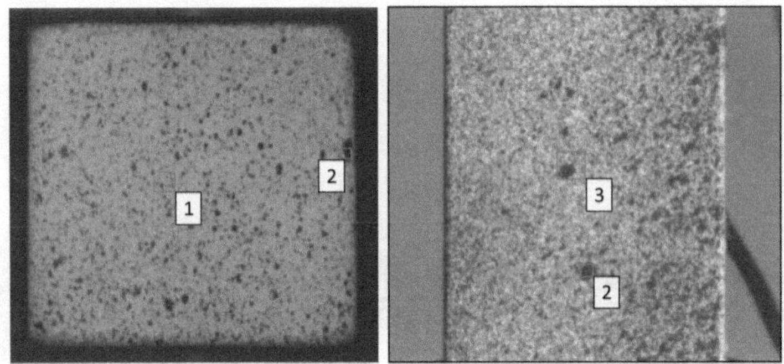

Figure 3.20: Examples of speckle patterns we used in preliminary tests for the application of DIC. In red, different theoretical subsets are represented to highlight the importance of choosing the subset size depending on the speckle: 1) correct subset size for the speckle, 2) subset too small for pattern recognition and 3) larger subset works but reduces gradients measurement.

Our application of DIC to a foamed structure aims at investigating to what extent the microstructure itself may act as a proper speckle for displacement correlation. This approach was called 'texture correlation' by Bay [51], but has not been further studied. Therefore, we performed DIC analyses of different samples which were divided into two groups: speckled and non-speckled. The speckle was created using two spray paints to create more contrast: first, a white paint was applied to specimen surface, followed by a subtle speckle addition using a black paint. The resulting speckle is depicted in Fig. 3.21. The results of the use of speckle as opposite to texture correlation are shown in section 3.2.4.4.

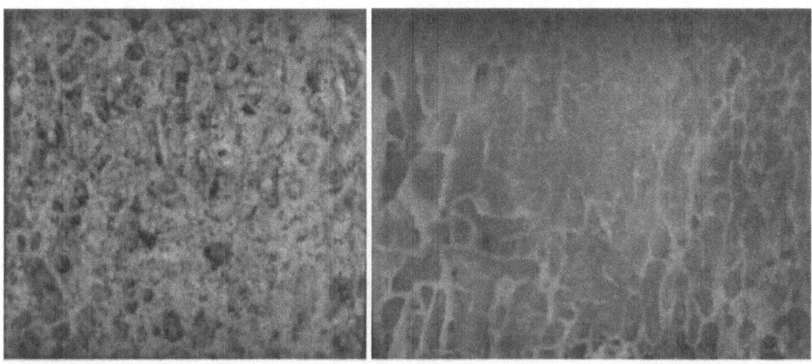

Figure 3.21: Speckled application to a cancellous bone specimen (left) and a non-speckled specimen (right).

3.2.4.2.4 Pattern matching criterion

Pattern matching criterion may have influence on the failure strain properties determination. We have introduced three of them: sum of squared differences (SSD), normalized sum of squared differences (NSSD) and zero-normalized sum of squared differences (ZNSSD). The first one assumes no changes in lighting during image acquisition, while the other two permit those changes and differ from the other on the photometric transformation applied to the deformed image.

However, the selection of any criterion leads to the same yield and failure strain values, so it does not affect the results in terms of the highest strain value in the failure zone. Specifically, a 0.062 yield strain and a 0.089 failure strain were estimated, considering a subset of 101 pixels and a step of 10 pixels. Furthermore, a representation of the strain values obtained for each criterion revealed no differences on the strain distribution results, Fig. 3.22.

We can conclude that, for our experiment set, the pattern matching criterion
is not relevant both in strain distribution and values. Nevertheless, we select
a normalized squared differences criterion for the following failure properties
estimation.

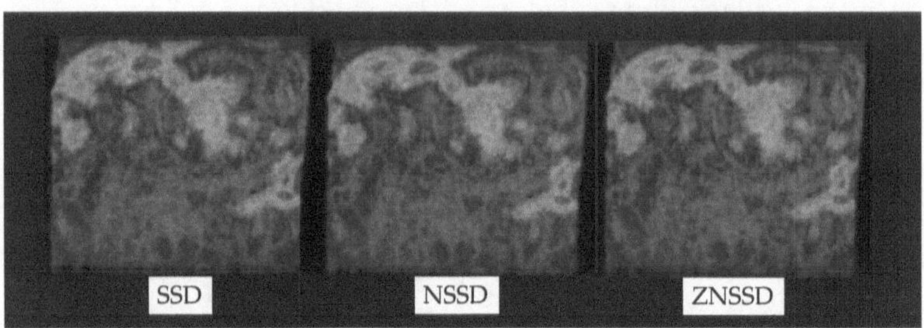

Figure 3.22: Representation of equivalent strain distribution considering squared differences (SSD), normalized squared differences (NSSD) and zero-normalized squared differences
(ZNSSD). The pattern matching criterion produce no differences in the strain distribution
for our experimental set.

3.2.4.2.5 Incremental vs non-incremental correlation

VIC-2D Digital Image Correlation software (v.6.0.2 Correlated Solutions Inc.,
US) incorporates an option to compare each image to the reference one, what
they call non-incremental correlation, and to compare each deformed image to
the previous one, an incremental correlation.

Regarding the failure strain values, this option had no significant effect,
as happened with pattern matching criterion. However, comparing each deformed image to the reference one leads to areas where the correspondence
problem is not properly solved and voids appear in the failure region, represented in in Fig. 3.23 for Specimen #A1. Therefore, it is recommended to
consider incremental correlation for a proper failure definition.

3.2.4.3 Fracture patterns using DIC

The analysis of the effect of DIC parameters on failure localization and failure
strains estimation permits to select the following options for our DIC application to cancellous bone failure characterization: subset size of 120 pixels, step

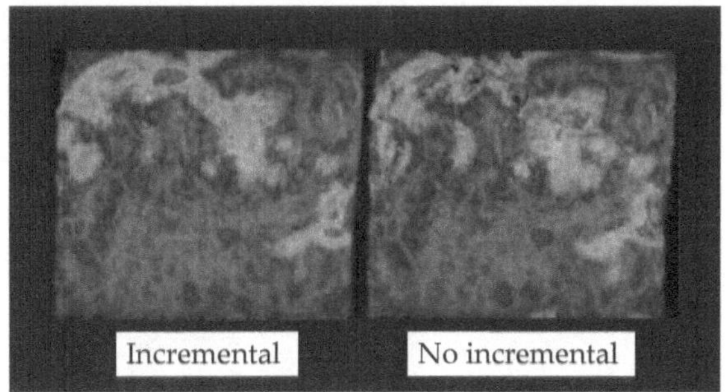

Figure 3.23: Representation of equivalent strain distribution considering incremental or non-incremental correlation in a post-yielding image. As it could be expected, comparing each image with the previous one enhances the accuracy of the correlation.

size of 10 pixels, incremental correlation and normalized squared differences pattern matching criterion.

In this section we aim at finding an accurate fracture pattern descriptor for cancellous bone using DIC. To determine the most suitable variable to characterize trabecular bone fracture, different strain fields were calculated: maximum principal strain ε_1 and shear strain γ_{12}, provided by the software VIC-2D, and equivalent strain, defined by Eq. (4.3), which was manually implemented.

The region of interest (ROI) was selected to analyze the whole specimen and ensuring a perpendicular relative position between the camera and the specimen to avoid out-of-plane displacements during testing. Here we performed a non-speckle approach, as specimen microstructure was used as a grid to compute displacements during testing.

The results obtained after applying DIC to specimens from set A are shown in Fig. 3.24, where column a) represents γ_{12}, b) ε_{eq}, c) ε_1 and d) is a digital image of each fractured specimen.

In the literature, there is agreement about the importance of shear properties in cancellous bone compression fracture, which is highlighted when shear bands and strain localization occur at the microscale [57, 230, 231]. As shown in Fig.3.24 a), γ_{12} provides an indication of failure location, but its definition seems to be spread or at least is less accurate than the other strain candidates.

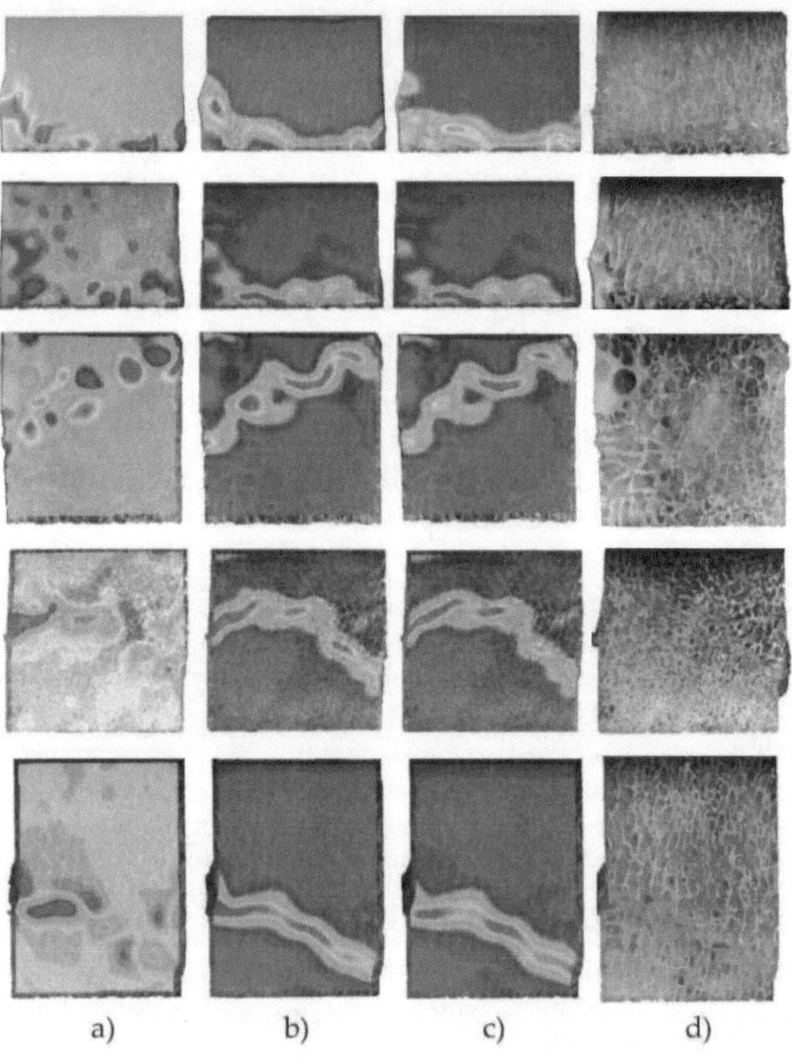

Figure 3.24: Computed strain fields using DIC for specimens from set A: #A1 (top) to #A5 (bottom). a) γ_{12}, b) $\varepsilon_{\mathrm{eq}}$, c) ε_1 and d) experimental fracture pattern.

Therefore, despite the fact that shear strain concentrations can be observed in the fracture zone, they do not fully represent the experimental fracture. Regarding γ_{12}, we conclude that is not the best variable to describe compression fracture with DIC. The homogenized nature of this technique may explain the spreading of this phenomenon compared to the patterns described by the other candidates.

Column b) in Fig. 3.24 shows ε_{eq} strain fields, which is a strain invariant accounting for the normal and shear contributions. Its fracture pattern prediction seems to be the most accurate compared to the experimental evidence. On the other hand, as it can be noted in Fig. 3.24 c), ε_1 also determines with accuracy the fracture area but, due to its non-invariant nature, it can detect tensile stresses in a region submitted to bending stresses (local buckling depicted in left bottom side of #2 Fig. 3.24, c)). Nonetheless, the failure that is occurring in this zone is not directly characterized by this variable. Therefore, ε_1 is suitable to distinguish tension/compression modes but it is not as representative as ε_{eq} to predict fracture patterns.

3.2.4.4 Failure properties estimation using DIC

We estimated cancellous bone failure properties using DIC. For each specimen, the maximum value of equivalent strains in the failure zone was registered for the yield and the fracture points. After the parametric study, we choose the following parameters for cancellous bone failure properties estimation using DIC: subset size of 125 pixels, step size of 10 pixels, strain filter size of 9 pixels, incremental correlation and normalized sum of squared differences pattern matching criterion.

Table 3.9 present the maximum strain values registered in the fractured area for the yield and ultimate points. Strains at the ultimate point ($\varepsilon_{eq,f}$) in the fractured area are found in the range [0.03-0.044]. On the other hand, the strains at the yield point ($\varepsilon_{eq,y}$) are between 0.021 and 0.03. A mean ultimate strain ($\varepsilon_{eq,f}$) of 3.66 % was found, while the yield strain presented a mean value of 2.42 %. It is important to note that those values are average strains in the failure region, not in a single trabeculae.

Table 3.9: Yield and failure strain measurement using DIC. The results are expressed as maximum values in the fracture area at yield and ultimate apparent points.

Specimen	$\varepsilon_{eq,f}$ [-]	$\varepsilon_{eq,y}$ [-]
#A1	0.031	0.024
#A2	0.044	0.021
#A3	0.034	0.025
#A4	0.044	0.030
#A5	0.030	0.022

We only found a work that provides specific yield and ultimate strain values at the failure region for cancellous bone measured using DIC [37]. In their work, Jungmann et al. [37] test a single trabeculae and detect local strain distribution during testing, which permit to estimate a 1.6 ± 0.9 % yield strain and a 12 ± 4 % ultimate strain, but do not provide information about the DIC parameters used. With regards to the yield strain, our estimations are similar but our maximum strain estimations at the ultimate point are around 4 %, which are lower than the reported in [37]. Other works, perform strain analysis to compare with FE results but do not report specific failure values [67, 232].

3.3 Numerical characterization

3.3.1 Introduction

In this section, we present the numerical models developed to characterize and reproduce cancellous bone elastic and failure behavior. The models have a high degree of discretization to account for an accurate microstructural description and were developed from the segmentation of micro-CT images. Our goals are: to estimate the tissue elastic properties, the apparent stiffness of the specimens, to calculate the whole stiffness matrix and failure properties. An inverse analysis method was used to estimate the tissue elastic and failure properties, while an elastic homogenization approach allowed the complete stiffness matrix calculation.

3.3.2 Experimental test reproduction

Finite element models of each specimen were generated from the micro-CT images, reproducing with great accuracy the heterogeneous microstructure of cancellous bone. Micro-FE meshes were created using ScanIp Software (Simpleware, UK), leading to meshes between 0.9M and 2.5M nodes and 2.8M and 8.2M 3D linear elements (C3D4 in Abaqus).

The behavior of cancellous bone tissue at trabecular level was modeled as a homogeneous isotropic linear-elastic material. This assumption is sufficient to estimate the apparent stiffness of cancellous bone [233]. Boundary conditions were defined to mimic the experimental unconfined compression tests, so the nodes in the lower surface were constrained in the test direction. The experimentally recorded displacement was prescribed at the nodes of the upper surface, see Fig. 3.25.

Table 3.10 presents the material bone mechanical properties used for the finite element simulations in this work. Note that calibrated values are inferred from FE models by inverse analysis. Young's modulus at tissue level were calibrated to match the experimental elastic response for each specimen and, similarly, the yield strain in compression was calibrated so that the numerical post-yield response matched the experimentally recorded one. Few specimens included a small portion of closed and mineralized bone growth plate. At these regions we define the same material properties than for cancellous bone.

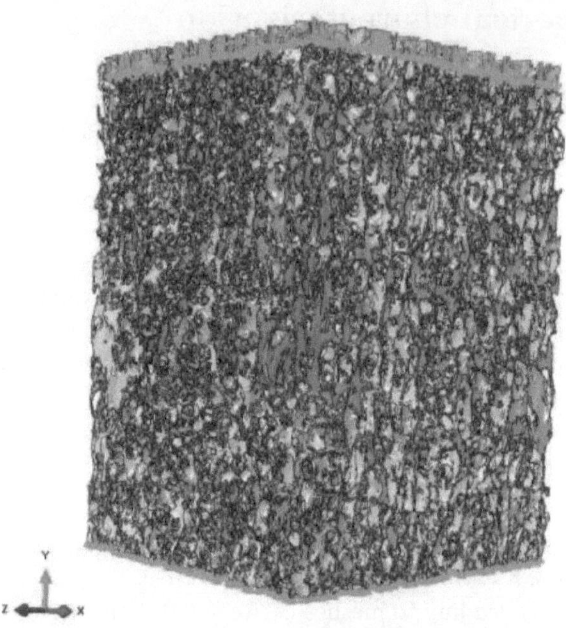

Figure 3.25: Boundary conditions scheme: experimentally measured displacement was prescribed at the upper face nodes of each model, while the bottom face nodes were constrained in the compression direction.

Table 3.10: Material properties defined to simulate fracture with image-based micro-FE models. Tissue Young's modulus expressed as mean $\pm$ SD.

Parameters	Notation	Value	Reference
Tissue Young's modulus	E [GPa]	11.09 ± 1.69	Calibrated
Poisson's ratio	ν [-]	0.3	Literature [78]
Yield strain in compression	$\varepsilon_{y,c}$ [%]	0.69 ± 0.086	Calibrated
Strain at compression fracture	$\varepsilon_{f,c}$ [%]	3.69 ± 0.91	Calibrated
Damage at compression fracture	D_c	0.95	Literature [142, 143]
Damage exponent	n	2	Literature [82]
Characteristic crack length	L_{frx} [mm]	0.075	Literature [234, 235]

3.3.3 Elastic homogenization

The homogenization of cancellous bone elastic properties is relevant to assess the influence of microstructure on the mechanical competence of its heterogeneous structure. Furthermore, those homogenized elastic properties may be used in multiscale models to take into account the underlying microstructure without defining it explicitly in the numerical models. Thus, we aim at calculating elastic homogenized properties of cancellous bone specimens through the estimation of the stiffness matrix associated to its microstructure. The methodology to calculate the homogenized elastic properties presented in this section will help to analyze cancellous bone surrogates in Chapter 4.

Our approach to estimate the homogenized elastic properties can be explained as follows, which was implemented in Matlab (MATLAB 2014a, The MathWorks Inc., USA) (pre- and post-processing) and Ansys (FE modeling). The Lamé-Hooke constitutive equation is given by:

$$\sigma = C\varepsilon \tag{3.15}$$

where $\sigma = (\sigma_{xx}\ \sigma_{yy}\ \sigma_{zz}\ \tau_{yz}\ \tau_{zx}\ \tau_{xy})^T$ is the stress vector, C is the stiffness matrix and $\varepsilon = (\varepsilon_{xx}\ \varepsilon_{yy}\ \varepsilon_{zz}\ \gamma_{yz}\ \gamma_{zx}\ \gamma_{xy})^T$ is the strain vector. The stiffness matrix C of cancellous bone RVE is calculated through the application of six independent unitary strain fields (3 axial and 3 shear strains) in combination with periodic boundary conditions (PBC) constraints, and then computing the equilibrium stress vector (σ^i) for each strain field (ε^i) from the finite element results. Each load case permits to assess one of the columns of C. Fig. 3.26 (b) depicts the application of the 6 unitary load cases for a cancellous bone specimen.

- Load case 1: $\varepsilon^1 = (100000)^T$, $C_{(:,1)} = \sigma^1$

- Load case 2: $\varepsilon^2 = (010000)^T$, $C_{(:,2)} = \sigma^2$

- Load case 3: $\varepsilon^3 = (001000)^T$, $C_{(:,3)} = \sigma^3$

- Load case 4: $\varepsilon^4 = (000100)^T$, $C_{(:,4)} = \sigma^4$

- Load case 5: $\varepsilon^5 = (000010)^T$, $C_{(:,5)} = \sigma^5$

- Load case 6: $\varepsilon^6 = (000001)^T$, $C_{(:,6)} = \sigma^6$

We consider each specimen as a unit cell or elementary representative volume (RVE) of the cancellous bone of each vertebra, to estimate its behavior as a heterogeneous material [236, 237, 238, 239]. Considering periodic boundary conditions (PBC) on the RVE permits its response to be representative of the whole structure. Two conditions must be fulfilled, following Reisinger et al. [240]:

- The stress field must be periodic $\sigma_{ij}^{+} = \sigma_{ij}^{-}$.

- The strain field must be periodic, so the deformed shape of opposite RVE faces must match.

Therefore, constraint equations were defined on RVE faces to fulfill the PBC displacement field requirements, considering the equations proposed by Hohe [237], summarized below.

$$u^{1+} = u^{1-} + a\varepsilon_1^i \tag{3.16}$$

$$v^{1+} = v^{1-} + \frac{1}{2}a\varepsilon_6^i \tag{3.17}$$

$$w^{1+} = w^{1-} + \frac{1}{2}a\varepsilon_5^i \tag{3.18}$$

$$u^{2+} = u^{2-} + \frac{1}{2}b\varepsilon_6^i \tag{3.19}$$

$$v^{2+} = v^{2-} + b\varepsilon_2^i \tag{3.20}$$

$$w^{2+} = w^{2-} + \frac{1}{2}b\varepsilon_4^i \tag{3.21}$$

$$u^{3+} = u^{3-} + \frac{1}{2}c\varepsilon_5^i \tag{3.22}$$

$$v^{3+} = v^{3-} + \frac{1}{2}c\varepsilon_4^i \tag{3.23}$$

$$w^{3+} = w^{3-} + c\varepsilon_3^i \tag{3.24}$$

where a, b, c define the RVE dimensions, $N^{+,-}$ define the external opposite faces at x (1), y (2) or z (3) directions and u, v and w represent displacement fields, Fig. 3.27. The super index i refers to the load case applied (1-6).

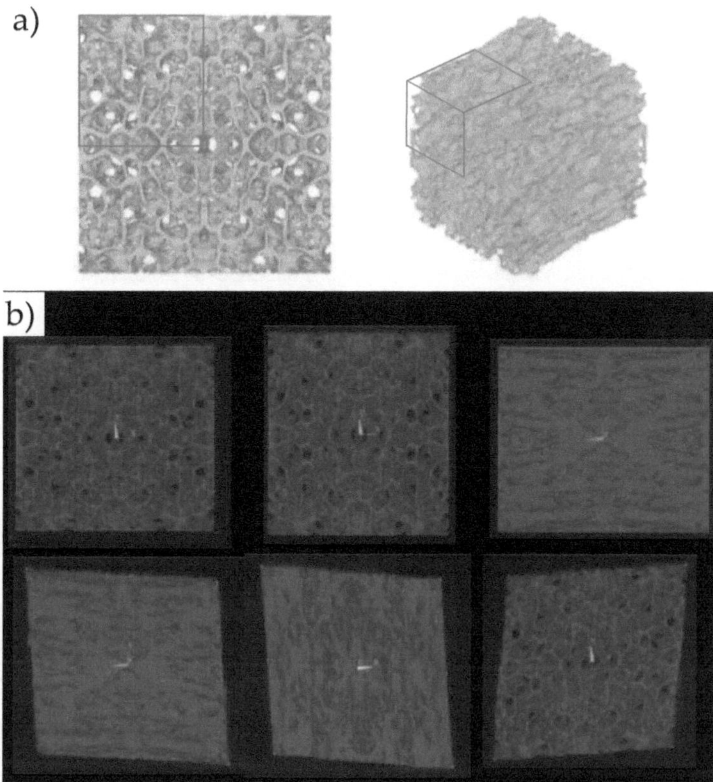

Figure 3.26: a) Mirroring the structure to be able to apply PBC (volume under analysis marked in red): 2D view (left) and 3D representation (right) and b) representation of the six load cases with periodic boundary conditions to calculate the stiffness matrix of a RVE: elongation load cases (top) and shear load cases (bottom).

The procedure followed has been successfully applied in the literature, for example, in a multiscale approach to estimate the elastic constants of lamellar bone [238, 239, 241] and cancellous bone specimens [133, 134].

It is known that cancellous bone is a heterogeneous non-periodic structure so, in order to be able to define PBC, the finite element mesh was mirrored against its three main directions, see Fig. 3.26 (a). This approach was already studied to analyze cancellous bone by Pahr and Zysset [134], who stated that it permits to calculate RVE effective elastic properties, while other approaches, such as applying kinematic or mixed uniform boundary conditions lead to upper and lower properties bonds estimation.

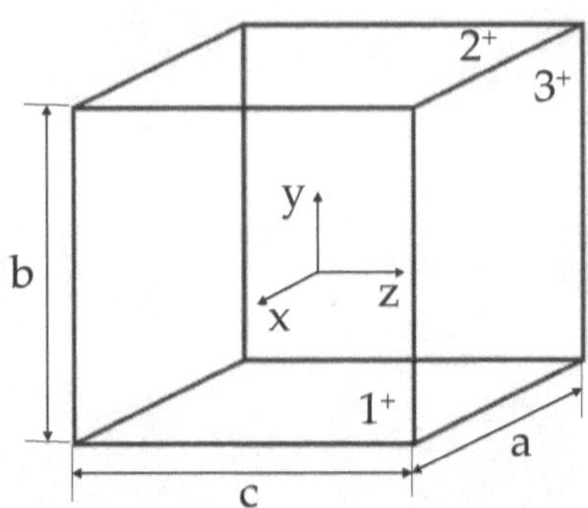

Figure 3.27: RVE notation scheme: a, b and c define the RVE dimensions, $1^{+,-}$ define the opposite faces on x direction.

In this section, we present the results of the elastic homogenization of different cancellous bone volumes. We divide our results between partial volume (cubic volumes of around 7 mm side) and whole specimens analysis. The results of the partial volumes are represented as function of its microstructural features to elucidate if there are mechano-morphometric significant relationships while the whole specimen analysis are compared to experimental measurements.

3.3.3.1   Stiffness matrix estimation for cancellous bone volumes

Here, we calculate the stiffness matrix of cancellous bone volumes. For this purpose, twenty-eight 7-mm cubic volumes of cancellous bone were extracted digitally, which were segmented and then served to generate finite element models. The elastic homogenization procedure described in section 3.3.3 was applied to each model and the complete stiffness matrix was calculated for each case. We assumed an effective isotropic tissue Young's modulus of 10 GPa and a Poisson's ratio of 0.3 for the specimens digitally extracted, so the variations in the terms of the stiffness matrix are only result from specimen-specific microstructure.

The constitutive elastic matrix C_{ij} is a 6x6 matrix which relates elastic stresses and strains through Hooke's law (Eq. 3.25). In the most general case, 36 non-zero components define material behavior (triclinic material case, Eq. 3.26). For materials with one or more planes of symmetry, some components become 0 (if calculated with respect to their oriented axis). Specifically, in case of orthotropic materials, only 12 are non-zero components (Eq. 3.27). In that case, only 9 of the 12 components are independent and can be expressed as a function of the so-called engineering constants. Those constants are the axial stiffnesses, shear stiffnesses and Poison's ratios for the different main directions and planes: E_x, E_y, E_z, G_{xy}, G_{xz}, G_{yz}, ν_{xy}, ν_{xz}, ν_{yz}. Cancellous bone can be assumed to have orthotropic material behavior, which is equivalent to the existence of 3 planes of symmetry. The engineering constants for an orthotropic material may be expressed as a function of the compliance matrix $(S_{ij} = C_{ij}^{-1})$ whose components are defined in Eq. 3.28.

$$\sigma_i = C_{ij}\varepsilon_j \tag{3.25}$$

$$C_{ij} = \begin{pmatrix} C_{11} & C_{12} & C_{13} & C_{14} & C_{15} & C_{16} \\ C_{12} & C_{22} & C_{23} & C_{24} & C_{25} & C_{26} \\ C_{13} & C_{23} & C_{33} & C_{34} & C_{35} & C_{36} \\ C_{14} & C_{24} & C_{34} & C_{44} & C_{45} & C_{46} \\ C_{15} & C_{25} & C_{35} & C_{45} & C_{55} & C_{56} \\ C_{16} & C_{26} & C_{36} & C_{46} & C_{56} & C_{66} \end{pmatrix} \tag{3.26}$$

$$
C_{ij} = \begin{pmatrix}
C_{11} & C_{12} & C_{13} & 0 & 0 & 0 \\
C_{12} & C_{22} & C_{23} & 0 & 0 & 0 \\
C_{13} & C_{23} & C_{33} & 0 & 0 & 0 \\
0 & 0 & 0 & C_{44} & 0 & 0 \\
0 & 0 & 0 & 0 & C_{55} & 0 \\
0 & 0 & 0 & 0 & 0 & C_{66}
\end{pmatrix}
\tag{3.27}
$$

$$
S_{ij} = \begin{pmatrix}
\frac{1}{E_x} & -\frac{\nu_{yx}}{E_y} & -\frac{\nu_{zx}}{E_z} & 0 & 0 & 0 \\
-\frac{\nu_{xy}}{E_x} & \frac{1}{E_y} & -\frac{\nu_{zy}}{E_z} & 0 & 0 & 0 \\
-\frac{\nu_{xz}}{E_x} & -\frac{\nu_{yz}}{E_y} & \frac{1}{E_z} & 0 & 0 & 0 \\
0 & 0 & 0 & \frac{1}{G_{yz}} & 0 & 0 \\
0 & 0 & 0 & 0 & \frac{1}{G_{zx}} & 0 \\
0 & 0 & 0 & 0 & 0 & \frac{1}{G_{xy}}
\end{pmatrix}
\tag{3.28}
$$

The non-orthotropic terms of the stiffness matrix have a value ranging between $[10^{-5} - 10^{-6}]$ in our estimations, which may be neglected compared to the rest of the stiffness matrix terms. Those coefficients are related to the first and second type of mutual influence coefficients and Chentsov coefficients for a general anisotropic behavior. In fact, cancellous bone may exhibit anisotropic behavior under multiaxial loading conditions not oriented with the material symmetry planes.

For representation purposes, we present the stiffness matrix estimation for the 28 specimens by plotting their non-zero components, highlighting the mean value of each component (Fig. 3.28). The range of variation of the results shows a strong influence of the microstructure of the specimens on the estimation of the elastic tensor, because only microstructure changes between specimens while material properties are maintained. A larger variation is found for the components which represent axial stiffness (C_{11}, C_{22}, C_{33}), compared to components related with shearing properties (C_{44}, C_{55}, C_{66}).

On the other hand, Table 3.11 summarizes the mean value of each component of C_{ij} and their standard deviation. Based on those values, an average value of the engineering constants is calculated for the data set analyzed using Eq. 3.28. $E_x = 382.66$ MPa, $E_y = 908.20$ MPa, $E_z = 361.04$ MPa, $G_{xy} = 183.77$ MPa, $G_{yz} = 185.89$ MPa, $G_{zx} = 119.34$ MPa, $\nu_{xy} = 0.1130$, $\nu_{yz} = 0.2887$, $\nu_{zx} = 0.2720$.

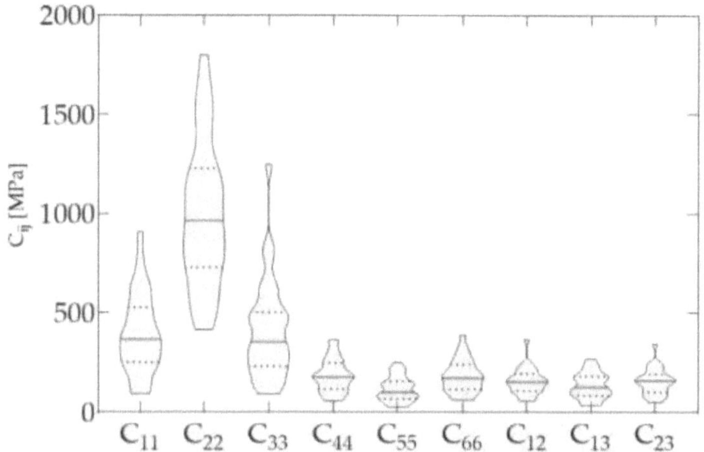

Figure 3.28: Summary of non-zero components of the elastic matrix represented as violin plots, estimated for the 28 cancellous bone volumes and median values (in red). The interquartile range is marked using dash lines.

The homogenized results of the 28 cancellous bone samples have revealed an orthotropic apparent behavior, which is close to be equivalent to a transversely isotropic material, because C_{11} and C_{33} values are very similar. Following that argument, directions x and z define the isotropy plane, while y is the main trabecular orientation direction.

Table 3.11: Mean values and standard deviation of the components of the constitutive elastic tensor C_{ij}.

C_{ij}	Mean value [MPa]	Standard deviation [MPa]
C_{11}	400.26	205.46
C_{22}	995.94	366.90
C_{33}	416.60	254.86
C_{12}	157.88	65.55
C_{13}	137.89	64.95
C_{23}	157.25	65.35
C_{44}	185.89	83.61
C_{55}	119.34	62.59
C_{66}	183.77	82.90

3.3.3.2 Investigation of morphometric and mechanical variables relationships on the 7 mm side cubic samples

The first statistical analysis that we conducted was about the estimation of linear relationships between morphometric and mechanical variables. In order to achieve this goal, first, we visualized the scatter plot of each pair of morpho-mechanic variables to find clear non-linear relationships which would not fit in the analysis. However, no clear non-linear representation was found. Then, we calculated the linear correlation coefficient matrix of the variables under study. Specifically, we estimated: BV/TV, BS/BV, Tb.Th, Tb.Sp, Tb.N, $D_{\text{2D-1}}$, $D_{\text{2D-2}}$, $D_{\text{2D-3}}$, D_{3D}, $DA_{\text{MIL,2D-1}}$, $DA_{\text{MIL,2D-2}}$, $DA_{\text{MIL,2D-3}}$, $DA_{\text{MIL,3D}}$ and Conn.D as morphometric variables and, E_{x}, E_{y}, E_{z}, ν_{xy}, ν_{xz}, ν_{yz}, ν_{yx}, ν_{zx}, ν_{zy}, G_{xy}, G_{yz}, G_{zx}, as mechanical variables. Half of the Poisson's ratio can be calculated using symmetry properties of the stiffness matrix. The correlation technique used in this section will help to evaluate similar relationships of cancellous bone surrogates in Chapter 4.

The correlation coefficient measures the linear dependence of two random variables (A,B). The Pearson correlation coefficient (ρ) is defined in Eq. 3.29:

$$\rho(A, B) = \frac{1}{N-1} \sum_{i=1}^{N} \frac{(A_i - \mu_A)(B_i - \mu_B)}{\sigma_A \, \sigma_B} \tag{3.29}$$

where N is the number of observations, μ_i and σ_i are the mean and standard deviation of each variable.

The correlation coefficients may be expressed in matrix form as the matrix of correlation coefficients (R), Eq. 3.30.

$$R = \begin{pmatrix} \rho(A, A) & \rho(A, B) \\ \rho(B, A) & \rho(B, B) \end{pmatrix} = \begin{pmatrix} 1 & \rho(A, B) \\ \rho(B, A) & 1 \end{pmatrix} \tag{3.30}$$

where obviously each variable correlates to themselves, so the entries in the diagonal are 1's.

A value of ρ close to 1 (or -1) indicates that there is a linear correlation between those variables.

Fig. 3.29 shows a visual representation of the linear correlation coefficients computed for the morphometric and elasto-mechanical variables. Dark red and blue colors represent a positive or negative linear correlation, while light colors represent no correlation. A total of n=28 samples are used for the analysis. The morphometric parameters, sorted as each row and column in the graph are: BV/TV, BS/BV, Tb.Th, Tb.Sp, Tb.N, $D_{2D\text{-}1}$, $D_{2D\text{-}2}$, $D_{2D\text{-}3}$, D_{3D}, $DA_{MIL,2D\text{-}1}$, $DA_{MIL,2D\text{-}2}$, $DA_{MIL,2D\text{-}3}$, $DA_{MIL,3D}$ and Conn.D. On the other hand, the mechanical parameters are the engineering constants estimated from the constitutive elastic tensor, which are sorted as follows in Fig. 3.29 scheme: E_x, E_y, E_z, ν_{xy}, ν_{xz}, ν_{yz}, ν_{yx}, ν_{zx}, ν_{zy}, G_{xy}, G_{yz}, G_{zx}.

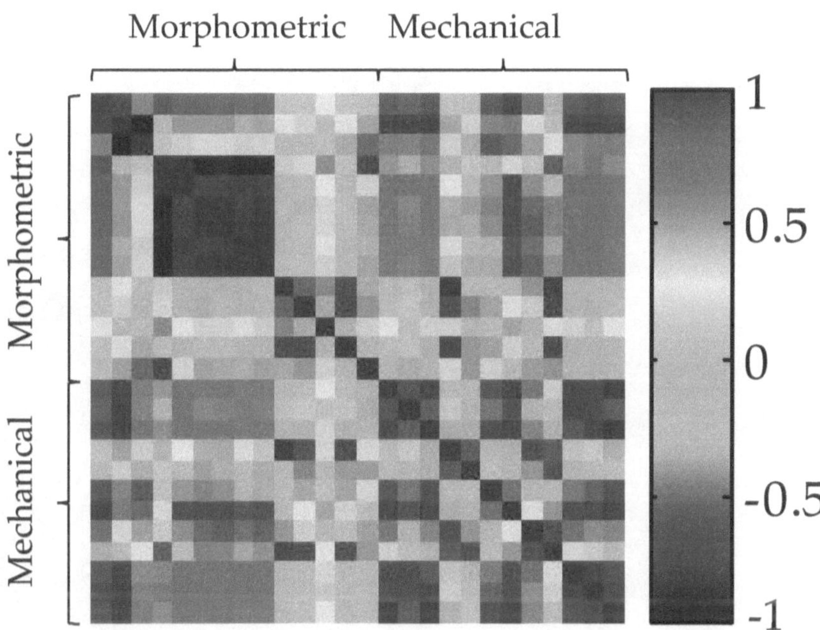

Figure 3.29: Linear correlation coefficient representation between morphometric and mechanical parameters. The positive or negative correlations are summarized numerically in Table 3.12.

Table 3.12: Linear correlation coefficients (ρ) between morphometric and mechanical parameters. The regressions of $|\rho| > 0.6$ are highlighted in the Table.

	BV/TV	BS/BV	Tb.Th	Tb.Sp	Tb.N	D_{2D-1}	D_{2D-2}	D_{2D-3}	D_{3D}	$DA_{MIL,2D-1}$	$DA_{MIL,2D-2}$	$DA_{MIL,2D-3}$	$DA_{MIL,3D}$	Conn.D
E_x	**0.902**	**-0.762**	**0.633**	-0.379	**0.736**	**0.692**	**0.701**	**0.672**	**0.672**	-0.264	-0.199	0.295	-0.228	-0.152
E_y	**0.864**	**-0.765**	**0.612**	-0.299	**0.709**	0.592	**0.614**	**0.653**	**0.614**	0.086	0.142	0.106	0.119	-0.327
E_z	**0.919**	**-0.787**	**0.700**	-0.404	**0.705**	**0.709**	**0.702**	**0.663**	**0.673**	-0.300	-0.310	0.211	-0.312	-0.135
ν_{xy}	0.425	-0.357	0.379	-0.320	0.305	0.463	0.481	0.340	0.408	**-0.810**	**-0.696**	0.205	**-0.755**	0.351
ν_{xz}	-0.294	0.169	-0.336	0.408	-0.151	-0.368	-0.334	-0.272	-0.339	0.432	**0.613**	-0.096	0.531	-0.385
ν_{yz}	-0.591	**0.620**	-0.564	0.090	-0.387	-0.428	-0.404	-0.287	-0.335	0.438	0.487	-0.216	0.496	0.200
ν_{yx}	**-0.763**	**0.655**	-0.493	0.336	**-0.666**	**-0.658**	**-0.655**	-0.572	**-0.607**	0.432	0.316	-0.354	0.357	0.051
ν_{zx}	-0.488	0.346	-0.364	0.39	-0.405	-0.496	-0.543	-0.476	-0.521	0.541	0.382	-0.299	0.430	-0.365
ν_{zy}	0.475	-0.260	0.266	-0.547	0.428	**0.615**	0.599	0.480	0.558	**-0.758**	**-0.720**	0.264	**-0.712**	0.539
G_{xy}	**0.904**	**-0.744**	**0.584**	-0.420	**0.779**	**0.703**	**0.729**	**0.733**	**0.711**	-0.124	-0.034	0.206	-0.064	-0.141
G_{yz}	**0.941**	**-0.767**	**0.634**	-0.448	**0.782**	**0.736**	**0.743**	**0.745**	**0.731**	-0.113	-0.100	0.113	-0.099	-0.140
G_{zx}	**0.920**	**-0.774**	**0.664**	-0.411	**0.731**	**0.719**	**0.715**	**0.677**	**0.685**	-0.309	-0.287	0.273	-0.297	-0.121

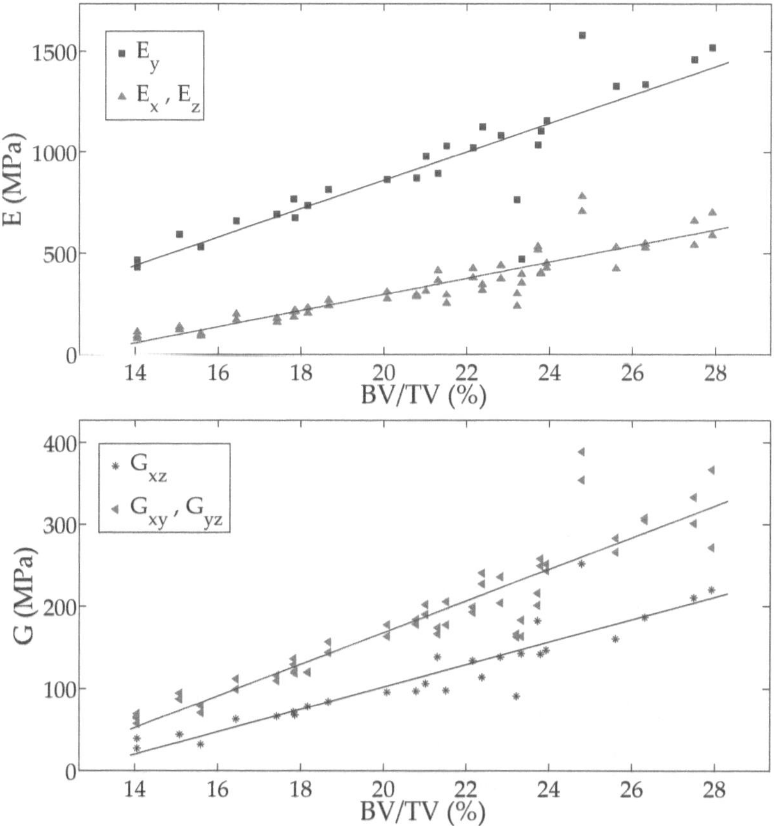

Figure 3.30: Scatter plot and linear correlations obtained for the axial (E) (top) and shearing (G) stiffnesses (bottom) in the preferred trabecular orientation (y) and transversal orientations (x,z) depending on the bone volume fraction (BV/TV).

Based on the results shown in Fig. 3.29, we summarize the correlation coefficients of morpho-mechanic relationships, highlighting the values greater than 0.6 in Table 3.12. Both the axial (E_x, E_y, E_z) and shearing stiffnesses (G_{xy}, G_{yz}, G_{zx}) in the three orthogonal directions show correlation to the same morphometric parameters: BV/TV, BS/BV, Tb.Th, Tb.N, $D_{2D\text{-}1}$, $D_{2D\text{-}2}$, $D_{2D\text{-}3}$ and D_{3D}. For those parameters, the linear correlation coefficients (ρ) range from 0.6 to 0.94 and the highest correlation is against BV/TV. BS/BV, Tb.Th,

Tb.N, $D_{2D\text{-}1}$, $D_{2D\text{-}2}$, $D_{2D\text{-}3}$ and D_{3D} show a similar degree of correlation both to E and G values. Regarding anisotropy degree parameters, a significant degree of correlation was found to ν_{xy}, ν_{zy} and ν_{xz}. On the other hand, no significant correlation was found to Tb.Sp nor Conn.D.

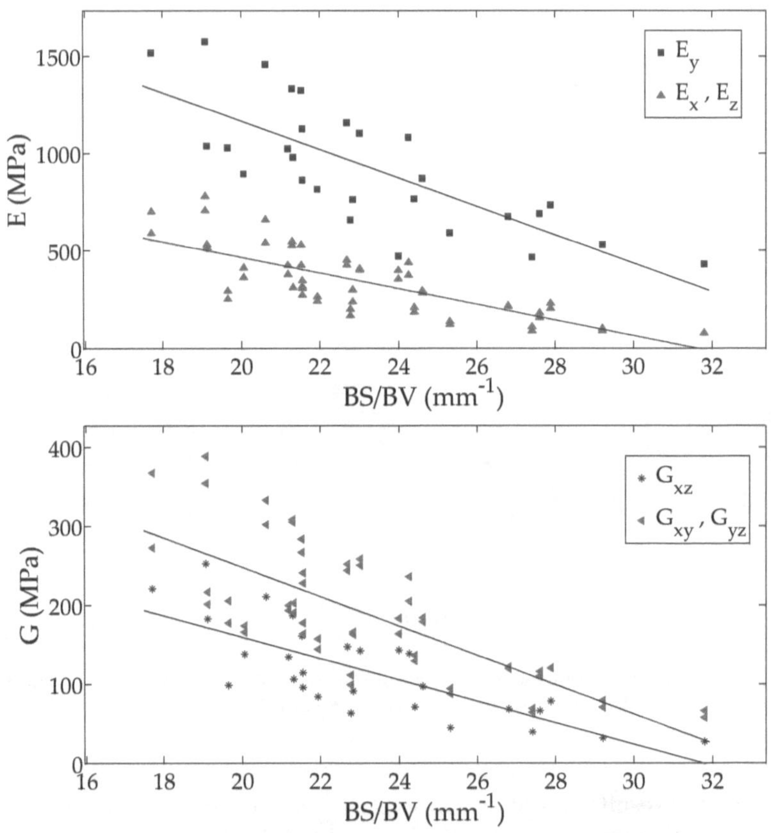

Figure 3.31: Scatter plot and linear correlations obtained for the axial (E) (top) and shearing (G) stiffnesses (bottom) in the preferred trabecular orientation (y) and transversal orientations (x,z) depending on the bone surface area to volume ratio (BS/BV).

The apparent behavior observed in the samples studied is close to be transversely isotropic, with a preferred direction of higher stiffness (y) and an isotropic transversal plane (xz). Therefore, in the plots we represent the values for axial stiffness in directions x and z, and the shearing stiffnesses G_{xy} and G_{yz} as two unique data sets. For each direction a linear correlation to each parameter is calculated and compared to the other direction. Looking at E and G values, sorted by directions, E values are between 2 and 5-fold larger in direction y than transverse directions (x and z). In case of G values, the transversal plane (xz) is around 1.5 times more flexible than planes xy and yz.

Starting with the linear analysis of morpho-mechano variable pairs, Fig. 3.30 shows the positive correlation of E and G to bone volume fraction. As the amount of bone increases, so do the axial and shearing stiffnesses in the 3 orthogonal directions or planes, respectively. The graph also stands out the existence of a main trabecular orientation with a higher axial rigidity, while the estimations about the other two directions (x and z) are similar, so they may define an isotropy plane, as stated before. Regarding G vs BV/TV relationships, lower differences between shearing planes are shown, compared to E values. However, two clearly different groups of points can be distinguished, defining planes with distinct shear properties. For both stiffnesses, a highly linear correlation is found, with a ρ mean value of approximately 0.9 for axial and 0.92 for shearing.

The relationship between E and G values to the bone surface area to volume ratio is presented in Fig. 3.31. For both rigidities modes (axial and shear), the correlation obtained is negative. As BS/BV increases, that is, bone is less dense (more rod-like, or more osteoporotic), E and G decrease. In this case, the results are more spread than for BV/TV ($\rho = -0.77$ for both E and G). Shearing stiffness scatter plot shows that, for BS/BV, the groups depending on the direction are less clearly distinguishable.

Fig. 3.32 shows the linear relationships between the rigidities calculated through homogenization and the mean trabecular thickness of each specimen. As for BV/TV, a positive correlation is found, whose correlation coefficient is approximately 0.7 for each stiffness. The results are coherent, because larger mean thicknesses produce larger axial and shearing stiffnesses values. Again, the scatter plot shows two groups of points for E and G, with the higher values for the main trabecular orientation direction. In this case, an increment of 55 μm in Tb.Th produces E_y to augment two-fold.

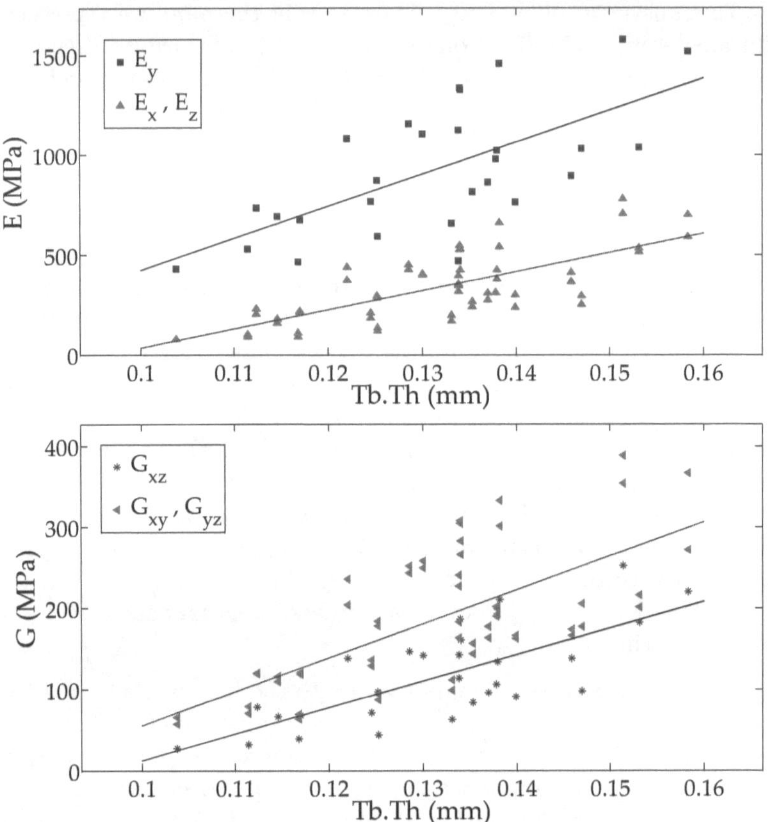

Figure 3.32: Scatter plot and linear correlations obtained for the axial (E) (top) and shearing (G) stiffnesses (bottom) in the preferred trabecular orientation (y) and transversal orientations (x,z) depending on the mean trabecular thickness (Tb.Th).

The correlations to the trabecular number (Tb.N) are presented in Fig. 3.33. A positive linear correlation was calculated for E and G on the three orthogonal directions or planes, respectively. The trends obtained are consistent with the physical meaning of Tb.N, which for a plate-like model is the BV/TV to Tb.Th ratio. The higher Tb.N is, the greater E and G values are found. Again, the correlation is not as robust as for BV/TV case, with ρ

values around 0.75.

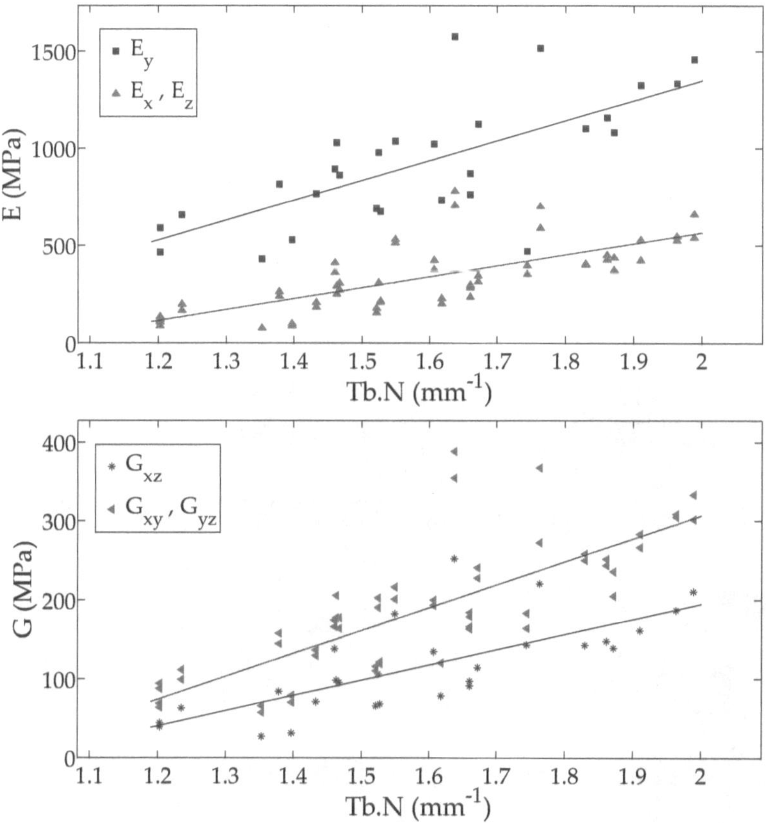

Figure 3.33: Scatter plot and linear correlations obtained for the axial (E) (top) and shearing (G) stiffnesses (bottom) in the preferred trabecular orientation (y) and transverse orientations (x,z) depending on the trabecular number (Tb.N).

The complexity of the specimens, measured by D_{2D} and D_{3D}, also correlated to both the axial and shearing stiffnesses. The 2D version of fractal dimension was applied to the three main orientations of each sample, two of them containing the main trabecular orientation (D_{2D-1}, D_{2D-2}) and the other one referred to the transversal plane ($D_{2D\text{-}3}$). The scatter plots and the linear correlations are shown in Figs. 3.34, 3.35, 3.36 and 3.37 respectively. For both versions of fractal dimension, the correlation is positive and therefore, an increment of D_{2D} or D_{3D} values is associated with larger stiffness values. In this case, the linear correlation coefficients are around 0.7 for the axial and shearing stiffnesses.

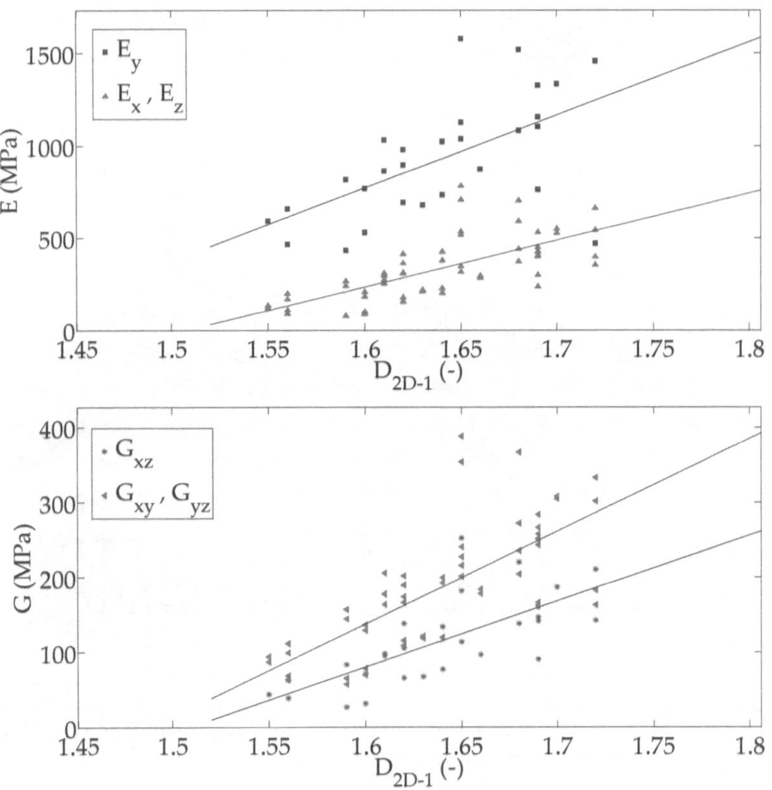

Figure 3.34: Scatter plot and linear correlations obtained for the axial (E) (top) and shearing (G) stiffnesses (bottom) in the preferred trabecular orientation (y) and transversal orientations (x,z) depending on the fractal dimension 2D calculated in planes containing the main trabecular orientation ($D_{2D\text{-}1}$).

The application of fractal dimension 2D to the directions containing the main trabecular orientation gives analogous results regarding the linear correlations calculated (Figs. 3.34 and 3.35). On the other hand, its application to the transversal plane lead to similar but significantly higher regression slope (around 20 % higher) (Fig. 3.36). These results confirm observations reported in the literature: the higher the fractal dimension is, the higher the axial stiffness [214, 221].

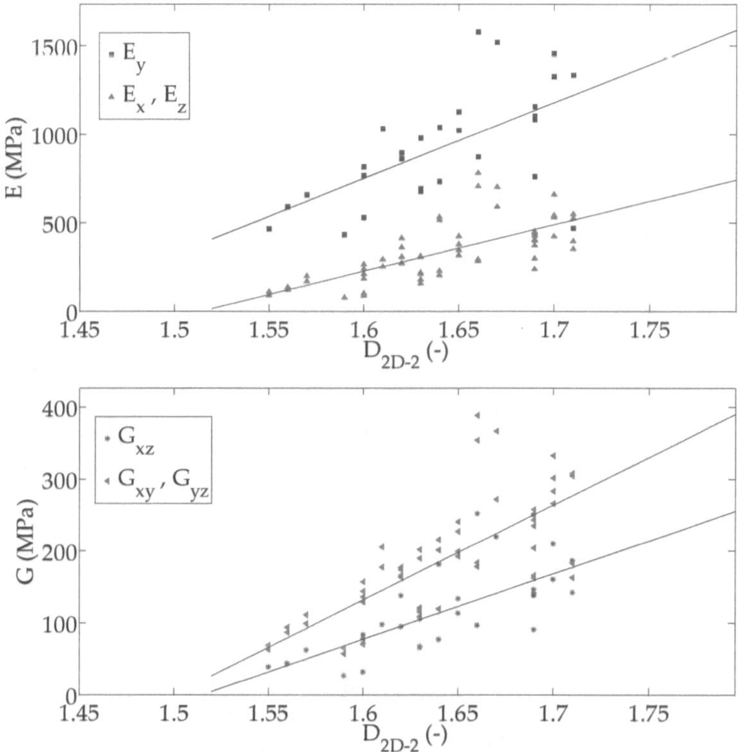

Figure 3.35: Scatter plot and linear correlations obtained for the axial (E) (top) and shearing (G) stiffnesses (bottom) in the preferred trabecular orientation (y) and transversal orientations (x,z) depending on the fractal dimension 2D calculated in planes containing the main trabecular orientation ($D_{2D\text{-}2}$).

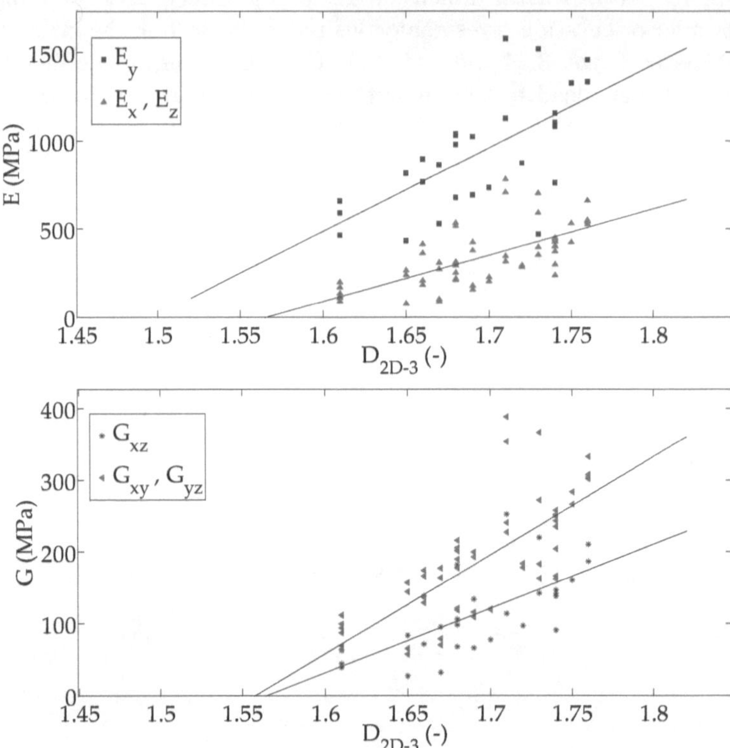

Figure 3.36: Scatter plot and linear correlations obtained for the axial (E) (top) and shearing (G) stiffnesses (bottom) in the preferred trabecular orientation (y) and transversal orientations (x,z) depending on the fractal dimension 2D calculated in the transversal plane direction (D_{2D-3}).

Table 3.12 reveals that Poisson's ratio values do not correlate to the same morphometric parameters, but some significant relationships were found. For example, from our results, ν_{yx} showed correlation to bone volume fraction (ρ=-0.76), displayed in Fig. 3.38 (top), a positive correlation to BS/BV and a negative correlation to Tb.N (Fig. 3.41) and fractal dimension, both 2D and 3D versions (Fig. 3.40).

In case of BS/BV, the correlation obtained against ν_{yx} follows an analo-

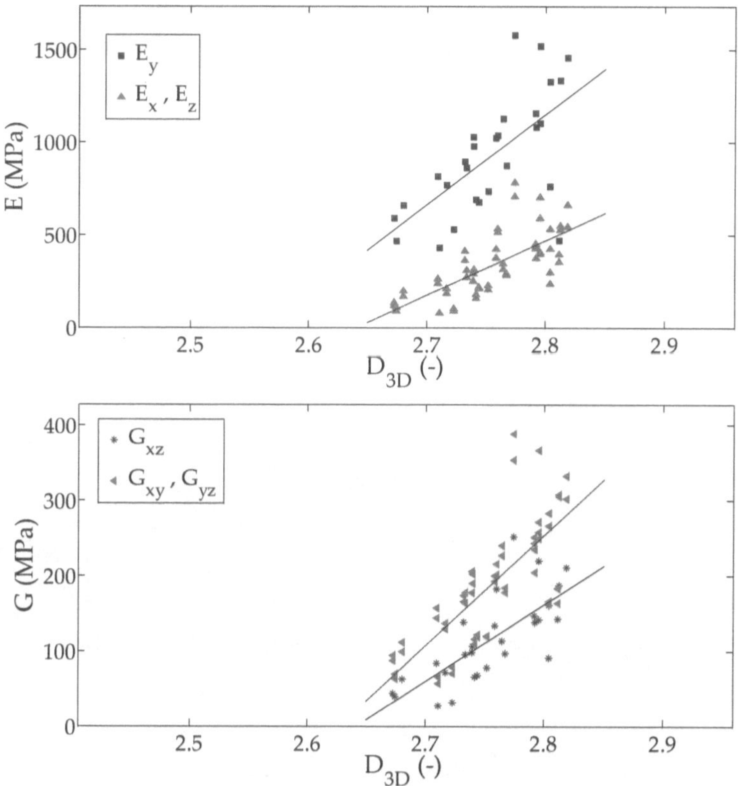

Figure 3.37: Scatter plot and linear correlations obtained for the axial (E) (top) and shearing (G) stiffnesses (bottom) in the preferred trabecular orientation (y) and transversal orientations (x,z) depending on the fractal dimension 3D (D_{3D}).

gous trend than the one obtained for ν_{yz}, which enforces the idea that BS/BV may have an influence on some of the Poisson's ratio estimations (Fig. 3.41).

DA$_{MIL3D}$ and its 2D version showed correlation to ν_{xy} and ν_{zy}, visualized in Fig. 3.38 (bottom) and Fig. 3.39. However, Fig. 3.38 (bottom) must not be considered a significant correlation. Two values of Fig. 3.38 (bottom) seem far from the rest of data and if discarded, ρ decreases until 0.5 and 0.3, respectively. Therefore, those correlations are less significant than the ones reported for the stiffness values. In case of ν_{yx} to BV/TV correlation, it is strange for us that only it correlates to bone volume fraction, so the correlation may be arbitrary (even with a p-value<0.001).

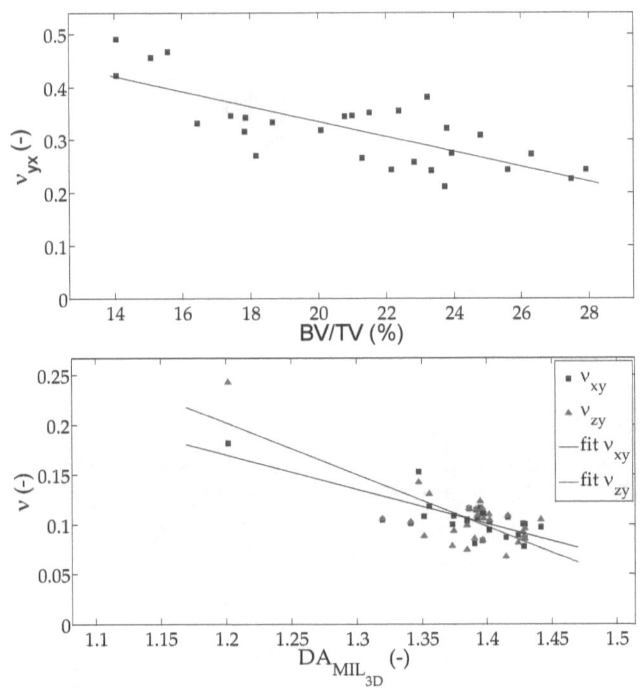

Figure 3.38: Scatter plot and linear correlations obtained for ν_{yx} as function of BV/TV (top) and ν_{xy} and ν_{zy} as function of DA_{MIL3D} (bottom).

The connectivity density (Conn.D) alone did not show any linear correlation to the mechanical parameters, as can be seen in Table 3.12.

On the other hand, taking into account the DA_{MIL3D} definition, we expected some degree of correlation to E_y/E_x or E_y/E_z and maybe also to shear stiffnesses ratios. However, only a weak correlation of about $\rho = 0.55$ was found to the axial stiffnesses ratios, while $\rho = 0.62$ for shearing rigidities ratios.

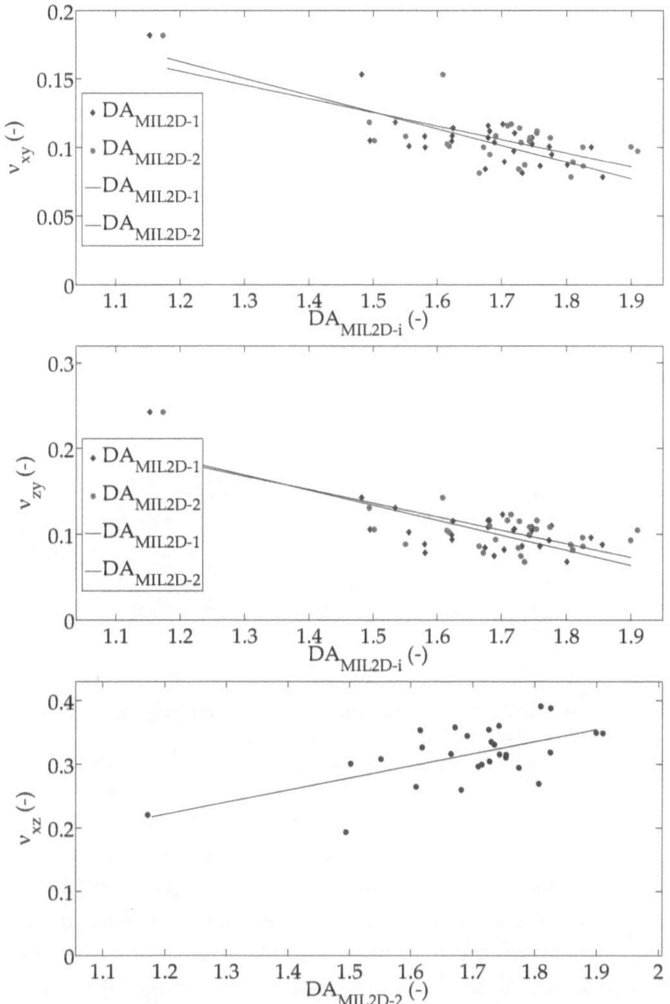

Figure 3.39: Scatter plot and linear correlations obtained for ν_{xy} and ν_{zy} depending on the $DA_{MIL2D\text{-}1,2}$ (top and centre, respectively) and ν_{xz} as a function of $DA_{MIL2D\text{-}2}$ (bottom).

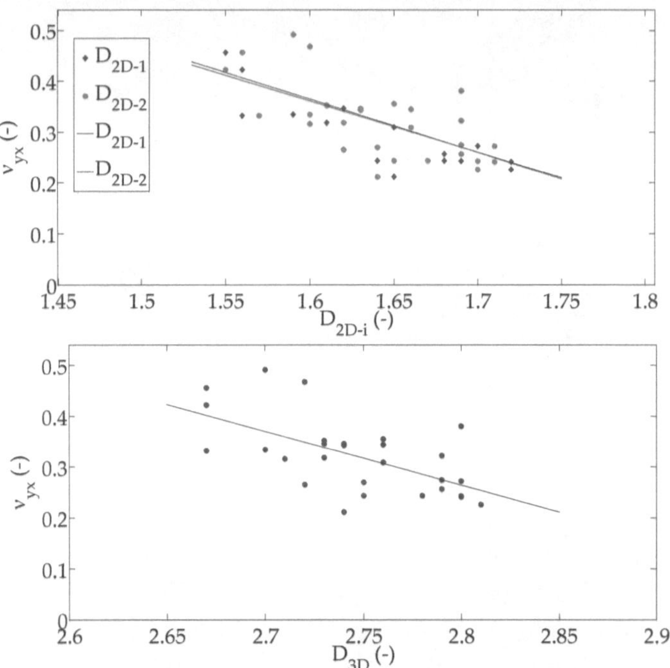

Figure 3.40: Scatter plot and linear correlations obtained for ν_{yx} as a function of fractal dimension in 2D ($D_{2D\text{-}1,2}$) (top) and 3D (D_{3D}) (bottom).

In [10], the concept of Strength to Anisotropy Ratio (SAR) is discussed, relating the yield strength of a sample to its main orientation and transverse directions. Keaveny et al. [10] presented SAR results as a function of the apparent density for compression, tension and shearing loading modes. Following that concept and applying it to axial and shearing stiffnesses, we calculate the ratio of axial or shear stiffnesses about the main and transversal directions (which we call Rigidity to Anisotropy Ratio, RAR), as function of the morphometric parameters with a significant correlation. RAR calculation was performed using the correlation functions obtained, and hence it is a ratio between the slopes and gives insight into how each direction is affected by each morphometric parameter. The results of the RAR are shown in Table 3.13. From the results, the higher RAR values for the axial stiffness than for shear-

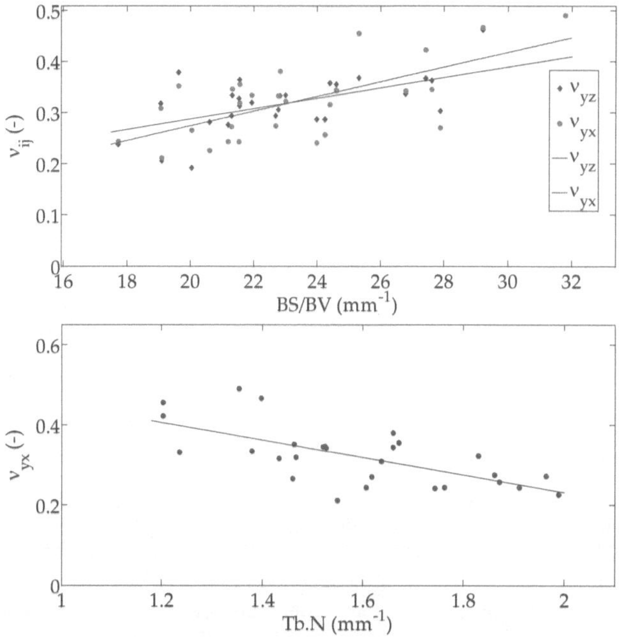

Figure 3.41: Scatter plot and linear correlations obtained for ν_{yx} and ν_{yz} as a function of BS/BV (top) and ν_{yx} as a function of Tb.N (bottom).

ing stiffness show a greater importance of the loading direction for the axial, and a less anisotropic behavior for the shearing stiffness. Further, the values of Table 3.13 permit to analyze which morphometric parameter describes the anisotropy of the stiffness of cancellous bone in a better way. In this case, BS/BV and Tb.N would be the best to differentiate axial anisotropy, while Tb.N would be for shearing stiffness.

Table 3.13: Rigidity to Anisotropy Ratio (RAR) between the preferred and transverse directions obtained for each morphometric parameter with a significant linear correlation, calculated as the ratio between the slopes of the correlations.

RAR	BV/TV	BS/BV	Tb.Th	Tb.N	D_{2D}	D_{3D}
$E_y/(E_x, E_z)$	1.76	1.83	1.67	1.82	1.67	1.65
$(G_{xy}, G_{yz})/G_{xz}$	1.41	1.37	1.28	1.51	1.43	1.44

The main aim of this section was to evaluate morpho-mechano relationships for cancellous bone. However, in the following, we will point out other relationships between morphometric and mechanical parameters separately, visualized in Fig. 3.29. The correlation coefficients between mechanical parameters are presented in Table 3.14, while the ones for morphometric parameters, in Table 3.15.

Table 3.14: Linear correlation coefficients (ρ) between mechanical parameters estimated through elastic homogenization, highlighting values greater than 0.7.

	E_x	E_y	E_z	ν_{xy}	ν_{xz}	ν_{yz}	ν_{yx}	ν_{zx}	ν_{zy}	G_{xy}	G_{yz}	G_{zx}
E_x	1	**0.919**	**0.962**	0.427	-0.155	-0.603	**-0.754**	-0.460	0.372	**0.955**	**0.944**	**0.987**
E_y	**0.919**	1	**0.876**	0.156	-0.007	-0.461	-0.617	-0.302	0.098	**0.953**	**0.947**	**0.890**
E_z	**0.962**	**0.876**	1	0.461	-0.329	-0.678	**-0.734**	-0.423	0.440	**0.899**	**0.955**	**0.989**
ν_{xy}	0.427	0.156	0.461	1	-0.573	-0.263	-0.318	-0.697	**0.898**	0.407	0.382	0.465
ν_{xz}	-0.155	-0.007	-0.329	-0.573	1	0.086	-0.040	0.539	-0.658	-0.118	-0.239	-0.240
ν_{yz}	-0.603	-0.461	-0.678	-0.263	0.086	1	**-0.788**	0.029	-0.209	-0.440	-0.520	-0.657
ν_{yx}	**-0.754**	-0.617	**-0.734**	-0.318	-0.040	**-0.788**	1	0.270	-0.386	-0.636	-0.659	**-0.762**
ν_{zx}	-0.460	-0.302	-0.423	-0.697	0.539	0.029	0.270	1	-0.641	-0.463	-0.407	-0.431
ν_{zy}	0.372	0.098	0.440	**0.898**	-0.658	-0.209	-0.386	-0.641	1	0.335	0.375	0.435
G_{xy}	**0.955**	**0.953**	**0.899**	0.407	-0.118	-0.440	-0.636	-0.463	0.335	1	**0.959**	**0.929**
G_{yz}	**0.944**	**0.947**	**0.955**	0.382	-0.239	-0.520	-0.659	-0.407	0.375	**0.959**	1	**0.953**
G_{zx}	**0.987**	**0.890**	**0.989**	0.465	-0.240	-0.657	**-0.762**	0.431	0.435	**0.929**	**0.953**	1

Table 3.14 summarizes ρ values between mechanical parameters, estimated through elastic homogenization. Each axial stiffness correlates both to the other axial and shearing stiffnesses, with ρ values around 0.95. The same trends were found for shearing stiffnesses. On the other hand, ν_{zy} shows a positive correlation to ν_{xy}, while ν_{yx} presents a negative linear correlation to the axial stiffnesses and to ν_{yz}.

The results in Table 3.15 reveal some relationships between morphometric parameters. For example, BV/TV correlates to BS/BV negatively and to Tb.Th, Tb.N, D_{2D} and D_{3D}, positively. Other variables, such as Tb.N, D_{2D} and D_{3D} and Conn.D follow a negative correlation to the mean trabecular separation. On the other hand, DA_{MIL3D} did not correlate with any other parameter except for the 2D version of anisotropy degree applied to the planes containing the main trabecular orientation.

Finally, summarizing, the morphometric parameter that better correlates to the mechanical variables is bone volume fraction (BV/TV). From results resumed in Tables 3.12 and 3.14, we can say that an accurate estimation of E_x, E_y, E_z, G_{xy}, G_{yz} and G_{zx} can be derived from specimen BV/TV measurement. Similarly, but with lower accuracy expectations, the estimation can be done by measuring any of the morphometric variables with a significant correlation: BS/BV, Tb.Th, Tb.N, D_{2D} or D_{3D}.

Other works in the literature have addressed the problem of evaluating relationships between morphometry and elastic properties [8, 9, 103, 214, 217, 221, 222, 227]. Our results confirm most of the observations from those works, except for the relationship between anisotropy degree and modulus [217, 227]. However, as it will be discussed in next section, a multivariate linear regression analysis reveals that anisotropy degree, in combination with other parameters, permits to increase the accuracy on the elastic properties estimation, as stated by Maquer et al. [217]. On the other hand, our results about fractal dimension match other from the literature [221], while the lack of a direct relationship between conncctivity density and apparent elastic properties was already reported in the literature [9].

Table 3.15: Linear correlation coefficients (ρ) between morphometric parameters, highlighting values greater than 0.7.

	BV/TV	BS/BV	Tb.Th	Tb.Sp	Tb.N	D_{2D-1}	D_{2D-2}	D_{2D-3}	D_{3D}	$DA_{MIL2D-1}$	$DA_{MIL2D-2}$	$DA_{MIL2D-3}$	DA_{MIL3D}	Conn.D
BV/TV	1	**-0.771**	0.640	-0.585	**0.865**	**0.864**	**0.863**	**0.843**	**0.852**	-0.238	-0.229	0.269	-0.205	0.03
BS/BV	**-0.771**	1	**-0.939**	-0.012	-0.384	-0.379	-0.390	-0.339	-0.356	0.255	0.179	-0.059	0.247	0.502
Tb.Th	0.640	**-0.939**	1	0.110	0.188	0.243	0.232	0.178	0.209	-0.293	-0.295	0.043	-0.345	-0.502
Tb.Sp	-0.585	-0.012	0.110	1	**-0.811**	**-0.879**	**-0.860**	**-0.886**	**-0.893**	0.150	0.218	-0.414	0.083	**-0.740**
Tb.N	**0.865**	-0.384	0.188	**-0.811**	1	**0.956**	**0.965**	**0.975**	**0.965**	-0.106	-0.086	0.310	-0.037	0.360
D_{2D-1}	**0.864**	-0.379	0.243	**-0.879**	**0.956**	1	**0.986**	**0.966**	**0.985**	-0.293	-0.327	0.366	-0.245	0.497
D_{2D-2}	**0.863**	-0.390	0.232	**-0.860**	**0.965**	**0.986**	1	**0.975**	**0.988**	-0.304	-0.269	0.361	-0.224	0.483
D_{2D-3}	**0.843**	-0.339	0.178	**-0.886**	**0.975**	**0.966**	**0.975**	1	**0.989**	-0.116	-0.107	0.322	-0.040	0.456
D_{3D}	**0.852**	-0.356	0.209	**-0.893**	**0.965**	**0.985**	**0.988**	**0.989**	1	-0.215	-0.211	0.377	-0.139	0.496
$DA_{MIL3D-1}$	-0.238	0.255	-0.293	0.150	-0.106	-0.293	-0.304	-0.116	-0.215	1	**0.857**	-0.423	**0.937**	-0.341
$DA_{MIL3D-2}$	-0.229	0.179	-0.295	0.218	-0.086	-0.327	-0.269	-0.107	-0.211	**0.857**	1	-0.337	**0.945**	-0.390
$DA_{MIL2D-3}$	0.269	-0.059	0.043	-0.414	0.310	0.366	0.361	0.322	0.377	-0.423	-0.337	1	-0.288	0.367
DA_{MIL3D}	-0.205	0.247	-0.345	0.083	-0.037	-0.245	-0.224	-0.040	-0.139	**0.937**	**0.945**	-0.288	1	-0.273
Conn.D	0.030	0.502	-0.502	**-0.740**	0.360	0.497	0.483	0.456	0.496	-0.341	-0.390	0.367	-0.273	1

3.3.3.3 Multivariate analysis of mechano-morphometric relationships

After exploring single linear regressions between specimen microstructure and elastic variables which define an orthotropic apparent behavior, we study multivariate relationships between those variables that may improve the estimation of the mechanical competence of trabecular bone samples. Specifically, we aim at finding multivariate linear regressions (in the form of Eq. 3.31) that improve the estimations provided by single factor analysis, developed in the previous section. We used the software Statgraphics Centurion XVII to perform the multivariate analysis. A total of n=28 samples are used for the analysis.

$$Mech, var_i = f(morph_1, morph_2, ..., morph_j) \tag{3.31}$$

$$\begin{aligned} Mech, var_i = {} & C + a_1 \text{BV/TV} + a_2 \text{BS/BV} + a_3 \text{Tb.Th} + a_4 \text{Tb.Sp} \\ & + a_5 \text{Tb.N} + a_6 \text{D}_{\text{2D-1}} + a_7 \text{D}_{\text{2D-2}} + a_8 \text{D}_{\text{2D-3}} + a_9 \text{D}_{\text{3D}} \\ & + a_{10} \text{DA}_{\text{MIL2D-1}} + a_{11} \text{DA}_{\text{MIL2D-2}} + a_{12} \text{DA}_{\text{MIL2D-3}} \\ & + a_{13} \text{DA}_{\text{MIL3D}} + a_{14} \text{Conn.D} \end{aligned} \tag{3.32}$$

From the data set observations of morphometry and homogenized elastic behavior, we calculated multiple regression following a forward step by step procedure: First, none of the independent morphometry variables is considered in the correlation and the p-values are computed for each variable. At each step, the variable with the highest significant correlation (minimum p-value < 0.05) is included. Then, the multiple regression is checked again, until it only depends on variables with a significant correlation (p-value< 0.05). We applied the procedure to each of the mechanical variables. The results are summarized in Table 3.16, where the coefficient multiplying each morphometric parameter and the correlation coefficient (R^2) are presented for each multiple regression, following Eq. 3.32. The relationships obtained with this method for each variable are in all cases statistically significant with a confidence interval of 95%.

As a first conclusion about the multiple regressions, we can say that all the predictions were improved compared to the ones comprising only one independent factor. For example, E_x correlation increased from $R^2 = 0.8136$

Table 3.16: Multiple regression linear analysis of mechanical variable dependence on morphometric parameters and linear correlation coefficient (R^2) for each multiple regression.

	C	a_1	a_2	a_3	a_4	a_5	a_6	a_7	a_8	a_9	a_{10}	a_{11}	a_{12}	a_{13}	a_{14}	R^2
E_x	-2713.75	76.362	29.343	-	1480.530	-	-	-	-	-	-	-	-	-	-	0.8733
E_y	1587.34	146.862	59.6782	-	-	-	-7364.22	-	4323.9	-	-	-	-	-	-27.616	0.9591
E_z	-1698.30	116.59	76.644	-	-	-617.471	-	-	-	-	-499.667	-	-	-	-28.667	0.9664
ν_{xy}	0.2301	-	-	-	-	-	-	-	0.1484	-	-0.1309	-	-	-	-	0.7215
ν_{xz}	-0.00696	-	-	-	-	-	-	-	-	-	-	0.1902	-	-	-	0.3725
ν_{yz}	-0.1407	-	0.0091	-	-	-	-	-	-	-	-	0.1473	-	-	-	0.5286
ν_{yx}	0.3591	-0.013	-	-	-	-	-	-	-	-	0.1412	-	-	-	-	0.6486
ν_{zx}	0.6094	-	-	-	-	-	1.099	-	-1.428	-	0.186	-	-	-	-	0.5546
ν_{zy}	0.7969	-	-	-	-0.2301	-	-	-	-	-	-0.1821	-	-	-	-	0.7700
G_{xy}	-396.357	19.550	-	-	-	-	-	-	-	-	-	102.76	-	-	-	0.8478
G_{yz}	-490.355	26.096	9.1445	-	-	-	-	-	-	-	-	-	-	-	-6.166	0.9314
G_{zx}	625.921	33.778	21.127	-	-	-	-	-764.733	-	-	-207.757	-	-	-	-8.0898	0.9613

to 0.8733. In other cases with even a less significant relationship for a one factor analysis, like ν_{yx}, increased from 0.5822 to 0.6486. For other correlation comparisons, we refer to Tables 3.12 and 3.16.

As happened with single factor regression analysis, both the axial and shearing stiffnesses have greater correlation to morphometry variables. In all those cases, a high degree of correlation is achieved ($R^2 = [0.8478 - 0.9664]$). Regarding Poisson's ratios lower degree of correlations were found, ranging from 0.3725 to 0.77.

Table 3.16 shows that Tb.Th, D_{3D}, $DA_{MIL2D-3}$ and DA_{MIL3D} did not contribute to any multiple regression, so they were not significant within the data set analyzed, or their contribution was already included by other variables. For example, in case of Tb.N, Tb.Th is accounted, $D_{2D-1,2}$ are equivalent calculations than D_{3D} or $DA_{MIL2D-1,2}$ presented analogous values than DA_{MIL3D}.

In case of E_x, E_y and E_z, a dependence on the amount of bone (BV/TV) and the surface area to volume ratio (BS/BV) was found. Other parameters also contribute to the regressions, like Tb.Sp for E_x, Conn.D and fractal dimension for E_y, or Conn.D, Tb.N, and anisotropy degree $DA_{MIL2D-1}$ for E_z. Regarding Poisson's ratio regressions, less significant correlations were found. However, they are all influenced by the anisotropy degree. Furthermore, some of them (ν_{xy} and ν_{zx}) show dependence to fractal dimension, while others seem to be influenced by Tb.Sp, BV/TV or BS/BV, following the results presented in Table 3.16. Shear stiffnesses had similar dependences than axial ones. BV/TV influences the three mechanical shear stiffnesses, while BS/BV, anisotropy degree, fractal dimension and Conn.D present a significant contribution, depending on the shearing plane.

As a general qualitative conclusion, the amount of bone (BV/TV), BS/BV, fractal dimension, anisotropy degree and the connectivity density have a greater influence on the axial and shear stiffnesses estimation. In case of Poisson's ratios, from our results, anisotropy degree and fractal dimension are the parameters that major influence the estimations.

Our multivariate analysis results are in line with other reported in the literature. For example, Kabel et al. [9] studied the capabilities of Conn.D to explain variations of mechanical properties and reported a negative correlation, as we do in Table 3.16. They claimed that Conn.D permits to explain little variation, which in our results vary between a 3 % to a 13 %. On the other hand, Ulrich et al. [8] reported that, in conjunction with BV/TV, anisotropy degree was the parameter that most increased the correlations. However, they pointed out that the variables dependence varied for different cancellous bone locations, and other parameters like BS/BV, Tb.Th, Tb.Sp or Tb.N had significant contributions to estimate mechanical parameters.

This study has some limitations that should be mentioned: first, the results are limited to the 28 samples analyzed, so the conclusions about variables dependence would need to be confirmed with larger datasets. Secondly, the specimens analyzed were extracted from two pigs skeletally mature and the trabecular structures observed are more plate-like, so the results could be referred to as a normal healthy population. To be able to relate the regressions to fracture risk evaluation, the procedure should be applied to specimens out of the range from our dataset, in terms of microarchitecture. This could be achieved by varying the segmentation threshold in our data set. For example, increasing it would result in trabecular thinning and loss of connectivity, which would simulate osteoporotic cancellous bone. A strength of this study, is that we analyze the influence of the microarchitecture, without accounting for material density, because we use the same material properties for each sample-specific finite element model.

Furthermore, we applied a forward procedure to evaluate the combination of morphometric variables that permit accurate estimation of mechanical variables. It is possible that, considering a backward procedure, which a priori includes all the variables and excludes at each step the less significant one, may lead to other regressions. However, we chose the first procedure because we aimed at using a low number of variables, even penalizing the degree of correlation, which was higher for the backward procedure.

3.3.3.4 Stiffness matrix estimation for cancellous bone specimens: comparison to experimental measurements

In this section, we present the stiffness matrix estimation for cancellous bone specimens of set C. Then, we compare the estimation of the engineering constants, calculated from the stiffness matrix, to experimental measurements of the apparent elastic modulus, estimated through compression testing about the three main directions. The definition of x, y and z directions is analogous to the previous section: x and z directions define the transversal plane, while

y direction refers to the preferred trabecular orientation.

The stiffness matrices C for each specimen from set C are presented in Eqs. 3.33, 3.34, 3.35, 3.36 and 3.37, expressed in MPa. The small differences between x and z directions both in terms of axial and shearing stiffnesses make possible to approximate plane xz as a plane of isotropy, while the stiffest direction belongs to the trabecular orientation. The zero values of the stiffness matrix estimations were not exactly 0, but less than 10^{-6}, so we neglected them.

$$C_{\mathrm{C\#1}}\;[\mathrm{MPa}] = \begin{pmatrix} 349.9 & 148.1 & 140.9 & 0 & 0 & 0 \\ 148.1 & 1048.2 & 148.0 & 0 & 0 & 0 \\ 140.9 & 148.0 & 380.8 & 0 & 0 & 0 \\ 0 & 0 & 0 & 174.7 & 0 & 0 \\ 0 & 0 & 0 & 0 & 98.0 & 0 \\ 0 & 0 & 0 & 0 & 0 & 176.8 \end{pmatrix} \tag{3.33}$$

$$C_{\mathrm{C\#2}}\;[\mathrm{MPa}] = \begin{pmatrix} 698.8 & 289.8 & 275.6 & 0 & 0 & 0 \\ 289.8 & 1646.6 & 309.8 & 0 & 0 & 0 \\ 275.6 & 309.8 & 793.7 & 0 & 0 & 0 \\ 0 & 0 & 0 & 350.7 & 0 & 0 \\ 0 & 0 & 0 & 0 & 214.5 & 0 \\ 0 & 0 & 0 & 0 & 0 & 327.3 \end{pmatrix} \tag{3.34}$$

$$C_{\mathrm{C\#3}}\;[\mathrm{MPa}] = \begin{pmatrix} 612.3 & 246.7 & 211.6 & 0 & 0 & 0 \\ 246.7 & 1192.7 & 245.7 & 0 & 0 & 0 \\ 211.6 & 245.7 & 596.2 & 0 & 0 & 0 \\ 0 & 0 & 0 & 262.8 & 0 & 0 \\ 0 & 0 & 0 & 0 & 174.4 & 0 \\ 0 & 0 & 0 & 0 & 0 & 270.6 \end{pmatrix} \tag{3.35}$$

$$C_{\mathrm{C\#4}}\;[\mathrm{MPa}] = \begin{pmatrix} 434.6 & 182.0 & 181.0 & 0 & 0 & 0 \\ 182.0 & 1172.5 & 198.8 & 0 & 0 & 0 \\ 181.0 & 198.8 & 488.9 & 0 & 0 & 0 \\ 0 & 0 & 0 & 215.9 & 0 & 0 \\ 0 & 0 & 0 & 0 & 123.7 & 0 \\ 0 & 0 & 0 & 0 & 0 & 202.2 \end{pmatrix} \tag{3.36}$$

$$C_{\text{C\#5}} \ [\text{MPa}] = \begin{pmatrix} 543.7 & 222.2 & 210.8 & 0 & 0 & 0 \\ 222.2 & 1238.3 & 218.7 & 0 & 0 & 0 \\ 210.8 & 218.7 & 530.2 & 0 & 0 & 0 \\ 0 & 0 & 0 & 235.7 & 0 & 0 \\ 0 & 0 & 0 & 0 & 152.2 & 0 \\ 0 & 0 & 0 & 0 & 0 & 246.5 \end{pmatrix} \tag{3.37}$$

The engineering constants (E_{x}, E_{y}, E_{z}, G_{xy}, G_{yz}, G_{zx}, ν_{xy}, ν_{yx}, ν_{xz}, ν_{zx}, ν_{yz}, ν_{zy}) were calculated from C matrices using the expressions for an orthotropic material (Eq. 3.28), and are shown in Table 3.17. The numerical homogenization predicts a y direction between 2 and 3.2-fold stiffer, depending on the specimen. Shearing stiffness is about 1.6-fold more flexible in the transversal plane than the planes containing the preferred orientation. Regarding Poisson's ratio, the coefficients of the transversal plane xz have a relatively constant value of 0.3, while ν_{yz} and ν_{yz} are approximately 0.1 for the set of specimens analyzed, Table 3.17.

Table 3.17: Engineering constants calculated from stiffness matrix for each specimen of set C.

	C#1	C#2	C#3	C#4	C#5
E_{x} [MPa]	288.96	581.33	513.82	356.81	443.90
E_{y} [MPa]	961.39	1470.60	1044.1	1059.8	1108.3
E_{z} [MPa]	316.13	659.93	499.51	399.67	433.14
ν_{xy} [-]	0.094	0.119	0.146	0.099	0.118
ν_{xz} [-]	0.333	0.301	0.295	0.330	0.349
ν_{yz} [-]	0.273	0.285	0.307	0.298	0.296
ν_{yx} [-]	0.314	0.302	0.297	0.295	0.294
ν_{zx} [-]	0.365	0.341	0.287	0.370	0.341
ν_{zy} [-]	0.090	0.128	0.147	0.112	0.116
G_{xy} [MPa]	176.83	327.31	270.59	202.21	244.47
G_{yz} [MPa]	174.71	350.66	262.82	215.86	235.69
G_{zx} [MPa]	98.02	214.47	174.39	123.65	152.24

Furthermore, we compare the experimental results of the stiffness along the three main directions to the engineering constants estimated, Figs. 3.42 and 3.43. The numerical predictions tend to overestimate the measurements at a certain degree, as can be seen in Figs. 3.42 and 3.43, where the points

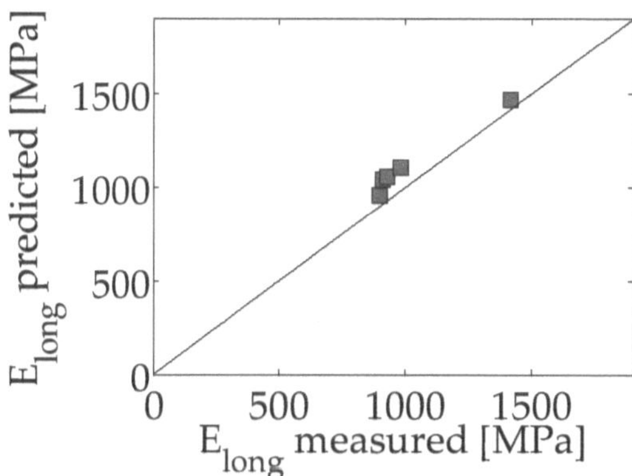

Figure 3.42: Comparison between stiffness measurements and FE predictions along the preferred trabecular orientation direction (E_{long}).

lie in the prediction side of the graph. The preferred orientation apparent modulus (E_{long}) is well predicted by the finite element models, with mean differences of about a 10 %, while the transversal direction has more prediction error compared to the experiments, with a mean difference of 25 % and 40% for each direction.

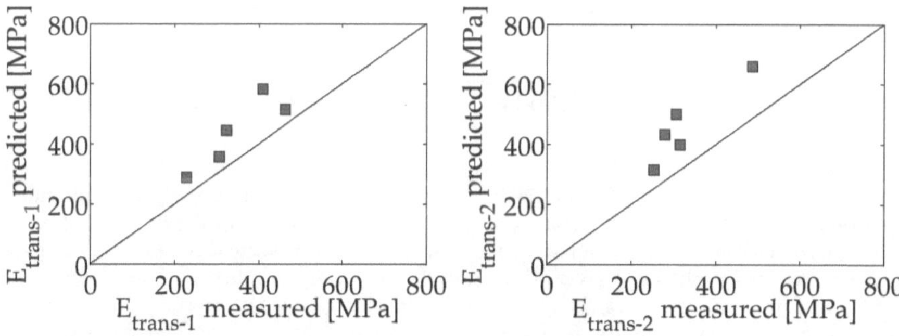

Figure 3.43: Comparison between stiffness measurements and FE predictions along the transverse directions ($E_{\text{trans}-1}$ and $E_{\text{trans}-2}$).

The greater error on the transversal plane prediction may be due to experimental measurement underestimation. The experimental apparent stiffness in the preferred orientation as a function of the compression strain applied increases up to 0.4 % strain and it stabilizes up to 0.8% strain, see blue square markers in Fig. 3.44. An analogous behavior is expected for the other testing directions. The testing protocol that we have used, which is commonly reported in the literature, defines that the apparent stiffness need to be estimated as a linear fit in the last preconditioning cycle. The four first points in the plot are estimations in the last preconditioning cycle region, while the red and green circle markers in Fig. 3.44 are the estimation of the apparent stiffness of the transverse directions in the last preconditioning cylce. This apparent stiffness evolution may be the reason of the differences between predictions and measurements in the transversal plane directions. In case of Specimen C#1 depicted in Fig. 3.44, the difference between the four first points and the stable region ranges between 22 to 30 %, in the range of differences observed between predictions and measurements in the transversal direction.

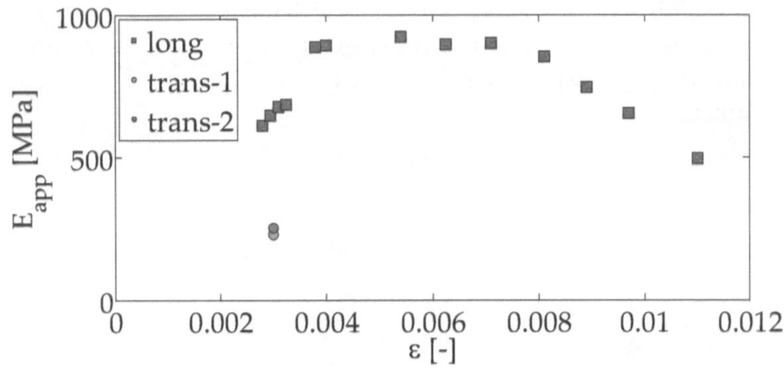

Figure 3.44: Representation of the experimental apparent modulus in the preferred trabecular orientation direction (long) from the preconditioning cycles until pre-yielding region (blue square markers), and the apparent modulus in both transverse directions (trans-1 and trans-2) measured in the las preconditioning cycle (red and green circle markers) for Specimen C#1. The strain values in the graph are the mean strain where the slope is calculated. It can be seen that the estimations at low strains provide a lower value than the stable one, which in case of Specimen C#1 occurs between 0.3 and 0.8 % for the preferred trabecular orientation direction. Then, before yielding, the apparent modulus decreases a 50 % from the stable value.

3.3.4 Failure in cancellous bone modeled using finite elements

3.3.4.1 Damage and fracture model implemented for cancellous bone

In this section, compression failure is modeled following a continuum damage mechanics approach. Complete fracture at the microscale subsequent to damage is modeled by means of the element deletion technique. In the framework of a continuum damage approach, failure is modeled as the degradation of the mechanical properties when critical values are reached. This is accomplished through an Abaqus user's subroutine (USDFLD), whereby a material degradation is introduced to describe the progressive loss of stiffness due to the propagation and coalescence of microcracks, microvoids and similar defects. These changes in the microstructure lead to a material stiffness degradation observed in the macroscale [242]. Bone failure process is controlled by strains, as reported in [243], so our approach is based on an equivalent strain, Eq. (4.3).

In the quasi-static regime, the isotropic relation of elasticity under a damage mechanics approach is expressed by [144]:

$$\sigma_{ij} = (1 - D)C_{ijkl}\varepsilon_{kl} \tag{3.38}$$

where D is the damage variable, σ_{ij}, ε_{kl} are the stress and strain tensors and C_{ijkl} is the constitutive elastic tensor.

Following [44, 138], at the tissue level we consider an isotropic damage law experimentally fitted, that is be expressed in a power form:

$$D = \begin{cases} 0 & \varepsilon_{\text{eq}} \leq \varepsilon_{\text{y,c}} \\ D_c(\frac{\varepsilon_{\text{eq}}}{\varepsilon_{\text{f,c}}})^n & \varepsilon_{\text{y,c}} < \varepsilon_{\text{eq}} < \varepsilon_{\text{f,c}} \\ D_c & \varepsilon_{\text{eq}} \geq \varepsilon_{\text{f,c}} \end{cases} \tag{3.39}$$

based on an equivalent strain, Eq. (4.3)

$$\varepsilon_{\text{eq}} = \sqrt{\frac{2}{3}\varepsilon_{ij}\varepsilon_{ij}} \tag{3.40}$$

In order to avoid mesh dependence on damage propagation, we performed a linear weighting of the strain at fracture as a function of the characteristic micro-FE length (L_{FE}) and the characteristic crack length for cancellous bone

(L_{frx}) [138], see Eq. (3.41). L_{FE} is computed at each iteration for each element during simulation and it is provided by Abaqus (referred as CELENT Abaqus code variable). As average crack lengths reported in the literature for cancellous bone range from 50 to 100 μm, we take the characteristic crack length as $L_{\text{frx}} = 0.075$ mm [234, 235]. Then, for computing purposes, the strain at fracture ε_{f} at each element is considered as:

$$\varepsilon_{\text{f}} = \varepsilon_{\text{f,c}} \left(\frac{L_{\text{frx}}}{L_{\text{FE}}} \right) \tag{3.41}$$

3.4 Cancellous bone fracture characterization results by combination of FEM and DIC

The results of fracture characterization combining FEM and DIC for specimens from sets A and C are presented in this section.

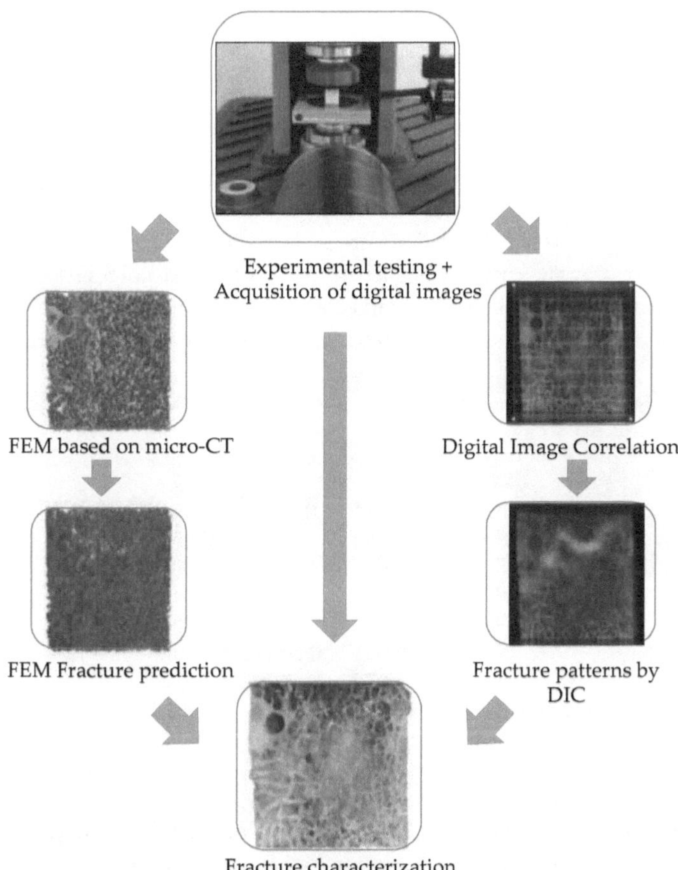

Figure 3.45: Scheme of cancellous bone fracture characterization procedure combining FEM based on μCT images and DIC.

Fig. 3.45 summarizes the methodology proposed to characterize compression fracture. Images are recorded during quasi-static compression testing. DIC technique is then applied to those images and the displacement field is calculated on the visible surface. Different strain fields are computed to evaluate the one that better represents fracture. DIC strain contour field is used to validate the FE models specimen-specific. Then, FE models based on micro-CT images are used to simulate specimen's fracture, imposing the testing boundary conditions. By inverse analysis, elastic and failure properties are estimated while the failure model proposed is validated. Both DIC and FEM approaches are also evaluated comparing their results with visual evidences.

3.4.1 Fracture properties estimation using micro-FE models

Quasi-static compression simulations were performed using the micro-FE models of each sample. To extract the optimal fracture parameters (compression yield strain $\varepsilon_{y,c}$ and strain at fracture $\varepsilon_{f,c}$) to reproduce the experimental response, a parametric study was carried out. The best correlation between the experimental force-displacement curve and the simulated one was achieved by applying the parameters summarized in Table 3.18.

Table 3.18: Fracture parameters obtained from micro-FE simulations of quasi-static compression.

	$\varepsilon_{y,c}$	$\varepsilon_{f,c}$
Specimen #A1	0.0068	0.0410
Specimen #A2	0.0068	0.0525
Specimen #A3	0.0068	0.0320
Specimen #A4	0.0068	0.0450
Specimen #A5	0.0068	0.0290
Specimen #C1	0.00925	0.0455
Specimen #C2	0.006	0.040
Specimen #C3	0.0065	0.028
Specimen #C4	0.0065	0.0265
Specimen #C5	0.0068	0.0295

The yield strain values calculated are similar for all the samples, except for Specimen #C1 that presents a higher yield strain value, Table 3.18. On the other hand, tissue fracture strain shows a wider variation, in a range between 2.65 to 5.25 % for the specimens analyzed. Our failure strain estimations are analogous to other reported in the literature (Table 1.4). For example,

Nagaraja [75] estimated a compression yield strain in the range 0.46 to 0.63 %, Niebur et al. [72] 1.01 % and a value of 0.83 % was estimated by Bayraktar et al. [50]. Similarly, Hambli [44] used a yield strain value of 0.0081 in a continuum damage approach which was obtained in [88]. Regarding the ultimate strain ($\varepsilon_{f,c}$) estimation values in the range 2.4 to 8.2 % have been reported [37] and are also of the order of the proposed by Wolfram et al. [82] for unconfined axial compression.

Our estimations about tissue yield and ultimate strains from FE modeling support the hypothesis that yield strain is relatively constant over a range of densities, while ultimate strain presents more scattering [10, 50, 73]. This supports that failure in cancellous bone is controlled by strains and it is essentially independent of density or microarchitecture.

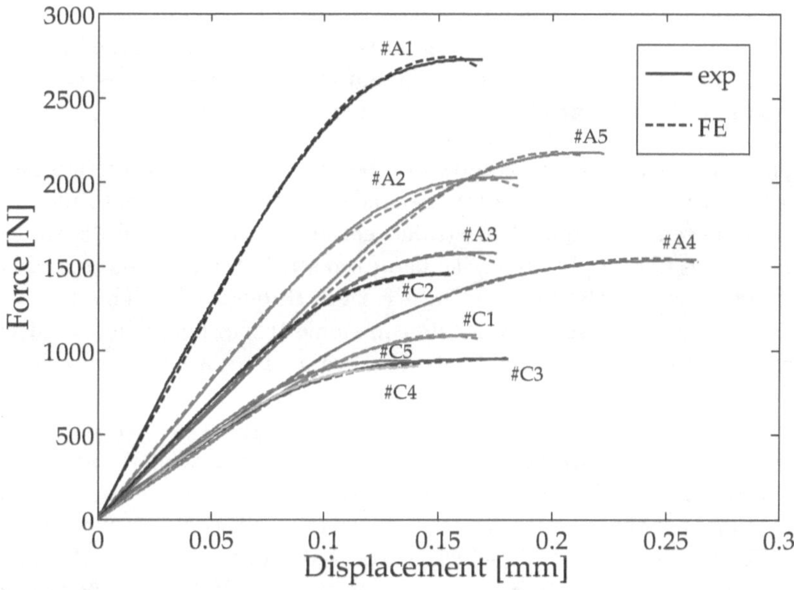

Figure 3.46: Force-displacement compression response comparison between experiments and finite element models for each specimen.

Fig. 3.46 presents a comparison between the experimental and the numerical force-displacement response until the ultimate point. It can be observed that our approach to model compression failure is capable to follow the experimental curve with a good level of accuracy. However, the use of element deletion technique is responsible of the slight force drop visible in Fig. 3.46. Toughening mechanisms should be included in the model to reproduce the non-linear behavior after the ultimate point. For example, Harrison et al. [141] used a similar approach to ours but also included stress correction in the elements adjacent to the deleted ones which were delayed in the subsequent steps to model cohesive effects in the crack tip. These enhanced the reproduction of the post-yield behavior observed experimentally. They used that cohesive force parameter to control brittle/ductile fracture of specimens.

The failure model considered in this work is dependent on both $\varepsilon_{y,c}$ and $\varepsilon_{f,c}$. The ductility of the sample within this model has proved to be dependent on the difference between $\varepsilon_{y,c}$ and $\varepsilon_{f,c}$ values. As mentioned, this permitted to control the response up to the ultimate point and further cohesive parameters should be included to accurately model post-yielding. As each of the specimens presents a different ductile behavior, different fracture strain values were back-calculated in order to reproduce the experimental response.

Figs. 3.47 and 3.48 show a comparison between the two methods studied in this work for fracture estimation for specimens in set A and C. Both micro-FE and DIC represent the equivalent strain field at fracture both in distribution and peak values. In the five cases studied from set A, the maximum predicted ε_{eq} at fracture is slightly higher using FE than through DIC. This finding is coherent as peak FE strains are located in single trabeculae, whereas in DIC the area of fracture is wider and, thus, the strain values are averaged (less local). These differences on peak strain range from 10 to 24 % depending on the specimen, Fig. 3.47. It can be observed that a fairly good correlation between simulations, DIC and experiments is achieved. However, a more precise estimation of the fracture is obtained with micro-FE as it is capable of predicting isolated failures at the microscale (note the isolated trabecular failure in specimen 1, Fig. 3.24, middle, (left), which is observed experimentally in the middle region of the lattice but it is not clearly detected by DIC. This phenomenon can be explained because the DIC technique performs a homogenization on the whole specimen, which implies a 3D to 2D conversion and an interpolation at a lower resolution. This averaging was also detected and reported elsewhere [51]. If fracture does not occur in the visible surface, the method may detect high strains at surfaces through specimen thickness. This phenomenon could

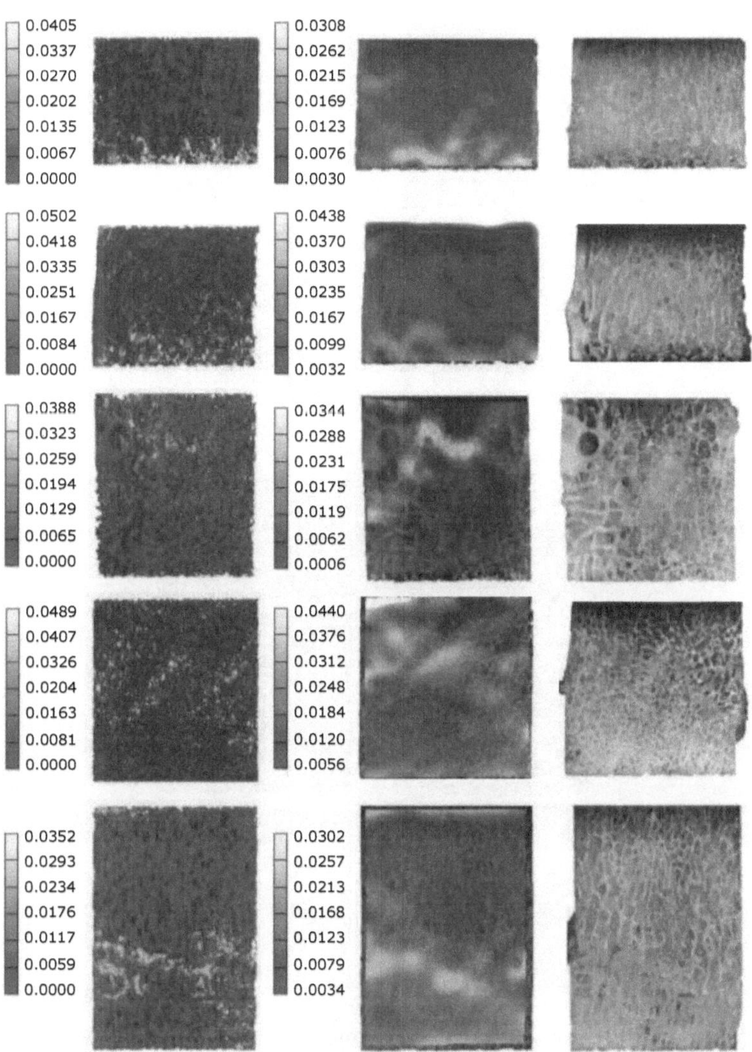

Figure 3.47: Predicted fracture pattern of specimen #A1 (top) to #A5 (bottom) by means of a) micro-FE models, b) DIC and c) experimental fracture under compression testing.

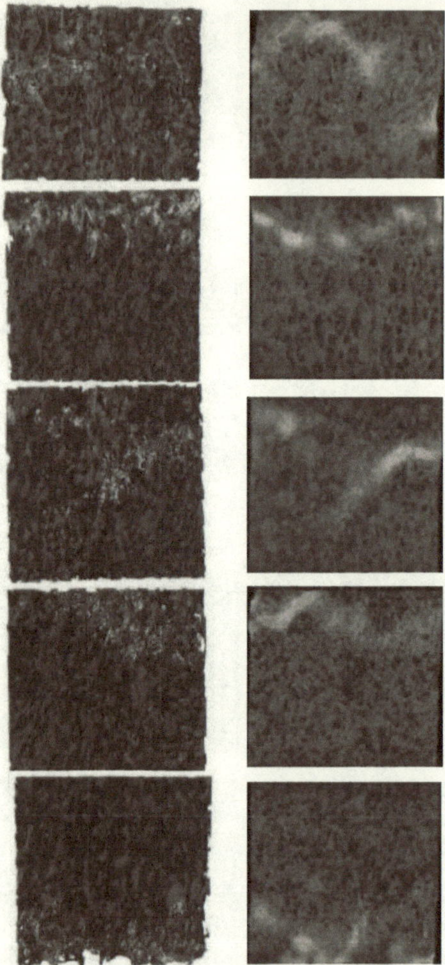

Figure 3.48: Predicted fracture pattern of specimen #C1 (top) to #C5 (bottom) by means of micro-FE models (left) and DIC (right). A high level of correlation between fracture patterns is achieved.

be minimized by using thinner samples [51]. However, buckling may happen and 2D DIC cannot distinguish out-of-plane displacements [61].

Nevertheless, DIC offers a qualitative fracture pattern characterization reducing computation time compared to the high cost of the micro-FE simulations. DIC may be used as a simple tool for experimental validation of numerical models which has not been deeply studied in the literature. For example, Cyganik et al. [232] used DIC to validate FE models in terms of displacement measurement. However, their results about strain distribution are noisy and do not represent failure. Furthermore, they did not provide any failure strain estimation using DIC.

The use of cancellous microstructure as a pattern for the application of digital image correlation was validated against manual surface marker analysis at low discretization by Bay [51]. Surface marker analysis implied the action of a technician and was impractical to evaluate the validate the method for a high discretization. A limitation of texture correlation method is that it needs for relatively high nominal strains, because, in other cases, the noisy strain contours appear [51].

Our non-speckle application of DIC went a step further in the study of fracture pattern detection, because we evaluated strain metrics that describe the compression fracture on cancellous bone specimens.

3.5 Conclusions

In this chapter, we have addressed the problem of cancellous bone mechanical characterization and the influence of the underlying microstructure. Our approach is experimental, through compression testing and applying DIC to images taken during testing, and numerical, through finite element modeling based on images acquired by micro-CT and their analysis.

Quasi-static compression tests permitted to assess the elastic and failure behavior at the apparent or macro level. With regards to the elastic properties, the specimens presented an orthotropic behavior with a direction of higher stiffness, aligned with the main trabecular orientation, the other two directions showed similar stiffness values, but significantly different. We reported yield and ultimate properties values in line with other values from the literature. Moreover, a linear relationship between stiffness and strength was observed, confirming some works of the literature.

We analyzed the dependence of mechanical parameters (E_{app}, σ_{y}, ε_{y}, σ_{f} and ε_{f}) measured in quasi-static compression tests to specimen-specific morphometric parameters. We have estimated single parameter linear regressions that have permitted to find which morphometric descriptors explain variations of mechanical properties. Specifically, bone volume fraction (BV/TV), bone surface to volume ratio (BS/BV), mean trabecular thickness (Tb.Th) and fractal dimension (D) presented the best linear correlations. However, the number of samples used (n=10) limit the significance of the regressions reported. Another limitation concerns the correlation coefficients obtained in the regressions, which were not as high as necessary to consider the relationships as significant (R^2 0.6). Therefore, it is more correct to denote the relationships reported as tendencies, which need to be confirmed in other data sets.

On the other hand, both the yield and failure strains did not show correlation to any morphometric parameter, except for the case of anisotropy degree calculated over the transversal plane (DA_{MIL2D} 3), which we considered as a spurious correlation because of the nearly isotropic values obtained for this parameter. This can be explained because yield and failure strains depend essentially on local tissue properties and not much on the morphology of the sample. Therefore, our observations regarding yield and failure strains confirm other results from the literature that claim that they are almost independent from density and microstructure.

Furthermore, we estimated tissue elastic properties of cancellous bone. A Young's modulus of 11.09 ± 1.69 GPa was estimated through a back calculation approach, using finite element models based on micro-CT images and the compression curve registered in the experiments. On the other hand, we used a modulus-density relationship from Morgan et al. [130] for vertebral cancellous bone to calculate tissue elastic properties. This phantom-based approach provided similar estimations to the ones using the previous approach.

In addition, the complete stiffness matrix of cancellous bone specimens was calculated for two purposes. The first one was to evaluate the influence of the microstructure on the elastic response, while the second one was to validate the methodology by a direct comparison between experiments and numerical predictions. We used an homogenization approach that consisted in the application of periodic boundary conditions and the application of 6 unitary strain cases, three normal and three angular. An orthotropic, close to transversely isotropic, behavior was observed for the samples analyzed.

Some morphometric parameters, such as BV/TV, BS/BV, Tb.Th and fractal dimension, presented linear correlation to the axial and shear stiffnesses, so their assessment may be used to estimate those properties which are difficult to measure experimentally. Moreover, multiple parameter linear regressions were shown to improve the correlation for the elastic properties prediction. For example, including BV/TV, BS/BV and fractal dimension improved the correlation for axial stiffness to R^2=0.9.

On the other hand, regarding the second purpose, the stiffness matrix was also estimated for 5 of the cancellous bone specimens tested and the results were compared to the measurements finding accurate numerical predictions for the main trabecular orientation direction, but the numerical overestimation occurred for the transversal directions. However, we hypothesize and confirmed for the main direction that the estimation about the transversal directions were performed under a strain range level lower than the one where stiffness is stable, prior to failure onset.

Digital image correlation was used to estimate surface displacements and failure strains on the fractured areas. First, we reported accurate displacement metric compared to the precision displacement gauge signal, with a maximum difference of 0.03 mm. Then, we assessed the influence of DIC parameters variation on strain estimation at the failure region. Facet and step sizes have a relevant effect on the failure strain estimation, and an increment of both parameters reduces the strain estimation up to 40 %. Besides, several parameters combinations led to correct failure pattern detection, so values reported in the literature should be referred to the parameters used. On the other hand, for our experimental setup, the pattern matching criterion had no influence on the strain estimation, which shows that no relevant lighting changes occurred during images acquisition. In case of incremental correlation, its consideration was relevant to properly solve the correspondence problem and control the presence of voids in the solution.

Furthermore, shear strain (γ_{12}), equivalent strain (ε_{eq}) and principal strain

(ε_1) were evaluated as variables for failure pattern description and ε_{eq} emerged as the more accurate one. Finally, using a facet size of 125 pixels, 10 pixels of step size, normalized sum of squared differences pattern matching criterion, incremental correlation and a filter strain size of 15 pixels led a mean value of the maximum equivalent strain at the fracture region of 3.66 % at the apparent ultimate point and 2.42 % at the apparent yield point.

Our numerical approach to estimate cancellous bone failure strain properties using finite element models consisted of a combination of elastic properties degradation, under a damage approach, and the elimination of finite elements at fracture conditions through the element deletion technique. The damage law used was suitable to reproduce the experimental force-displacement curve until the ultimate point and allowed the estimation of a tissue yield strain close to 0.7 %. Only one specimen presented a higher yield strain value of 0.925 %, so the values obtained were relatively constant for the specimens analyzed. In case of the ultimate strain $(\varepsilon_{f,c})$, more scattering was found in the results. Values in the range 2.8 to 5.25 % were calculated. The behavior of yield and failure strains estimated numerically supports observations reported in the literature that state that yield strain values are relatively constant, while ultimate strain values present a wider scattering.

Chapter 4

Trabecular bone surrogate: Open cell polyurethane foam characterization

4.1 Introduction

In this chapter, we aim at characterizing open-cell rigid polyurethane foams manufactured by Sawbones of three different densities from mechanical and morphometric perspectives. The mechanical characterization of open-cell rigid polyurethane foam is conducted experimentally, through compression testing combined with the application of DIC. This optical technique is used to estimate full-field surface displacements and to describe compression fracture patterns. On the other hand, FE models developed from micro-CT images of some of the tested samples are generated and simulated under the experimental loading conditions, which enables the estimation of elastic and failure parameters to be used for numerical modeling. In addition, a morphometric analysis is performed for each foam density grade, which is then related to the mechanical properties of the samples.

This study may give insight into the effect of microstructure and its variation within a specimen on the mechanical response of open cell polyurethane foams from three different densities. Moreover, we provide estimation of failure strains from experiments and FE modeling.

To our knowledge, no previous work in the literature has characterized open-cell PUR foams from experimental tests, by application of DIC and through the FE method. The detailed information about morphometry, elastic constants and strength limits provided in this work is not found in the manufacturer's data sheets. These parameters can be useful for researchers and practitioners that make use of these polyurethane foams in orthopedic implants and cement augmentation evaluations.

4.2 Description of specimens: open cell polyurethane foams

Three different grades of open-cell polyurethane foams (Sawbones, Sweden) are analyzed in the current study. The structure of the open cell polyurethane foam resembles that of human cancellous bone, so it is commonly used as a research surrogate [150, 156, 157, 158].

The grades are denoted as follows: Low density foam (LD, Ref. #1522-507), medium density foam (MD, Ref. #1522-524) and high density foam (HD, Ref. #1522-525) [244]. Each foam grade is sold in a block of 13x18x4 cm, from which a series of specimens are machined. The manufacturer provides some mechanical and morphological properties for each foam grade, like the apparent compressive Young's modulus (E_{app}), i.e. the Young's modulus of the foam as it is provided, the compressive strength (σ_f) and foam volume fraction (FV/TV). The structure is over 95% open cell and the cell size is between 1.5 to 2.5 mm. The manufacturer acknowledges a wide scattering on the mechanical properties, but they report average properties of each foam grade blocks, summarized in Table 4.1.

Table 4.1: Mechanical and morphological properties provided by the manufacturer for each open cell graded foam from [244].

Foam grade	Density [g/cm^3]	FV/TV [%]	σ_f [MPa]	E_{app} [MPa]
# LD	0.12	10.6	0.28	18.6
# MD	0.24	15.4	0.67	53
# HD	0.48	30.8	3.20	270

4.3 Preparation of specimens

A series of parallelepiped specimens (35, 11 of HD, 10 of MD and 14 of LD) were extracted from the initial open-cell polyurethane foam blocks. The specimens were chosen to maintain the initial block thickness and to have quadrilateral base, as it is shown on Fig. 4.1. The average specimen dimensions are 25 mm base-side and 40 mm height. The foam blocks were first traced with an indelible marker and then machined using a table saw, with constant water irrigation and low advance velocity to reduce the cutting effects. In any case, the disruption of the reticular microstructure due to specimen machining has a relevant effect on the mechanical properties as it happens for cancellous bone [23, 43, 53, 54]. In case of cancellous bone, a reduction from 20 to 50 % on the apparent modulus has been reported due to the so-called side artifacts, and a similar effect may be expected for other foamed structures. Some procedures are recommended to reduce side artifacts, like embedding the specimen ends in PMMA or applying preconditioning cycles [23, 30, 52, 56].

Table 4.2: Mean apparent density (ρ_{app}) measured for each density grade.

Foam grade	ρ_{app} [g/cm^3]
LD	0.107
MD	0.239
HD	0.442

In addition, special attention was taken to maintain parallel faces at each specimen to avoid point loads and stress concentration during compression testing due to uneven surfaces [22]. Each specimen was weighted and the apparent volume was estimated, which allows to estimate the apparent density, summarized in Table 4.2. It can be noted that foam blocks heterogeneity and specimen machining result in a slightly apparent density reduction compared to the values reported by the manufacturer in Table 4.1. Testing directions were defined as follows, see Fig. 4.3: 1 (or axial) is the initial foam block depth direction, while 2 and 3 are the transverse directions.

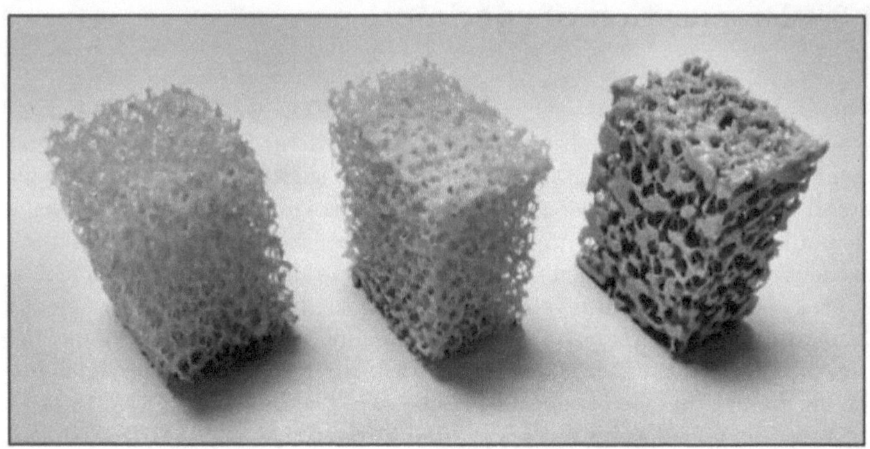

Figure 4.1: Specimens of different apparent densities analyzed in this chapter: Low density foam (LD) (left), medium density foam (MD) (middle) and high density foam (HD) (right).

4.4 Micro-Computed Tomography (μCT) and segmentation

Six specimens (two of each density) were scanned using a micro-CT (V|Tome|X s 240, GE Sensing and Inspection Technologies) through the CENIEH (Burgos, Spain) micro-CT service, with an isotropic voxel resolution of 24 μm (voltage 80kV, intensity 200 μm, integration time 200 ms). Then, the micro-CT images were segmented using ScanIp software (Simpleware, UK), following a manual image thresholding method combined with mask connectivity analysis, Fig. 4.2.

In Fig. 4.3, a 3D reconstruction of the three grades of foam samples generated from micro-CT images is shown. The resulting 3D segmented masks were analyzed to estimate morphometric parameters in the next section.

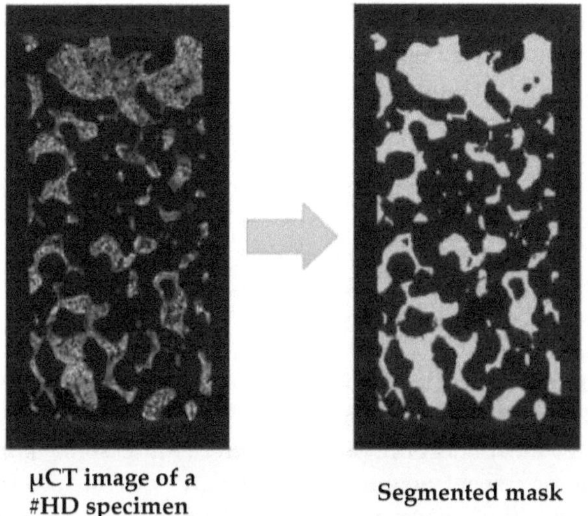

Figure 4.2: Segmentation of a μCT image of a HD specimen through a manual thresholding approach.

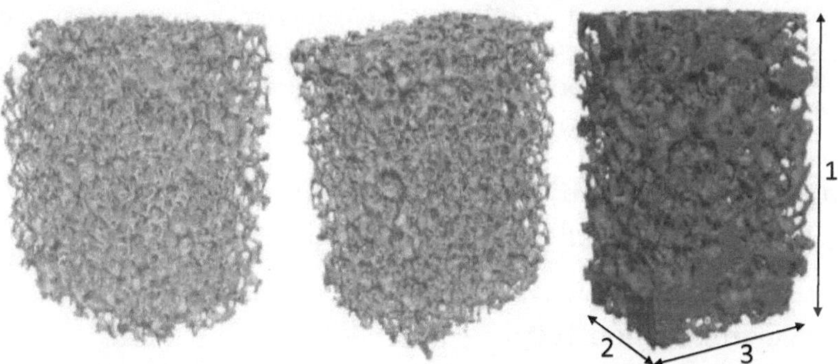

Figure 4.3: 3D reconstruction of each foam grade generated from μCT images: LF (left), MF (centre) and HF (right). Testing directions are defined as 1 (axial) and 2,3 (transverse).

4.5 Morphometric characterization

In order to characterize the microstructure of the different open cell foam specimens, a morphometric analysis of the segmented masks was carried out. We define the following parameters: foam volume fraction (FV/TV), foam surface area to total volume ratio (FS/TV), foam surface area to material (PUR) volume ratio (FS/FV), mean strut thickness (Str.Th), mean void dimension or mean strut separation (Str.Sp), strut number (Str.N), fractal dimension (D_{2D}, D_{3D}), degree of anisotropy based on mean intercept length (DA_{MIL3D}) and connectivity density (Conn.D). These parameters are commonly used for cancellous bone microstructure characterization [8, 245] and its definition is analogous to the description in section 2.5 for cancellous bone.

We remark that these parameters are average measurements for each region of interest. Having further information of the foam morphology is important for the study of local effects in the structure as in case of damage, fracture, screw insertion or cement augmentation. To give insight into the variation of those morphometric parameters, we also calculated them in slices of about 5 mm of thickness along specimen height.

4.6 Experimental characterization

We performed mechanical non-destructive compression tests to estimate the apparent Young's modulus ($E_{app,i}$) of the different graded foams in their 3 main directions (i=1,2,3 or axial(ax)/transverse(trans)) and destructive compression tests to characterize fracture behavior in the axial direction.

In addition, we applied DIC to images acquired during testing in order to analyze the inhomogeneous strain distribution and estimate failure parameters.

4.6.1 Compression tests

Quasi-static compression tests were conducted following this protocol: A 10 N pre-load was defined; then, after 5 preconditioning cycles, an increasing load was applied with a displacement rate of 1 mm/min between 0.5 % and 1 % strain levels to avoid damage in the specimens.

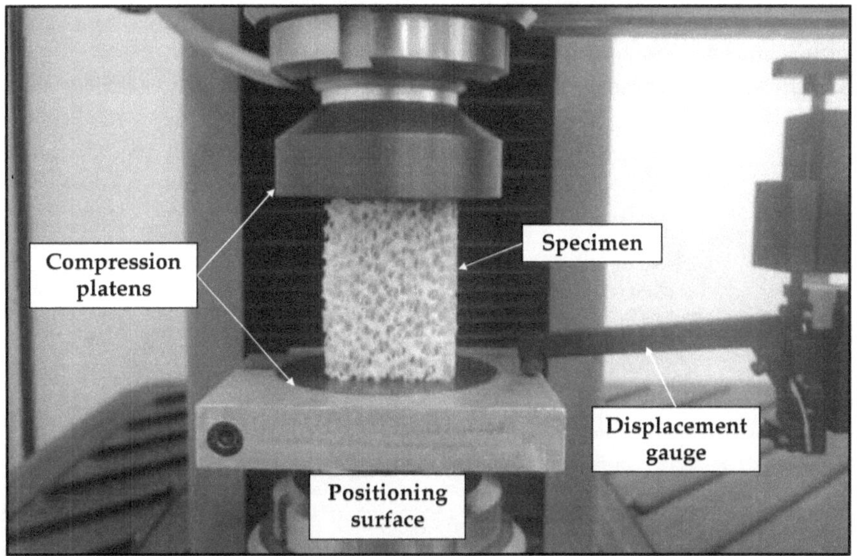

Figure 4.4: Testing set up for compression of foam samples. A local displacement gauge is used to measure the displacement between compression platens so as to avoid any compliance effect of the load chain.

Tests were carried out using an electromechanical testing machine (MTS Criterion C42), with aluminum compression platens (MTS ref.: FYA502A) for the compression tests and measuring the displacement between compression platens using a displacement gauge (MTS ref.:632.06H-20). The apparent stiffness ($E_{\mathrm{app,i}}$) of each specimen in its 3 main directions was determined from the linear response after the last preconditioning cycle, while failure stress (σ_f) was defined as the peak value following the elastic response and the failure strain (ε_f) was defined as the strain at σ_f. Yield stress (σ_y) and strain (ε_y) were estimated through the 0.2% convention. The compression test rig is shown in Fig. 4.4.

4.6.1.1 Testing machine performance checkup

The preliminary results obtained for compression testing of the open cell polyurethane foams motivated us to test out the performance of the electromechanical testing machine MTS Criterion c42, because of the differences between our measurements and the compressive stiffness values reported by the manufacturer for each foam grade in their catalog [244]. We tested each foam grade with three independent sources of displacement metrics, shown in Fig. 4.5: a displacement gauge from MTS which measures displacement between compression platens, a standard dial gauge used in metrology labs and an Instron extensometer attached to the compression platens.

Table 4.3: Comparison of the compressive stiffness measurements from different sources, expressed as MTS displacement gauge value and percentage differences to the other metrics: Instron extensometer attached to compression platens and dial gauge. The three different foam grades studied in this chapter were used for the validation.

Specimen	MTS E_{compr}[MPa]	Dial gauge $\Delta E_{\mathrm{compr}}$[%]	Instron $\Delta E_{\mathrm{compr}}$[%]
#HD1	93.15	1.8	1.6
#HD2	121.72	2.1	1.75
#MD1	21.71	0.09	0.12
#MD2	23.56	0.58	0.71
#LD1	9.36	0.8	0.85
#LD2	5.39	0.02	0.08

The results of the metrics comparison between the aforementioned sources are presented in Table. 4.3, expressed as MTS displacement gauge value and percentage differences to other sources, where it can be noted that the measurement differences are negligible. This procedure permits to validate our compressive stiffness values obtained through testing. On the other hand, we contacted the Sawbones support team by email asking for information about their reported values. They provided us valuable information about the testing protocol used and the results obtained.

As a transcription of the information provided by the manufacturer: they tested *'foam blocks of 20 mm length x 20 mm width x 40 mm height with molded bondo (a filler resin) end plates about 2 mm thick at a rate of 4 mm/min. Strain measurements were based on crosshead displacement which might be a source of error if you have better way of testing strain on these specimens under compression. We've found modulus highly variable in this foam and we think it might be based on its structure'.*

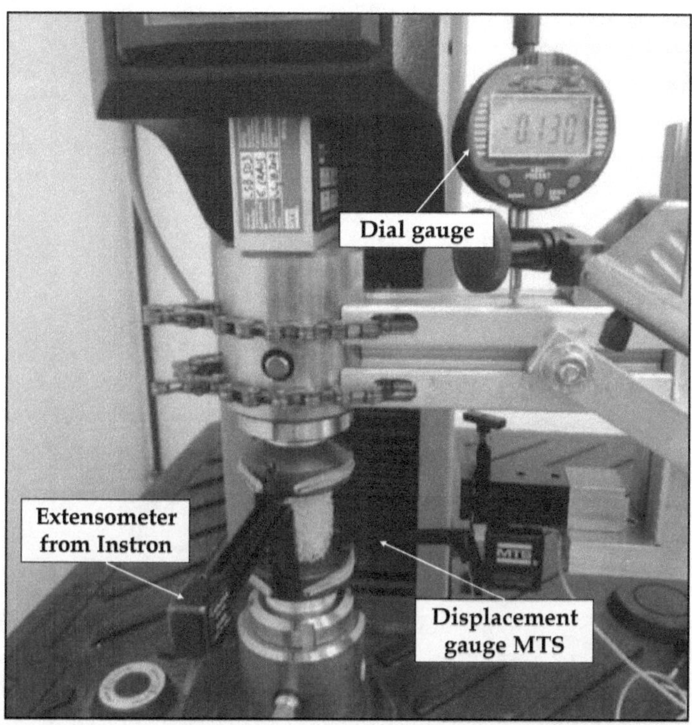

Figure 4.5: Testing set up to ascertain the measures from MTS Criterion c42 electromechanical testing machine. Three different sources were tested out: A displacement gauge from MTS, a dial gauge and an extensometer connected to an Instron external testing machine.

To discard sources of differences to the reported values, we tested one specimen with and without molded methacrylate end caps and at a displacement rate of 4 mm/min. The results of the comparative study are summarized in Table 4.4 in terms of % differences from the testing protocol defined in section 4.6.1. Sawbones testing protocol tends to stiffen the compressive modulus results. Adding methacrylate molded end caps increases 14.9 % E_{compr} from a non-end cap protocol, while a 4 mm/min displacement rate makes the results a 2.1 % greater than a 1 mm/min displacement rate. Therefore, differences between the values reported by the manufacturer and our results are not consequence of the testing protocols but the microstructural characteristics of each sample that induces potential damage due to specimen machining.

Table 4.4: Comparison of the compressive stiffness measurements using Sawbones' testing protocol and the one defined in sec. 4.6.1 for a #HD specimen.

Protocol	$\Delta E_{\mathrm{compr}}[\%]$
Resin molded end caps 1 mm/min	14.9
No resin molded end caps 4 mm/min	2.1

4.6.2 Full-field displacement measurement using Digital Image Correlation (DIC)

The objective of our DIC application to open cell foams is to characterize the strain field during testing and to detect fracture patterns from speckle and non-speckle approaches. The results will be used to validate the finite element models predictions and the failure model proposed.

We used VIC-2D Digital Image Correlation software (v.6.0.2 Correlated Solutions Inc., US), a high resolution fixed focal lens (HF7518V-2, Myutron, Japan) with 12 Mpx resolution, 10 mm extension rings, 65 mm focal length and a spotlight. Perpendicular camera-specimen relative position was ensured to avoid out-of plane displacements during testing. A region of interest (ROI) that covered the whole specimen was defined.

Moreover, we used a normalized squared differences pattern matching criterion and an incremental correlation, where each image is compared with the previous one instead of with the reference image. A high sub-pixel accuracy was ensured using a high order interpolation spline method (8-tap) [229]. A squared facet (the grid in which ROI is divided) of 81 mm pixels size, a step size of 5 pixels and a strain filter size of 21 pixels were defined for the strain field calculation. Those parameters were defined based on noise minimization and failure pattern localization accuracy.

Moreover, we study the influence of DIC parameters on the fracture pattern definition and failure properties estimation. Specifically, we study the following parameter variation:

- Facet (or subset) size: 31, 51, 81, 101, 125, 151 pixels size.

- Step size: 5, 10, 15, 20 pixels size.

- Speckle vs non-speckle

- Pattern matching criterion: SSD, NSSD, ZNSSD.

- Incremental vs non-incremental correlation

4.7 Numerical characterization

4.7.1 Finite element modeling

We developed finite element models based on high resolution micro-CT to reproduce the elastic and fracture behavior of the open cell foam specimens registered in the experiments. Then, the elastic and failure properties for each specimen are estimated by inverse analysis. The objective is to estimate the elastic properties at the so-called tissue level (i.e. the PUR material level) and the failure properties that make the simulations match the experimental force-displacement curve.

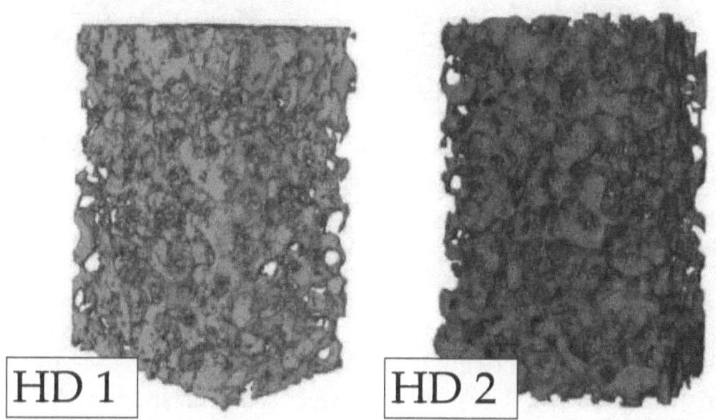

Figure 4.6: Finite element models developed for the high density open cell foams (HD) scanned using micro-CT. The finite element mesh of one of the models is shown.

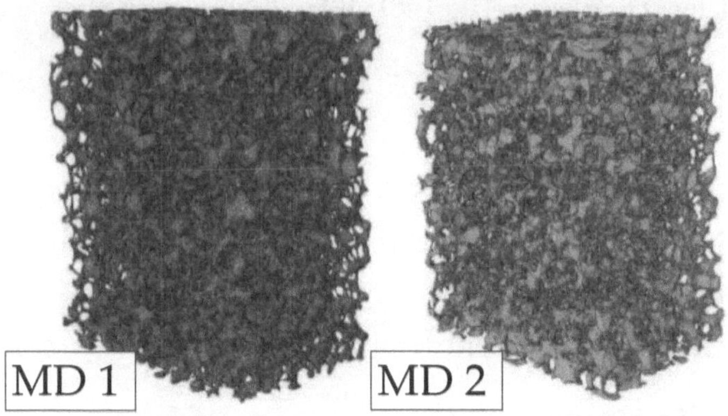

Figure 4.7: Finite element models developed for the medium density open cell foams (MD) scanned using micro-CT. The finite element mesh of one of the models is shown.

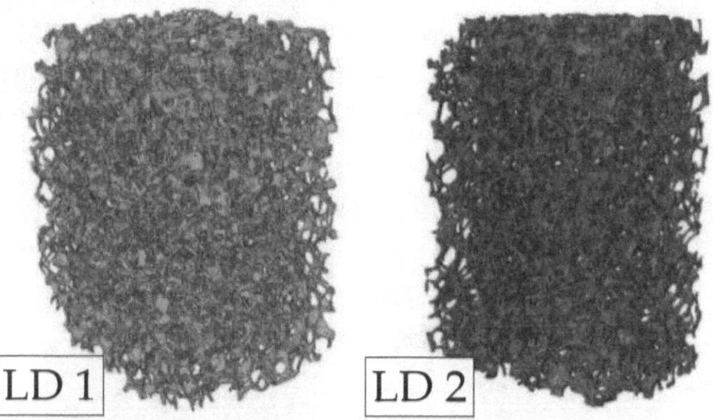

Figure 4.8: Finite element models developed for the low density open cell foams (LD) scanned using micro-CT. The finite element mesh of one of the models is shown.

Finite element meshes were generated from the micro-CT segmented masks using ScanIp (Simpleware, UK). The models were meshed with linear tetrahedral elements (coded C3D4 in Abaqus), resulting in finite element models of about 3 million elements and one million nodes for LD and MD grades and about 6 million elements and 1.5 million nodes for HD grade.

The finite element models generated for each specimen are shown in Figs. 4.6, 4.7 and 4.8. Linear-elastic isotropic material properties were assigned in the simulations, calibrated using the experimental data. A Poisson's ratio of 0.3 was assumed from the literature [160]. Boundary conditions were defined to mimic the experimental tests, imposing the displacement registered in the experiments on top face nodes and constraining the displacements in the load direction on the bottom surface. Lateral surfaces are free (unconfined compression).

4.7.2   Elastic properties homogenization

The estimation of the stiffness matrix that represents the apparent behavior of a heterogeneous structure is relevant to be able to analyze the effect of the underlying microstructure on the mechanical properties, which on the contrary are often assessed experimentally. Experiments may involve compliance effects or less controlled boundary conditions that may affect the measurements. So, numerical models permit great control of the boundary conditions and avoid other experimental issues and have been proved to accurately determine those apparent properties.

Our approach to calculate the effective apparent properties of foamed structures is analogous than the used for cancellous bone. It implies two main steps: the first one is to apply periodic boundary conditions, while the second is to solve displacement-controlled simulations to calculate the stiffness matrix (C). In order to be able to define PBC in a heterogeneous structure like foams, the mesh was mirrored against its three main directions, see Fig. 4.9 (top). Then, the compliance matrix was calculated through Hooke's law and applying 6 unitary strain cases (3 for normal strains and 3 for shear strains, see Fig. 4.9 (bottom)) and computing the stress at the structure surfaces nodes for each strain case. Further methodology explanations may be found in section 3.3.3.

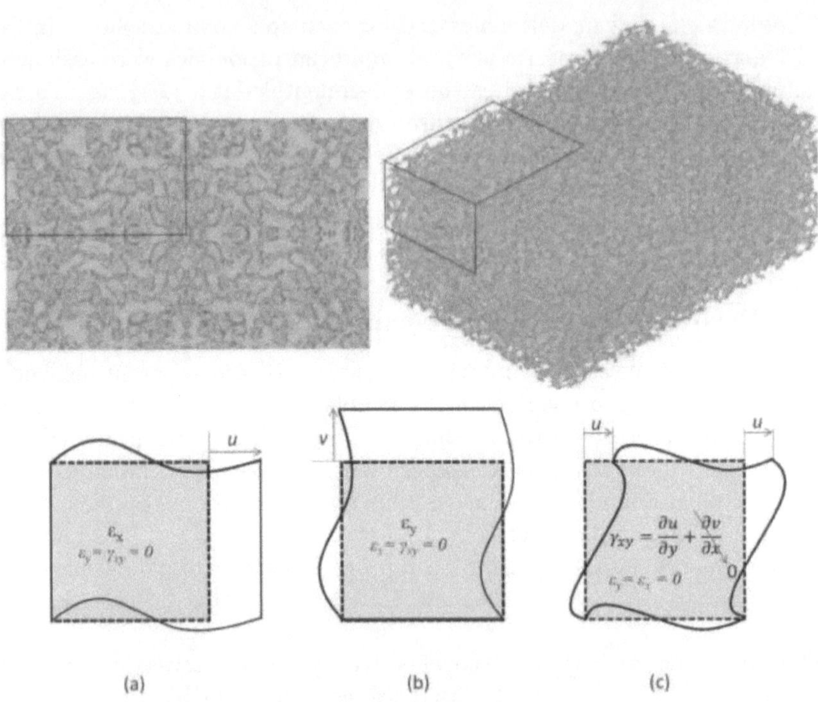

Figure 4.9: Mirroring the structure to be able to apply PBC (top) (volume under analysis marked in red): 2D view (left) and 3D representation (right) and a schematic representation of the load cases with periodic boundary conditions to calculate the compliance matrix of a region of interest (bottom): elongation load cases a),b) and shear load case c). The PBC have been generalized for the three-dimensional problem.

4.7.3   Compression failure modeling

In this study, we consider that foam failure at the strut level occurs in two phases: first the stiffness is reduced in the damage phase, following a continuum damage approach, and then the complete fracture of the struts is modeled using the element deletion technique. This approach has been used to model compression fracture in foam-like structures as cancellous bone [44, 141, 245]. These damage and fracture approaches were implemented using an Abaqus user's subroutine (USDFLD).

In the quasi-static regime, the isotropic relation of elasticity under damage mechanics approach is expressed by Eq. 4.1 [144]:

$$\sigma_{ij} = (1 - D)C_{ijkl}\varepsilon_{kl} \tag{4.1}$$

where D is the damage variable, σ_{ij}, ε_{kl} are the stress and strain tensors and C_{ijkl} is the constitutive elastic tensor. We propose D to vary following an isotropic damage law experimentally fitted (Eq. 4.2) for cancellous bone based on an equivalent strain (Eq. 4.3), because of its similarity to foam structure [245]. Material properties are reduced from compression yield strain ($\varepsilon_{y,c}$) until its 5 % at $\varepsilon_{f,c}$. At this point, the finite element is deleted.

$$D = \begin{cases} 0 & \varepsilon_{eq} \leq \varepsilon_{y,c} \\ 0.95\left(\frac{\varepsilon_{eq}}{\varepsilon_{f,c}}\right)^2 & \varepsilon_{y,c} < \varepsilon_{eq} < \varepsilon_{f,c} \\ 0.95 & \varepsilon_{eq} \geq \varepsilon_{f,c} \end{cases} \tag{4.2}$$

$$\varepsilon_{eq} = \sqrt{\frac{2}{3}\varepsilon_{ij}\varepsilon_{ij}} \tag{4.3}$$

The yield strain ($\varepsilon_{y,c}$) and ultimate strain ($\varepsilon_{f,c}$) parameters need to be back calculated from the simulation, so this approach enables the estimation of failure strains.

4.8   Results

4.8.1   Stress-strain relationships from quasi-static compression tests

After the five preconditioning cycles, the stress-strain response registered for three foam densities may be divided in an approximately linear part, followed by a non-linear stiffness decrease until the ultimate point, Fig. 4.10. Then, a softening region is observed within post-yielding until material stacks and the load bearing capacity increases (not shown in Fig. 4.10). The preconditioning cycles effect is clearly seen as a significant difference between the initial slope and the one after the cycles, helping to reduce the side artifacts [30, 23].

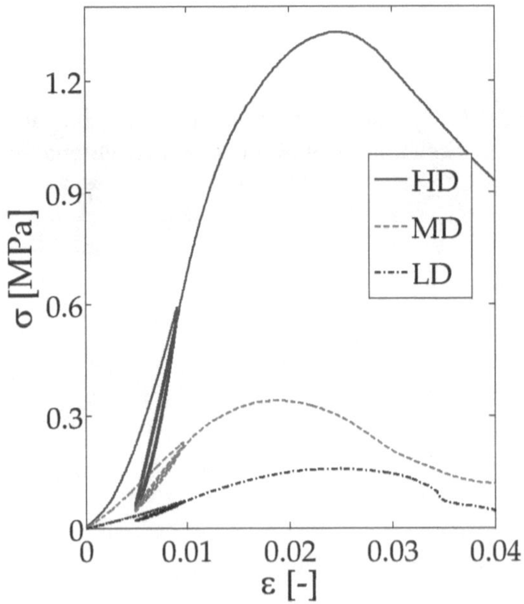

Figure 4.10: Stress-strain response registered in compression tests for three specimens of different densities.

4.8.1.1 Apparent Young's modulus

Compressive stiffness results along the axial and transverse directions are summarized in Table 4.5 as the mean value and the standard deviation for each foam density grade. The results show different compressive behavior for high, medium and low density grades. For the HD grade, the transverse direction is stiffer than the axial one, while for the MD and LD grades the axial direction is stiffer. To explain this distinct response depending on the foam apparent density, we refer to morphometric results presented in section 4.8.3. The morphometric analysis along specimens height reveal that, for HD specimens, the material distribution is not homogeneous and more material is placed near the upper and bottom surfaces. In those volumes, the foam volume fraction is around 40%, while in the center of the specimens it decreases to around 20%. Therefore, when the samples are compressed in the axial direction, the central part of the specimens is more compliant and governs the overall behavior (springs in series effect). In the transverse direction there is more material that stiffens the elastic behavior (springs in parallel effect). In case of MD and LD specimens, the variation of the foam volume fraction along the specimens is lower (from 20% to 12% and from 12% to 8 %, respectively) and specimens behave more isotropically.

Table 4.5: Mean and standard deviation (SD) values of compressive stiffness for each foam grade in their axial and transverse directions and yield and fracture stresses and strains measured through destructive testing in the axial direction.

	$E_{\text{app,ax}} \pm$ SD [MPa]	$E_{\text{app,trans}} \pm$ SD [MPa]	σ_y [MPa]	ε_y [%]	σ_f [MPa]	ε_f [%]
HD	108.37±27.04	160.56±63.65	1.00 ± 0.28	1.5 ± 0.2	1.09 ± 0.32	1.9 ± 0.3
MD	32.59±4.45	29.45±12.03	0.34 ± 0.05	1.6 ± 0.2	0.38 ± 0.06	2.1 ± 0.3
LD	8.94±1.2	6.14±1.75	0.11 ± 0.02	1.8 ± 0.1	0.13 ± 0.02	2.5 ± 0.2

For the HD specimens, the apparent modulus ranges between 70 and 140 MPa in the axial direction and between 70 and 320 MPa in the transverse direction. MD and LD samples present less scatter than HD. The apparent modulus values ranges between 27 and 40 MPa in the axial direction and between 17 and 65 MPa in the transverse one for MD foams, whereas for LD group, it ranges from 7 to 11 MPa in the axial and from 5 to 8 MPa in the transverse direction. The mean value and standard deviation for each density grade and testing direction is given in Table 4.5.

The manufacturer reports stiffness values for each foam grade (Table 4.1), but the testing conditions, directions or the standard deviation of the values provided are not specified in the catalog. For each foam density, the reported values are significantly greater than our measurements. After querying the manufacturer for further details about the testing protocol and results, they confirmed that specimen dimensions are similar to the ones in this work but their measurement system is global instead of local. The manufacturer observed a wide scattering of the results, not reported in the catalog. In addition, specimen machining may also be responsible for some of the scattering in the mechanical properties due to side artifacts resulting from connectivity disruption.

Other works in the literature have provided stiffness values very similar to our measurements. Jonhson and Keller [150] studied the static and dynamic behavior of LD samples from Sawbones and reported a stiffness value in the axial direction of approximately 6 MPa, three-fold less than the manufacturer value, which is similar to our measurements. However, they associate the differences to specimen dimensions and hypothesize that the manufacturer tested the whole foam blocks.

As a conclusion, the foams analyzed present apparent modulus directly related to density, but with a significant scattering. This may be attributed to microstructural differences and lattice disruption due to machining. Axial and transverse directions show higher differences for the HD group, whereas MD and LD groups are more isotropic.

4.8.1.2 Yield and ultimate stresses and strains

The estimation of yield and ultimate properties is also given in Table 4.5. The HD group presents a mean yield stress of 1 MPa and a mean ultimate stress of 1.09 MPa. The latter is about one third of the value (3.2 MPa) reported by the manufacturer. On the other hand, a mean yield strain of 1.5 % and a mean ultimate strain of 1.9 % were measured for HD specimens. The MD group presents mean values for the yield and ultimate stresses of 0.34 and 0.38 MPa, respectively, which are about half the value reported by Sawbones. As happened to the HD group, the yield strain values tend to concentrate around 1.6 %, while the ultimate strain are about 2.1 %. Similarly, approximately half the reported values by the manufacturer were measured for the LD ultimate stresses (0.127 MPa) and a mean yield stress of 0.111 MPa, as summarized in Table 4.5. In this case, a mean yield strain of 1.8 % and a mean ultimate strain of 2.5 % were measured.

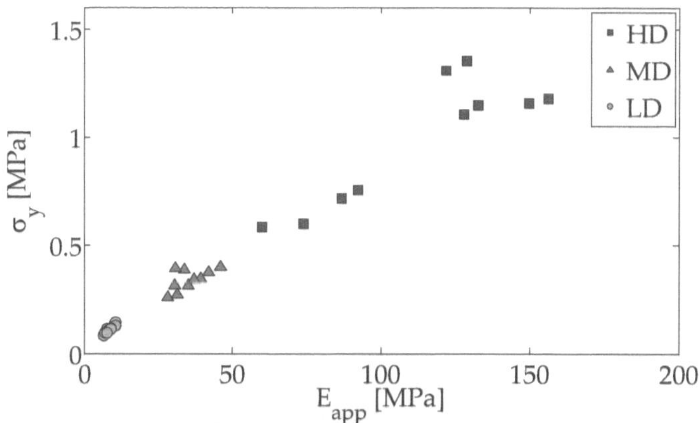

Figure 4.11: Representation of the yielding stress (σ_y) as a function of the apparent modulus (E_{app}) for the three foam grades.

Yield and ultimate stresses show a linear relationship with the apparent modulus, see Figs. 4.11 and 4.12, despite the scatter of E_{app}. Other authors, like Fürst et al. [147] reported similar linear relationships between ultimate strain and modulus and, in this sense, the open cell foams resemble cancellous bone strength-modulus dependence, which has been the reported in the literature [26, 10, 86]. From our results, this linear relationship is σ_y=0.008332 E_{app}+0.04376, with a correlation coefficient (R^2) of 0.967. The following linear expression was found between ultimate stress and modulus: σ_f=0.009079 E_{app}+0.04947, (R^2=0.98).

In the case of yield and ultimate strain values, there is no increasing relationship with the apparent modulus, see Figs. 4.13 and 4.14. Yield strain values show little scattering and they seem to be less dependent on microstructure and govern the failure process. The plot reveals that yielding is relatively constant in terms on strain for a wide range of densities. Nevertheless, LD samples have a yield strain value a bit higher than for HD samples. In the case of ultimate strain (ε_f), a larger scatter is found, with an incremental difference of 30 % between LD and HD groups, Fig. 4.14. Then, a foam of lower density is expected to fail at a higher strain than a denser foam, so the first one undergoes a greater deformation prior to compression failure.

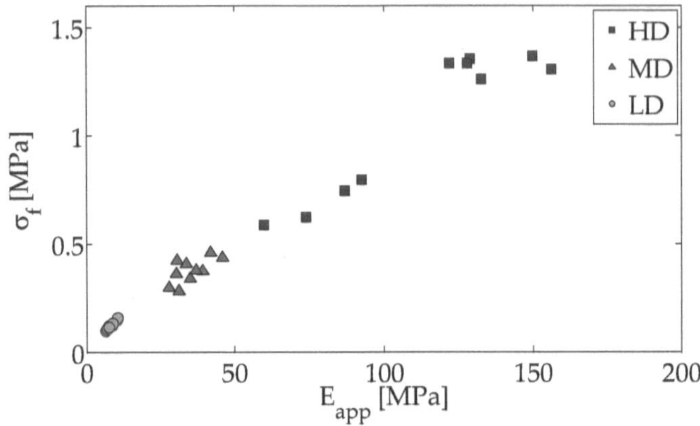

Figure 4.12: Representation of the failure stress (σ_f) as a function of the apparent modulus (E_{app}) for the three foam grades.

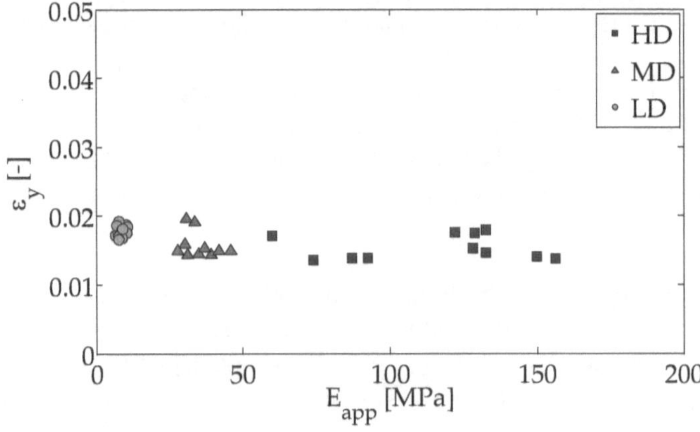

Figure 4.13: Representation of the yielding strain (ε_y) as a function of the apparent modulus (E_{app}) for the three foam grades.

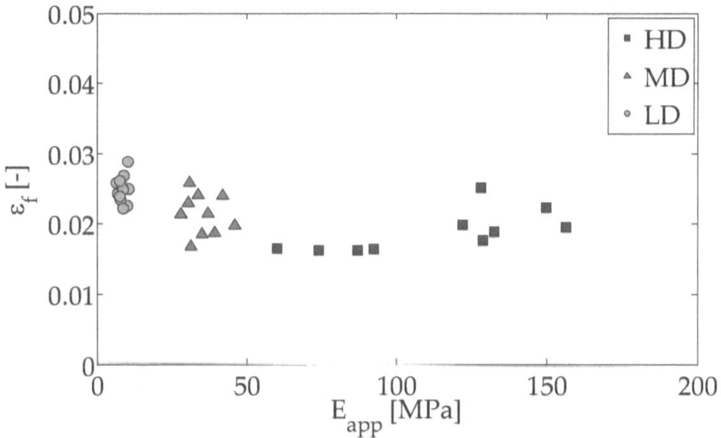

Figure 4.14: Representation of the failure strain (ε_f) as a function of the apparent modulus (E_{app}) for the three foam grades.

These results reveal that strains may control failure of open cell polyurethane foams, as it happens for cancellous bone [10, 26, 72, 50]. Moreover, the wide scatter of ultimate strain values has been also reported in the literature for cancellous bone [50, 73]. However, a small but significant dependence on modulus, volume fraction or microstructure may exist because yield and ultimate strains increase with decreasing density.

4.8.2 DIC application to compression fracture characterization of open cell polyurethane foams

The results of our application of DIC to compression fracture characterization of open cell polyurethane foams are divided in three main parts. First, we present a parametric study about DIC variables and procedure options. Secondly, we report the estimation of the maximum strain value at the apparent yield and ultimate points. Finally, DIC capability to determine fracture patterns is analyzed. The latter will be compared to finite element models results in section 4.8.5.3.

4.8.2.1 Parametric study

With regards to the parametric study, for subset size, step size, correlation criterion and considering incremental or non-incremental correlation, we analyzed 2 samples, speckled and non-speckled, of each density grade and we refer the results to the maximum equivalent strain value measured in the fracture zone.

Our criterion for choosing appropriate parameters is based on failure pattern detection accuracy and absence of voids in the solution. As we will see in the results, some parameters lead to accurate results for our criterion, so we will refer the failure properties estimation to a certain set of DIC parameters and assume them to be in a range based on the parametric analysis variation results.

4.8.2.1.1 Subset size

Regarding subset size, we analyzed its influence on failure strain estimation for 31, 51, 81, 101, 125, and 151 pixels size. The results for the the maximum equivalent strain ($\varepsilon_{\mathrm{eq,f}}$) for each foam grade, speckled and non-speckled, can be seen in Fig. 4.15. Higher maximum strains at failure were registered for the lowest density for the same combination of DIC parameters. The tendency observed is that the larger the subset size is, the lower the strain at failure, and the values tend to converge for increasing subset size.

The differences observed between speckle and non-speckle approaches are not consistent between foam grades, so they may result from specimen variability rather than because of the speckle or non-speckle approach. Differences up to 74 % were found between subset sizes for HD specimens, 100 % for MD specimens and 100 % for the LD specimens.

Failure is a local phenomenon, so subset size should be large enough to permit DIC to solve the correspondence problem but small enough to represent the local effect. Small subset sizes may lead to voids on the solution, while large subsets may homogenize the solution, as depicted in Fig. 4.16. A compromise is then needed to measure failure strains.

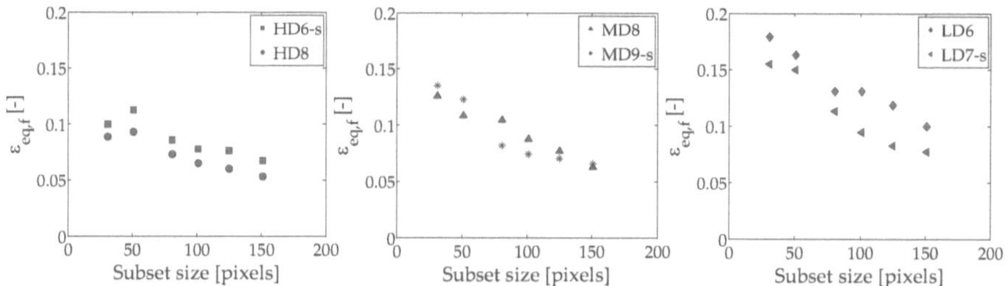

Figure 4.15: Subset size influence on the maximum equivalent strain in the failure region for HD (left), MD (middle) and LD specimens (right). The extension -s denotes speckled specimen.

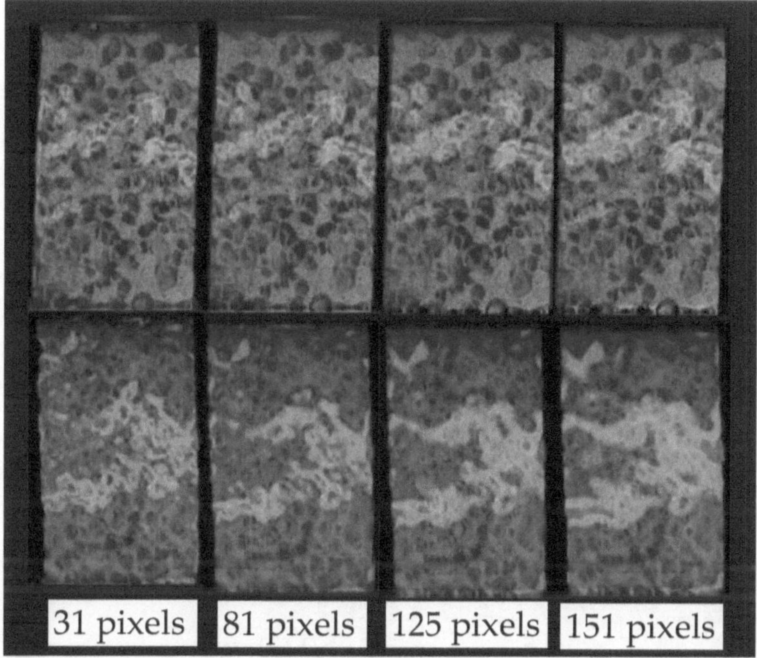

Figure 4.16: Subset size influence on the equivalent strain field for a HD (top) and a LD (bottom) specimens.

4.8.2.1.2 Step size

Step size parameter controls the number of pixels over which the correlation is made, so a low number is recommended to increase accuracy. Here we vary it between 5 and 20 pixels size for the six samples analyzed and two subset sizes (81 and 125 pixels). Figs. 4.17, 4.18 and 4.19 show the effect of subset size for the maximum equivalent strain at fracture for HD, MD and LD specimens, respectively. A clear influence is observed: a higher step size produces a lower equivalent strain at fracture with a greater difference for lower subset size.

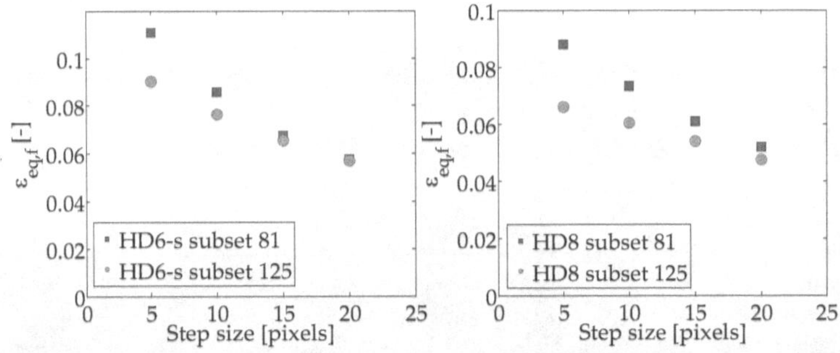

Figure 4.17: Effect of step size variation for HD6 specimen (left) anf HD8 (right) for 81 and 125 subset sizes.

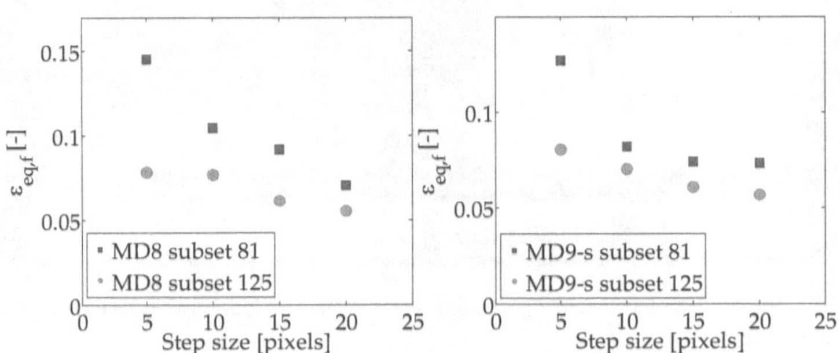

Figure 4.18: Effect of step size variation for MD8 specimen (left) anf MD9 (right) for 81 and 125 subset sizes.

For 81 pixels of subset size, a maximum difference of 93 % is observed for HD specimen, 100 % for MD and 124 % for LD specimens. A higher subset size of 125 pixels led to lower differences between step sizes. For example, a maximum difference of 59 % was found for HD, 41 % for MD and 45 % for LD specimens.

Larger step sizes homogenize the strain distribution, as depicted in Fig. 4.20 for a HD specimen. However, the step sizes analyzed describe with a good level of accuracy the experimental fracture pattern. Then, following the recommendation that a lower step size increases the accuracy of the solution, we chose a step size of 5 pixels to estimate failure strains.

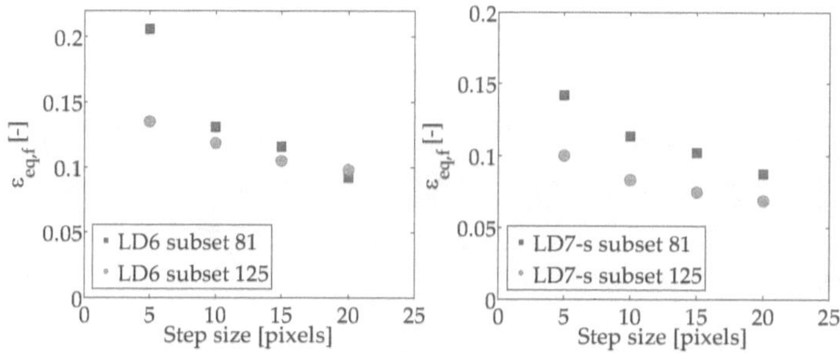

Figure 4.19: Effect of step size variation for LD6 specimen (left) anf LD7 (right) for 81 and 125 subset sizes.

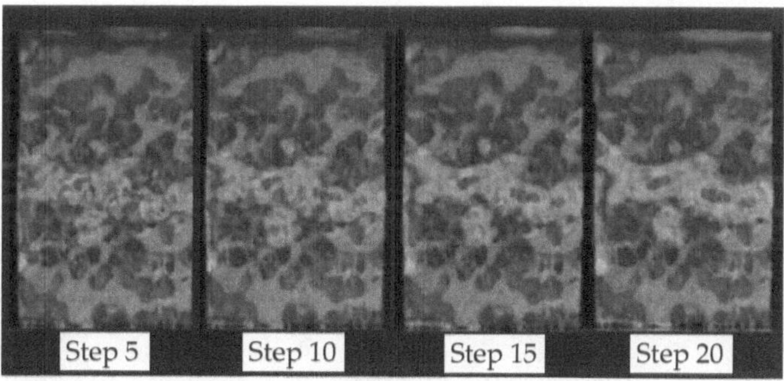

Figure 4.20: Influence of step size on the strain distribution. The larger the step size is, the more homogenized the strain distribution at the failure region.

4.8.2.1.3   Using speckle in a reticular structure

Speckle was applied to the visible surface of half of the specimens. First, a
white paint was used to increase contrast and then a black spray paint was
applied to ensure speckle randomness, Fig. 4.21. Here we present the effect of
a speckle/non-speckle approaches on the failure pattern description and strain
estimation, see Fig. 4.22 and Table 4.6.

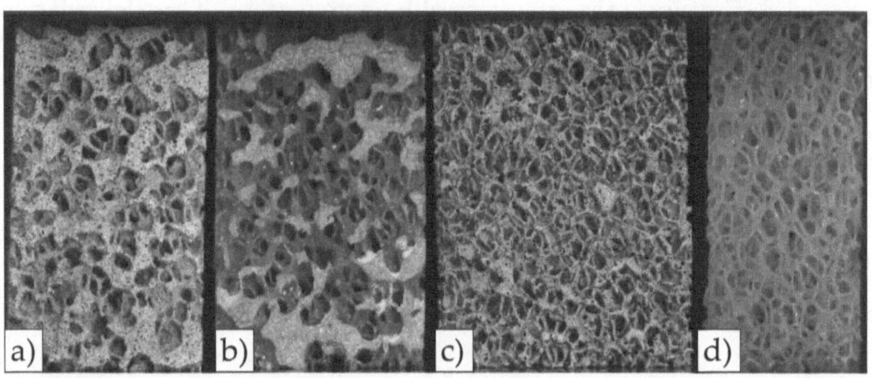

Figure 4.21: Speckled and non-speckled specimen examples: a) HD8 speckled, b) HD10
non-speckled, c) LD6 speckled and d) LD7 non-speckled.

Table 4.6: Mean and standard deviation (STD) values for speckle/non-speckle comparison
for the three densities analyzed.

Sample	Mean $\varepsilon_{eq,f}$ [-]	STD $\varepsilon_{eq,f}$ [-]
HD-s	0.131	0.044
HD	0.116	0.042
MD-s	0.093	0.029
MD	0.126	0.012
LD-s	0.119	0.025
LD	0.132	0.027

A mean value for the fracture strain for speckled HD foams of 0.13 was estimated, while for the non-speckled specimens a mean value of 0.12 was reported.
In case of MD specimens, a mean value of 0.09 was measured for speckle and

0.13 for non-speckle. LD speckled specimens presented a mean value of 0.12 while non-speckled gave 0.13, Table 4.6. Little differences were observed between speckle and non-speckle groups but no clear tendency was observed regarding failure strain values. So, those differences may be attributed to specimen characteristics rather than the speckle/non-speckle approach.

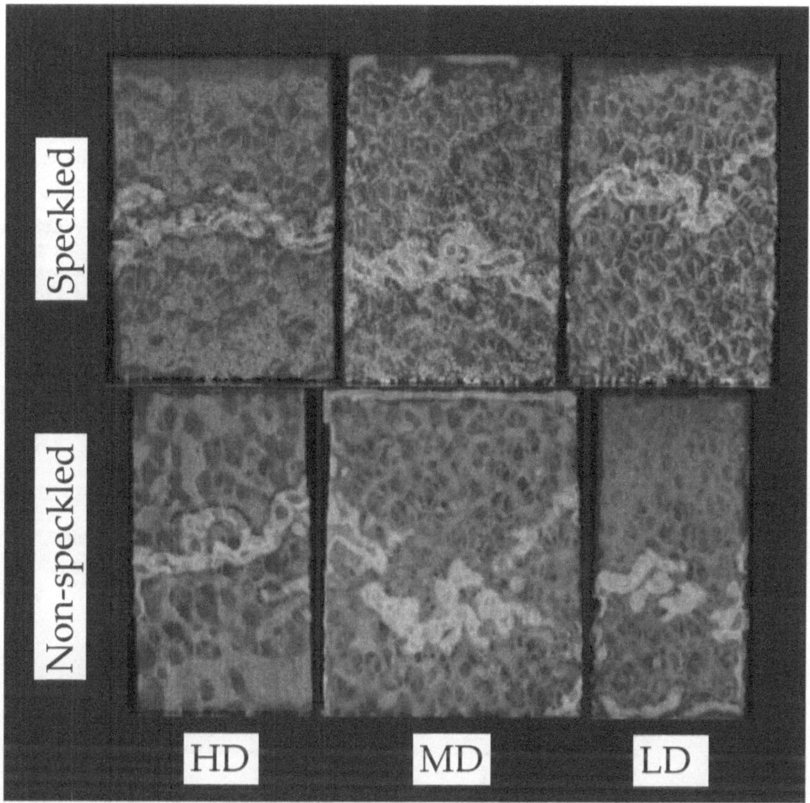

Figure 4.22: Equivalent strain distribution for speckled and non-speckled specimens. Slight differences are found between failure pattern criteria because in the non-speckle approach failure region is a bit more spread.

Fig. 4.22 depicts equivalent strain distribution for post-yield states of speckled (top) and non-speckled (bottom) specimens. Qualitatively, both approaches are equivalent regarding failure detection, but in case of non-speckled specimens it seems to be a bit more spread than for the speckle approach. It could be related to the greater contrast achieved using speckle that enhances pattern matching. Based on our results, speckled and non-speckled approaches are equivalent regarding failure strains measurement and their performance is similar about failure detection, but the speckle approach localizes more failure, which is slightly more spread in the non-speckle approach.

4.8.2.1.4   Correlation criterion

The influence of the pattern matching criterion in the equivalent strain in the fractured area is low and a maximum difference between criterion of 7 % was found, Fig. 4.23. It indicates that during the experiments no significant changes in lighting occurred.

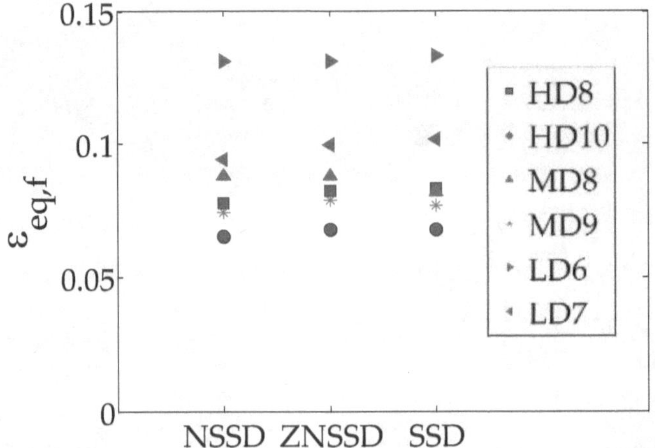

Figure 4.23: Representation of strain at the failure region variation as function of pattern matching criterion. Maximum differences of 7 % were found between criterion.

Choosing between squared differences (SSD), normalized squared differences (NSSD) or zero-normalized squared differences (ZNSSD) neither influenced the strain distribution, as can be noted in Fig. 4.24. No significant differences were found for both speckled (bottom) and non-speckled (top) approaches.

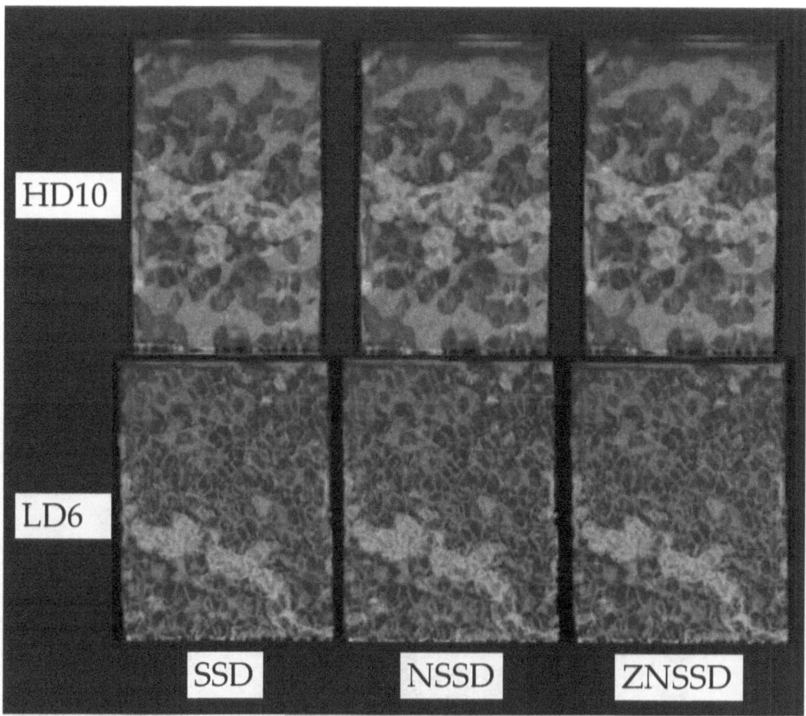

Figure 4.24: Equivalent strain distribution for a high density specimen (top) and a low density specimen (bottom), for a sum of squared differences (SSD) (left), normalized squared differences (NSSD) (centre) and zero-normalized squared differences (ZNSSD) pattern matching criteria (right).

4.8.2.1.5 Incremental vs non-incremental correlation

Considering incremental correlation, that is, comparing each deformed image to the previous one instead of to the reference image is relevant. In both cases, the strain values in the failure area do not differ much (Fig. 4.25), but voids appear in the latter case solution, so the correspondence problem is not properly solved, Fig. 4.26. In Fig. 4.25, there are slight differences on the maximum equivalent strain values but the presence of voids motivates to discard the non-incremental correlation values.

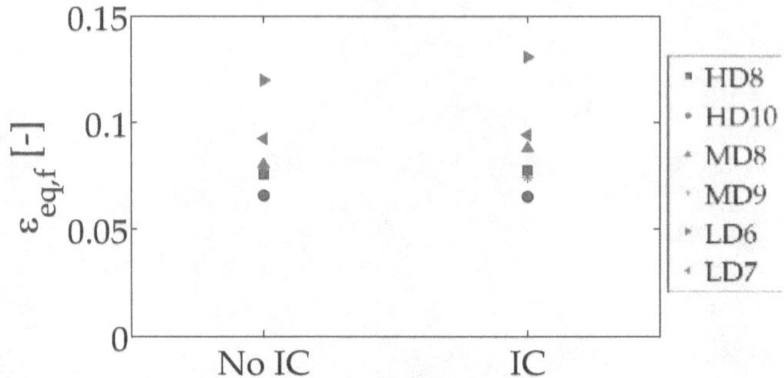

Figure 4.25: Influence of considering incremental correlation (IC) on the failure strain in the fracture area for 6 specimens of different densities.

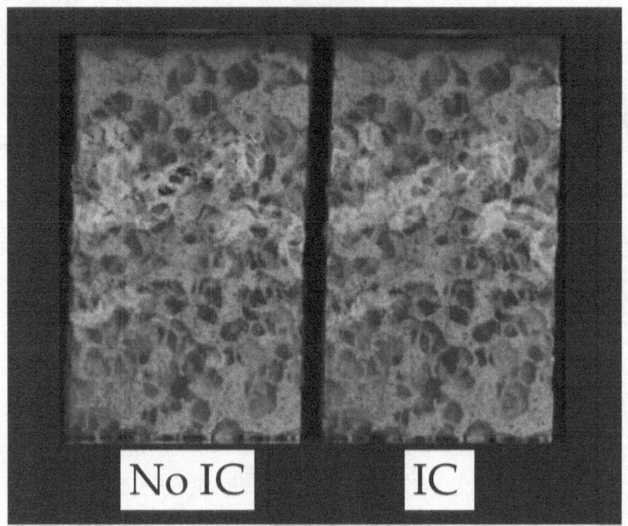

Figure 4.26: Example of the effect of considering incremental correlation (IC) for a HD specimen. Voids appear in the high strained areas of the no incremental correlation case.

4.8.2.2 Failure parameters estimation using DIC results

The parametric DIC results permit to give insight into the effect of DIC on the maximum equivalent strain measured in the fracture area and on the failure pattern definition. There was not a unique combination of parameters that gave the best results, so we refer our results to values registered at the fracture region for a combination of parameters.

The selection of those parameters depended on the absence of voids on the solution, minimization of noise and localization of failure pattern. Subset should be large enough to contain sufficient speckle/texture within it in order to solve the correspondence problem. Step size is recommended to be as lowest as possible to increase the solution accuracy. Incremental correlation, which compares each deformed image with the previous instead with the reference image, has major importance to avoid holes on the solution, while a filter size large enough must be selected to avoid strain blurring that makes the fracture pattern detection vanishes. Then, the following settings were selected: subset size of 81 pixels, step size of 5 pixels, incremental correlation and a filter size of 21 pixels.

Table 4.7: Maximum equivalent strain at yield and ultimate points measured in the region of failure. The results are presented as the mean value and standard deviation for each foam density.

Sample	$\varepsilon_{eq,y}$ [-]	$\varepsilon_{eq,f}$ [-]
HD	0.078 ±0.029	0.124 ±0.041
MD	0.062 ±0.025	0.109 ±0.027
LD	0.077 ±0.025	0.126 ±0.025

The results of the maximum equivalent strain at yield and ultimate apparent points in the fracture region are presented in Table 4.7 for each density grade. Mean and standard deviation values are reported. The values for each specimen are shown in Fig. 4.27. Yield and ultimate strain mean values for each foam grade were similar. HD foams had a mean maximum equivalent strain at the apparent yield point of 0.078, MD 0.062 and LD 0.077 and the same standard deviation was calculated for the three grades. Therefore, the maximum equivalent strain at the apparent yield point may be independent of foam density. Furthermore, it is important to note that failure strain estimations were performed on the fractured regions but not in a single strut, which may be also related to the scattering on failure strain estimation.

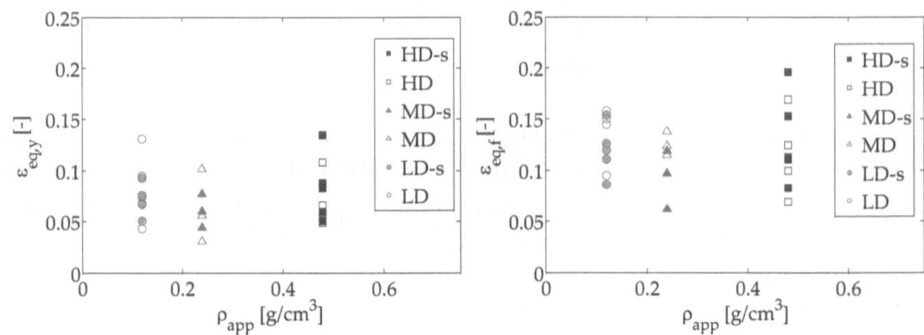

Figure 4.27: Scatter plot of the maximum equivalent strain values at the apparent yield point (left) and the apparent ultimate point (right) as a function of the apparent density group of the samples.

On the other hand, regarding ultimate strains, a mean value of 0.12 was estimated for HD group, 0.11 for MD and 0.13 for LD. Therefore, mean maximum equivalent strain values at the failure region at the apparent ultimate point are also relatively constant over the foam grades. Again, the scattering on the estimations may be a result from the approach to estimate the values. It could be interesting to apply this procedure to a single foam strut to calculate failure strains avoiding the homogenization performed by DIC in whole specimen testing, because we detected that failure tends to be highly localized.

Compression fracture tends to be localized in fracture bands rather than spread, Figs. 4.22 and 4.24. Speckle had no clear influence on failure strains determination, but it had a slight effect on the fracture pattern determination, being a bit more spread for non-speckled specimens.

We did not find any work in the literature that reports failure strains measured using DIC for open cell polyurethane foams. Wang et al. [174] studied deformation patterns on polymeric foams using DIC, reporting material densification but they did not provide any comparison with experimental observations. However, contrary to our observations, they claim that high density foams show no localization of deformation at any apparent deformation. On the other hand, [246] also analyzed strain heterogeneities using DIC and they reported failure to be localized in fracture bands rather than spread. They did not provide failure strain measurements.

4.8.3 Morphometric characterization results

Table 4.8 shows the morphometric parameters for the 6 specimens scanned by micro-CT, two for each foam grade. The first conclusion is that each foam grade is characterized by several parameters, except for Str.Sp, Str.N and DA_{MIL}, whose values are similar for all foam grades. In addition, we compare the morphometric values reported by the manufacturer (FV/TV and Str.Sp) to our measurements. As regards the foam volume fraction (FV/TV), all high and medium density foams specimens and LD2 match the manufacturer values, while LD1 volume fraction is lower than expected. This could be attributed to specimen cutting effects which are more important for the fragile LD foams. On the other hand, a mean cell size between 1.5 and 2.5 mm is provided, but they do not specify which value corresponds to each foam grade. Our estimations of the mean strut separation (Str.Sp) are in the upper range of the manufacturer values for all the foam densities and are more homogeneous. MD samples show the lowest Str.Sp value (2.16 mm), followed by HD (2.36 mm) and LD (2.45 mm). Therefore, Str.Sp does not correlate with the apparent density of the samples.

Table 4.8: Morphometric parameter results for each open cell polyurethane foamed specimen.

Sample	FV/TV [%]	FS/TV [mm^{-1}]	FS/FV [mm^{-1}]	Str.Th [mm]	Str.Sp [mm]	Str.N [mm^{-1}]	$D_{2D}[-]$	$D_{3D}[-]$	DA_{MIL3D} [-]	Conn.D [mm^{-3}]
HD1	30.83	1.08	3.61	1.82	2.38	0.169	1.71	2.73	1.11	0.059
HD2	30.81	1.20	3.89	1.81	2.34	0.171	1.71	2.72	1.10	0.093
MD1	15.40	0.93	6.04	0.69	2.15	0.223	1.55	2.56	1.13	0.212
MD2	15.39	0.89	5.77	0.73	2.17	0.210	1.56	2.58	1.11	0.168
LD1	8.01	0.83	10.35	0.34	2.34	0.234	1.43	2.45	1.15	0.507
LD2	10.60	0.86	8.07	0.51	2.57	0.208	1.47	2.49	1.12	0.240

The mean strut thickness (Str.Th) is quite homogeneous within each foam grade. As expected, HD specimens show the highest Str.Th value, 1.8 mm, which decreases to 0.7 mm for MD and about 0.4 mm for LD specimens. Regarding strut number (Str.N), lower differences between foam grades have been found: a 27% difference between HD and MD, while only a 2% difference between MD and LD. Hence, Str.N parameter seems to be better suited to characterize between high and medium or low density foams.

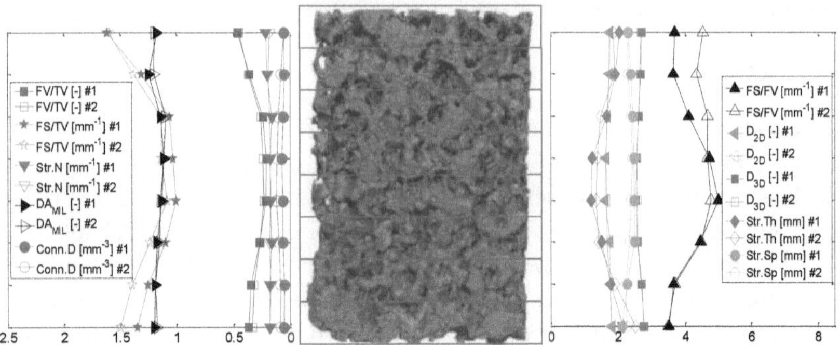

Figure 4.28: Results of the morphometric analysis along HD specimen thickness. For each subvolume, marked with red boxes, the parameters that define the microstructure were estimated after averaging in each subvolume.

The complexity of the structures, measured from D_{2D} and D_{3D} also makes it possible to distinguish between density groups. The degree of anisotropy values, estimated from the fabric tensor calculated through the mean intercept length method (DA_{MIL}), reveals the existence of a preferred orientation but of a low degree. Furthermore, the values are very similar for all the foam grades. This is indicative of a transversely isotropic mechanical behavior, containing a direction of higher stiffness.

On the other hand, connectivity density values (Conn.D) increase for decreasing foam density, and it is related to the amount of material in the region of analysis. Therefore, HD foams present a lower number of connections compared to MD and LD foams. This may be also visualized analyzing the 3D reconstruction of the samples, Fig. 4.3, because denser foams have more material but less connected.

The morphometric results estimated for subvolumes of approximately 5 mm height for the six specimens scanned by micro-CT are depicted in Figs. 4.28, 4.29 and 4.30 and resumed in Table 4.9. HD results show a greater concentration of material in the upper and bottom surfaces, see FV/TV values in Fig. 4.28. FV/TV changes from around 45% and 34% in the upper and lower surfaces to around 20% in the central volume. The relationship between the surface area and the total volume (FS/TV) shows the same trend with the lowest values in the mid-region of the sample (1-1.2 mm^{-1}) with increasing values at the surfaces (1.3-1.6 mm^{-1}). The opposite trend is found when considering the material (PUR) volume as a reference (FS/FV) instead of the total volume: the highest values in the center (5mm^{-1}) while the lowest near the surfaces (3.5mm^{-1}).

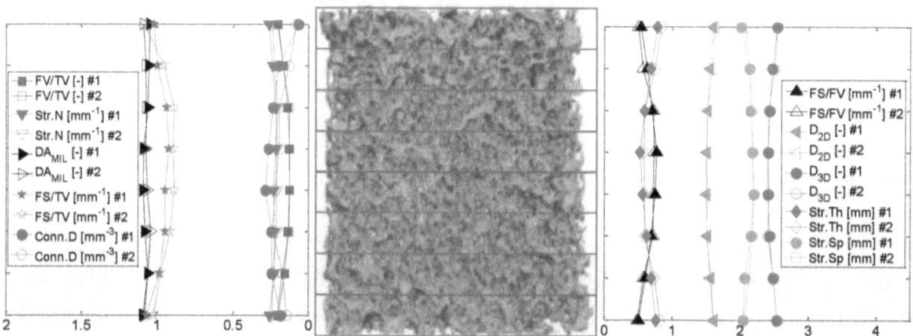

Figure 4.29: Results of the morphometric analysis along MD specimen thickness. For each subvolume, marked with red boxes, the parameters that define the microstructure were estimated after averaging in each subvolume.

The mean strut thickness (Str.Th) variation is in line with the foam volume fraction, the greatest values on the surfaces (1.9-2.5 mm) and the lowest in the middle of the specimen (1.2-1.4 mm). In contrast, a mean void size of between 2.1 and 2.3 mm near the surfaces increases up to 2.5 mm in the center. Other parameters, such as the anisotropy degree, Str.N, D_{2D}, D_{3D} and the connectivity density are quite homogeneous within the foam grade.

As regards the MD specimens, FV/TV, FS/TV and FS/FV present an analogous behavior to HD specimens, but with less variation. For example, foam volume fraction changes from 20% to approximately 12%. As for HD, DA$_{MIL}$ and fractal dimension show little variation along the sections: 3.8% for the anisotropy, and about 5% for the fractal dimension.

The mean strut thickness increases from 0.55 mm in the central section to 0.8 mm in the external sections. On the contrary, the mean void dimension

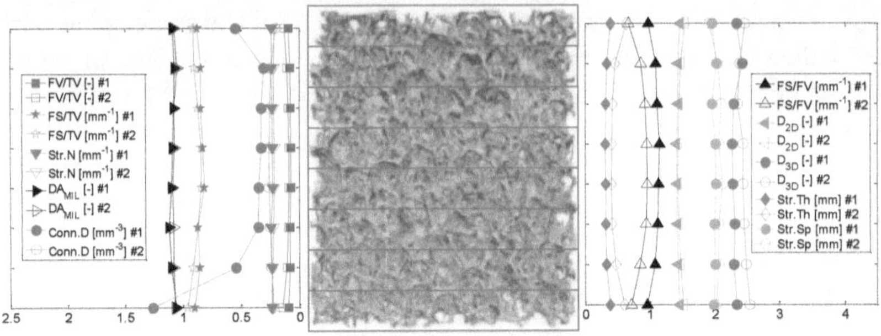

Figure 4.30: Results of the morphometric analysis along LD specimen thickness. For each subvolume, marked with red boxes, the parameters that define the microstructure were estimated after averaging in each subvolume.

takes a 2.2 mm value in the center while around 2.05 mm at the surfaces. Regarding connectivity density, the values estimated are higher than for HD specimens, which indicate that more connections per unit volume are found for MD specimens. Furthermore, more connectivity is found in one of the surfaces, resulting from the production process, and higher values are found in the areas presenting less material (0.28 mm^{-3} in contrast to 0.06 mm^{-3}).

The morphometry of the LD foams, resembling osteoporotic cancellous bone, is more homogeneous in terms of FV/TV, FS/TV, and FS/FV values, compared to the other foam grades, see Fig. 4.30. For example, volume fraction changes from 7-8.8 % to 9-12.8% near the surfaces. Again, parameters like Str.N, DA$_{MIL}$ and D$_{3D}$ show little variation in the section analysis. The connectivity density values are greater than for MD and HD foams, and present intra-specimen variation because higher values are found for specimen LD1, the one of lower FV/TV. In this low apparent density foams, the mean void dimension is more constant along the sections than for MD and HD specimens. The mean strut thickness also changes depending on the section and specimen analyzed. For the specimen LD1, Str.Th varies from 0.31 mm in the central sections to 0.39 in the external ones, while for LD2, greater values are found: 0.41 mm and 0.63 mm, respectively. In case of Str.Sp, the mean void size remains nearly constant through the sections analyzed. However, the mean void size increases in the inner central areas. This effect is more pronounced for increasing foam density.

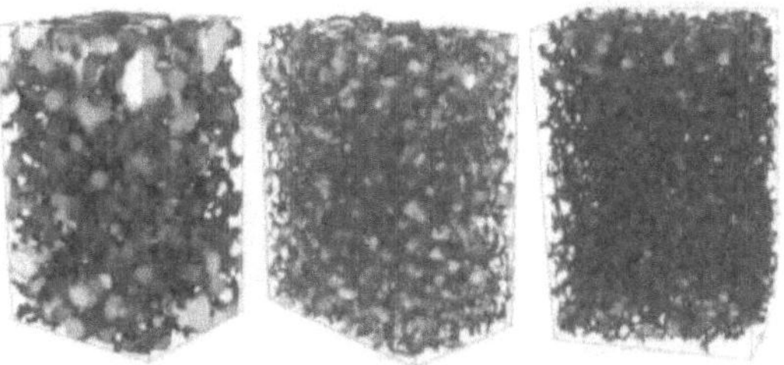

Figure 4.31: Struts thicknesses representation as the maximum sphere that fits within the segmented mask model: HD (left), MD (centre) and LD (right).

On the other hand, BoneJ software [112] allows to represent graphically the tissue level results of the mean strut thickness (Str.Th) and mean strut separation (Str.Sp), see Figs. 4.31 and 4.32. Higher Str.Th values can be noted near the top and bottom surfaces for the high density foams (Fig. 4.31 left), while the effect becomes lower for MD (Fig. 4.31 middle) and LD specimens (Fig. 4.31 right).

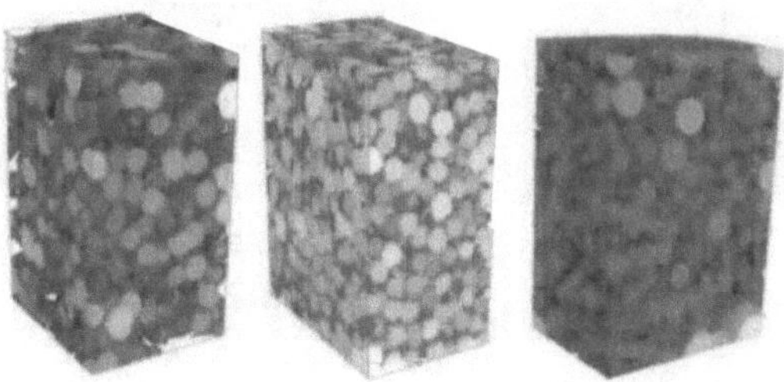

Figure 4.32: Voids dimensions representation, visualizing the maximum sphere that fits in the negative of the foam segmented masks: HD (left), MD (centre) and LD (right).

In case of Str.Sp values, as it can be noted quantitatively in Table 4.9 and visually in Fig. 4.32, the mean void size remains nearly constant. However, as happened with Str.Th, but inversely, the mean void size increases in the inner central areas. This effect is more pronounced for increasing foam density.

Table 4.9: Morphometry analysis results for slices of 5 mm thickness along each specimen (slices are numbered 1 (top) to 8 (bottom), top and bottom were chosen arbitrarily for MD and LD foams because they were almost symmetric but, for HD specimens, top slice was chosen to be the higher volume fraction one). A graphic representation of the data can be found in Figs. 4.28, 4.29 and 4.30.

Sample	Slice	FV/TV [%]	FS/TV [mm^{-1}]	FS/FV [mm^{-1}]	Str.Th [mm]	Str.Sp [mm]	Str.N [mm^{-1}]	D_{2D} [−]	D_{3D} [−]	DA_{MIL3D} [−]	Conn.D [mm^{-3}]
HD1	1 - top	45.92	1.62	3.52	2.15	2.12	0.213	1.82	2.78	1.17	0.053
	2	35.84	1.31	3.65	1.79	2.28	0.200	1.75	2.70	1.24	0.049
	3	23.80	1.06	4.46	1.51	2.50	0.158	1.77	2.58	1.14	0.058
	4	20.71	1.03	4.98	1.19	2.50	0.173	1.63	2.54	1.11	0.070
	5	21.28	1.00	4.72	1.22	2.49	0.174	1.63	2.56	1.13	0.061
	6	26.69	1.09	4.10	1.66	2.45	0.161	1.69	2.62	1.17	0.060
	7	34.44	1.25	3.64	1.93	2.39	0.179	1.75	2.69	1.19	0.051
	8 - bottom	36.65	1.35	3.68	2.04	2.31	0.180	1.75	2.69	1.19	0.051
HD2	1	44.77	1.60	3.48	2.54	2.26	0.176	1.81	2.78	1.19	0.052
	2	36.65	1.38	3.70	1.92	2.24	0.191	1.76	2.71	1.20	0.079
	3	25.34	1.13	4.48	1.42	2.34	0.179	1.67	2.60	1.09	0.101
	4	23.77	1.13	4.76	1.35	2.39	0.176	1.66	2.59	1.11	0.112
	5	23.15	1.08	4.67	1.38	2.44	0.168	1.65	2.58	1.14	0.120
	6	26.51	1.24	4.66	1.49	2.39	0.178	1.68	2.62	1.15	0.097
	7	32.131	1.39	4.34	1.90	2.31	0.169	1.73	2.68	1.19	0.085
	8	33.147	1.50	4.52	1.87	2.31	0.177	1.74	2.69	1.17	0.082
MD1	1	19.95	1.02	5.12	0.77	2.05	0.260	1.61	2.54	1.05	0.062
	2	16.23	1.00	6.14	0.69	2.07	0.234	1.56	2.49	1.06	0.194
	3	13.43	0.93	6.97	0.62	2.16	0.215	1.52	2.44	1.06	0.231
	4	12.21	0.92	7.55	0.57	2.21	0.214	1.50	2.41	1.09	0.264
	5	12.19	0.94	7.76	0.53	2.18	0.229	1.50	2.41	1.09	0.283
	6	13.32	0.94	7.10	0.60	2.15	0.223	1.52	2.44	1.08	0.241
	7	15.43	0.98	6.37	0.69	2.15	0.224	1.55	2.47	1.06	0.237
	8	19.68	1.07	5.44	0.78	2.01	0.252	1.60	2.54	1.09	0.179
MD2	1	19.74	1.08	4.97	0.83	2.06	0.238	1.61	2.55	1.09	0.077
	2	16.35	0.95	5.82	0.74	2.14	0.220	1.57	2.49	1.07	0.125
	3	12.24	0.89	7.25	0.60	2.18	0.204	1.51	2.41	1.07	0.191
	4	12.40	0.89	7.18	0.60	2.20	0.207	1.51	2.42	1.07	0.189
	5	12.02	0.89	7.37	0.58	2.19	0.207	1.51	2.41	1.06	0.219
	6	12.45	0.91	7.31	0.60	2.18	0.209	1.52	2.42	1.04	0.236
	7	17.05	0.98	5.73	0.75	2.14	0.229	1.58	2.50	1.06	0.163
	8	20.17	1.02	5.05	0.85	2.08	0.238	1.62	2.55	1.08	0.142
LD1	1	9.11	0.88	9.64	0.39	1.98	0.236	1.46	2.33	1.09	0.548
	2	7.79	0.85	10.87	0.33	2.01	0.236	1.43	2.29	1.07	0.303
	3	7.54	0.85	11.22	0.32	2.00	0.235	1.42	2.31	1.08	0.324
	4	7.28	0.83	11.38	0.32	2.02	0.229	1.41	2.28	1.09	0.322
	5	7.08	0.82	11.54	0.31	2.01	0.225	1.41	2.27	1.10	0.347
	6	7.80	0.87	11.17	0.32	1.96	0.244	1.43	2.29	1.12	0.348
	7	7.88	0.86	10.88	0.34	2.03	0.233	1.43	2.42	1.10	0.543
	8	9.20	0.90	9.78	0.39	1.96	0.236	1.46	2.34	1.06	1.260
LD2	1	12.84	0.91	7.10	0.60	2.02	0.213	1.52	2.54	1.07	0.204
	2	10.56	0.90	8.54	0.48	2.06	0.221	1.47	2.48	1.05	0.244
	3	9.198	0.87	9.49	0.42	2.06	0.221	1.45	2.45	1.07	0.253
	4	8.738	0.84	9.63	0.41	2.12	0.214	1.43	2.44	1.07	0.254
	5	8.809	0.84	9.55	0.42	2.07	0.212	1.44	2.44	1.09	0.254
	6	9.414	0.87	9.29	0.42	2.10	0.223	1.45	2.35	1.08	0.247
	7	10.57	0.91	8.64	0.46	2.05	0.229	1.47	2.38	1.08	0.237
	8	14.31	0.96	6.70	0.63	1.91	0.227	1.54	2.46	1.06	0.224

4.8.4 Relationships between microstructural parameters defining cancellous bone specimens and experimental compression tests

The importance of microstructure on the mechanical response of cancellous bone [8, 10, 103, 217, 223] motivated us to investigate relationships between morphometry and open cell foam mechanics. For simplicity, we calculated linear relationships between the morphometric parameters calculated (FV/TV, FS/TV, FS/FV, Str.Th, Str.Sp, Str.N, D_{2D}, D_{3D}, DA_{MIL3D} and Conn.D) and mechanical parameters from the experiments (E_{app}, σ_y, σ_f, ε_y and ε_f).

The correlation coefficients (R^2) of the morpho-mechano linear regressions are summarized in Table 4.10. Some morphometric parameters show a high degree of correlation to the mechanical response (E_{app}, σ_y, σ_f and ε_y), such as FV/TV, FS/TV, Str.Th, Str.N and D_{3D}. Other parameters (anisotropy degree, FS/FV and Conn.D) present a lower but significant degree of correlation, while mean void dimension (Str.Sp) shows no correlation to any of the mechanical variables. In addition, fracture strain (ε_f) does not correlate to morphometry. This lack of correlation is also found in cancellous bone morpho-mechano dependencies.

Table 4.10: Correlation coefficients (R^2) of linear regression between morphometry and mechanical response parameters. Values of R^2 greater than 0.9 are typed in bold. The regressions were significant with a p-value$<$0.05.

	σ_y	ε_y	σ_f	ε_f	E_{app}
FV/TV	**0.989**	**0.963**	**0.990**	0.496	**0.969**
FS/TV	**0.924**	0.836	**0.927**	0.431	**0.953**
FS/FV	0.786	0.771	0.779	0.402	0.727
Str.Th	**0.985**	**0.975**	**0.986**	0.531	**0.977**
Str.Sp	0.004	0.002	0.003	0.051	0.001
Str.N	0.850	**0.925**	0.843	0.690	0.864
D_{2D}	**0.964**	**0.934**	**0.960**	0.484	**0.928**
D_{3D}	**0.964**	**0.949**	**0.959**	0.510	**0.927**
DA_{MIL}	0.535	0.610	0.513	0.697	0.549
Conn.D	0.595	0.634	0.586	0.417	0.549

In the experimental results section, a linear relationship was observed between failure stresses (σ_y and $\sigma_{f)}$) and the apparent modulus. Therefore, it is expected that if any morphometric parameter correlates to one of them, it also will do to the other two. The results in Table 4.10 confirm this argument. Fig. 4.33 shows some of the linear regressions with high R^2 between morphometry and ultimate stress. These results evidence in a quantitative way the fact that microstructure controls the mechanical response of open cell foams of different densities.

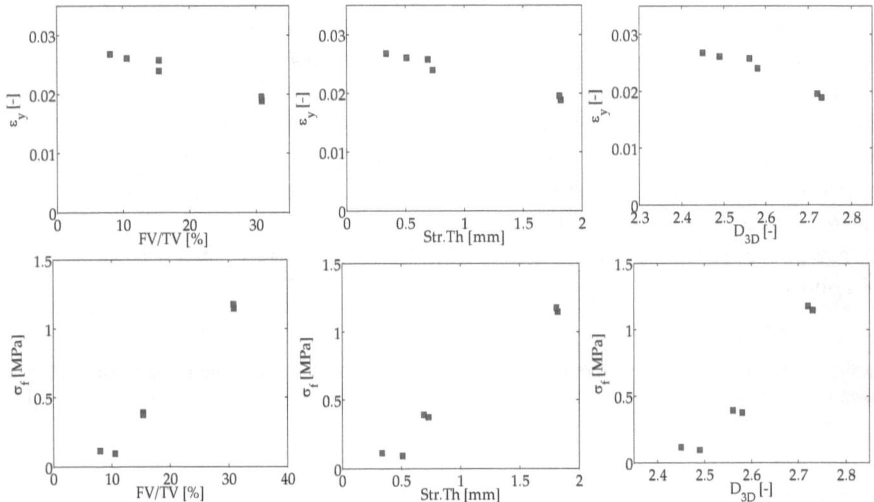

Figure 4.33: Some of the most significant relationships between morphometric parameters and yield strain and failure stress.

Other authors have investigated relationships between morphometry and mechanical properties for this type of structures [147]. Some of the reported relationships are in line with our observations, like is the case of FV/TV, Tb.N or a weak correlation of Conn.D with modulus or strength [147]. Other parameters that showed correlation in our results did not correlate to mechanical parameters in [147].

4.8.5 Finite element modeling results

4.8.5.1 Elastic modulus and failure properties estimation through FEM and testing

Table 4.11 shows the tissue Young's modulus (E_i) estimated for each specimen by inverse analysis using FEM and calibration with test results. The values estimated for the elastic modulus present differences according to the foam grade. This could be expected because in the manufacturer's catalog it is said that the material is a composite foam made of urethanes, epoxies and structural fillers, and the material composition may be different for each foam grade. A mean elastic modulus of 3 GPa was estimated for the material in high density foams, 2.7 GPa for the medium density foams and 1 GPa for the low density foams.

Table 4.11: Young's modulus (E_i), yield (ε_y) and fracture strains (ε_f) calculated for each specimen using finite elements after calibration with the experimental force-displacement curve.

	E_i[GPa]	ε_y [-]	ε_f [-]
HD1	3.290	0.050	0.070
HD2	2.809	0.040	0.058
MD1	2.119	0.03	0.070
MD2	3.358	0.03	0.070
LD1	1.543	0.0225	0.048
LD2	0.579	0.04	0.0775

The results of the back calculation of yield and failure strains for each specimen using experiments and finite element models are summarized in Table 4.11. Finite element models were simulated using Abaqus (6.14, Dassault Systems, US) and a user subroutine (USDFLD). The failure strain values obtained are quite homogeneous for each density grade and also between MD and LD groups. HD foams present a mean yield strain of 0.045, 0.03 for MD and 0.031 for LD. The slightly higher value reported for HD specimens may be related to its different composition, as it may contain more structural fillers. On the other hand, fracture strains were also considerably homogeneous between samples and density grades, as shown in Table 4.11. A mean ultimate strain of 0.064 was estimated for the HD group, 0.07 for MD and 0.063 for

LD specimens. Therefore, despite different density and microstructure, tissue yield and ultimate strains are relatively constant for the 6 samples analyzed.

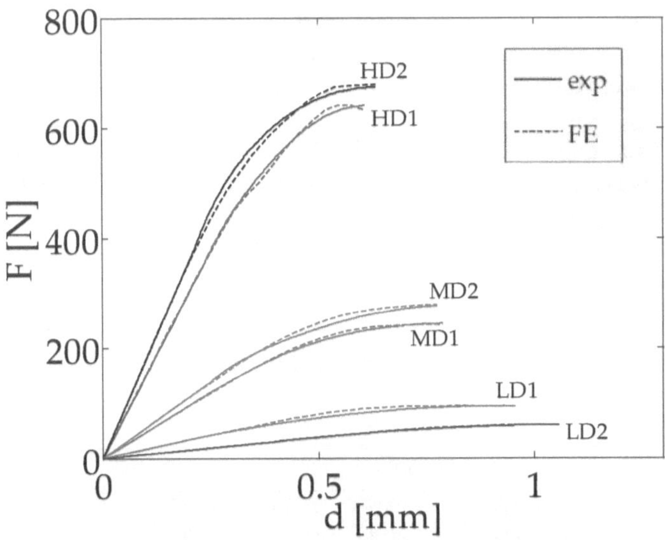

Figure 4.34: Comparison of the force-displacement curve obtained from experiments and simulations.

A comparison between the force-displacement curve from experiments and FE simulations after calibration is depicted in Fig. 4.34. The numerical models reproduce the elastic response and predict the failure load. However, a slight load overestimation is observed prior to the ultimate point. It could be related to the level of discretization of the models, which in our case is a compromise between accuracy and the computational resources available to solve the models. Another possible reason could be the damage law considered in the models, which was experimentally fitted for cancellous bone and used here due to its morphological similarity. Nevertheless, it is shown with the numerical models that the equivalent strain governs failure of the foamed structures and it describes with high accuracy the compression fracture pattern observed experimentally. A combination of material property degradation model following a power law and the element deletion technique based on equivalent

strain accurately describes compression failure of open cell polyurethane foams
of different densities.

4.8.5.2 Complete stiffness matrix estimation from a homogenization approach

The results of stiffness matrices estimation through a homogenization approach are summarized in the following for each specimen scanned. All the samples show an orthotropic material behavior, which is close to be transversely isotropic, Table 4.12. Therefore, the specimens present 2 or 3 planes of symmetry, defining their main directions. Moreover, the zero values of the stiffness matrix were not actually zero but negligible (between 10^{-6} and 10^{-7}). This material behavior supports our experimental observations of section 4.8.1, where transversely isotropic properties were measured for each foam grade.

$$C_{\text{HD1}} \ [\text{MPa}] = \begin{pmatrix} 165.7 & 37.5 & 23.9 & 0 & 0 & 0 \\ 37.5 & 186.2 & 22.7 & 0 & 0 & 0 \\ 23.9 & 22.7 & 89.2 & 0 & 0 & 0 \\ 0 & 0 & 0 & 29.0 & 0 & 0 \\ 0 & 0 & 0 & 0 & 33.2 & 0 \\ 0 & 0 & 0 & 0 & 0 & 62.5 \end{pmatrix} \tag{4.4}$$

$$C_{\text{HD2}} \ [\text{MPa}] = \begin{pmatrix} 201.1 & 49.0 & 42.6 & 0 & 0 & 0 \\ 49.0 & 191.9 & 40.6 & 0 & 0 & 0 \\ 42.6 & 40.6 & 165.0 & 0 & 0 & 0 \\ 0 & 0 & 0 & 45.6 & 0 & 0 \\ 0 & 0 & 0 & 0 & 51.0 & 0 \\ 0 & 0 & 0 & 0 & 0 & 66.5 \end{pmatrix} \tag{4.5}$$

$$C_{\text{MD1}} \ [\text{MPa}] = \begin{pmatrix} 22.5 & 8.0 & 12.3 & 0 & 0 & 0 \\ 8.0 & 30.9 & 14.1 & 0 & 0 & 0 \\ 12.3 & 14.1 & 42.6 & 0 & 0 & 0 \\ 0 & 0 & 0 & 10.3 & 0 & 0 \\ 0 & 0 & 0 & 0 & 9.4 & 0 \\ 0 & 0 & 0 & 0 & 0 & 8.1 \end{pmatrix} \tag{4.6}$$

$$
C_{\text{MD2}} \ [\text{MPa}] =
\begin{pmatrix}
28.6 & 8.0 & 11.1 & 0 & 0 & 0 \\
8.0 & 36.7 & 12.4 & 0 & 0 & 0 \\
11.1 & 12.4 & 42.7 & 0 & 0 & 0 \\
0 & 0 & 0 & 11.8 & 0 & 0 \\
0 & 0 & 0 & 0 & 11.0 & 0 \\
0 & 0 & 0 & 0 & 0 & 11.1
\end{pmatrix}
\tag{4.7}
$$

$$
C_{\text{LD1}} \ [\text{MPa}] =
\begin{pmatrix}
12.8 & 4.8 & 8.0 & 0 & 0 & 0 \\
4.8 & 9.4 & 6.8 & 0 & 0 & 0 \\
8.0 & 6.8 & 19.4 & 0 & 0 & 0 \\
0 & 0 & 0 & 3.5 & 0 & 0 \\
0 & 0 & 0 & 0 & 3.7 & 0 \\
0 & 0 & 0 & 0 & 0 & 2.9
\end{pmatrix}
\tag{4.8}
$$

$$
C_{\text{LD2}} \ [\text{MPa}] =
\begin{pmatrix}
7.3 & 2.7 & 4.0 & 0 & 0 & 0 \\
2.7 & 6.4 & 3.7 & 0 & 0 & 0 \\
4.0 & 3.7 & 10.4 & 0 & 0 & 0 \\
0 & 0 & 0 & 2.2 & 0 & 0 \\
0 & 0 & 0 & 0 & 2.2 & 0 \\
0 & 0 & 0 & 0 & 0 & 2.0
\end{pmatrix}
\tag{4.9}
$$

The engineering constants (E_x, E_y, E_z, G_{xy}, G_{yz}, G_{zx}, ν_{xy}, ν_{yx}, ν_{xz}, ν_{zx}, ν_{yz}, ν_{yz}) were calculated from C matrices using the expressions for an orthotropic material (Eq. 3.28), and are shown in Table 4.12. Half of the Poisson's ratio can be calculated using symmetry properties of the stiffness matrix. HD specimens showed a higher stiffness about x and y directions, which form the transversal plane, with values of around 170 MPa for the two specimens analyzed, and a less stiff direction z. The higher volume fraction near top and bottom surfaces makes the samples stiffer about x and y directions, while the lower FV/TV in the center of the samples makes it more flexible z direction. In case of MD and LD specimens, material distribution also controls the elastic response of the samples. In this case, they were more homogeneous regarding FV/TV so it is the material distribution anisotropy which controls stiffness. Then, for MD and LD specimens, z direction is stiffer than x and y directions, Table 4.12. Shear stiffnesses also represent an orthotropic material behavior.

Poisson's ratios were similar between samples for the same directions but varied among density grades. For example, a value of around 0.2 was estimated for ν_{xz} and HD specimens, which varied up to 0.22 for MD and to 0.3

for LD specimens. Other planes, like xy, presented similar values between foam grades (around 0.2).

Table 4.12: Engineering constants calculated from stiffness matrices for open cell polyurethane foam specimens.

	HD1	HD2	MD1	MD2	LD1	LD2
E_x [MPa]	153.8	181.9	18.4	25.0	8.9	5.5
E_y [MPa]	174.2	174.1	25.4	32.2	6.6	4.9
E_z [MPa]	84.1	150.8	32.4	35.9	12.5	7.3
ν_{xy} [-]	0.174	0.212	0.149	0.146	0.285	0.242
ν_{xz} [-]	0.223	0.207	0.240	0.217	0.313	0.296
ν_{yz} [-]	0.201	0.194	0.272	0.241	0.262	0.273
ν_{yx} [-]	0.197	0.202	0.206	0.187	0.212	0.215
ν_{zx} [-]	0.122	0.171	0.424	0.311	0.439	0.395
ν_{zy} [-]	0.097	0.168	0.347	0.269	0.496	0.412
G_{xy} [MPa]	62.5	66.5	8.1	11.1	2.9	2.0
G_{yz} [MPa]	29.0	45.6	10.3	11.8	3.5	2.2
G_{zx} [MPa]	33.2	51.0	9.4	11.0	3.7	2.2

4.8.5.3 Fracture patterns characterization using finite elements and DIC

In Figs. 4.35, 4.36 and 4.37, we compare the equivalent strain field obtained through the application of DIC to images taken during compression testing and the finite element predictions. Failure appeared at localized zones and dominated by microarchitecture. In general and as expected, DIC detects strain inhomogeneities and clearly localizes failure at the apparent level, while FEM results are more localized and sometimes present more difficulties to visualize failure patterns.

High density foams exhibit a failure pattern concentrated in the central region of the specimens, with a match between DIC and numerical predictions, even for the secondary fracture patterns. Several struts broke up, conforming a fracture pattern through the specimens, see Fig. 4.35. On the other hand, medium density specimens present a main fracture in the central part of the specimen and other secondary inclined failure patterns detected by DIC and also predicted by the finite element models, Fig. 4.36.

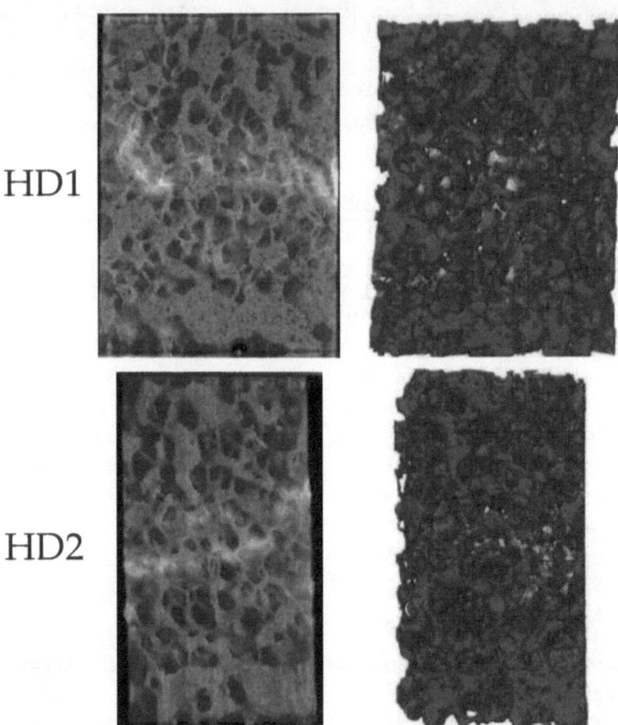

Figure 4.35: Representation of equivalent strain field for HD specimens using DIC (left) and FE results (right). Cold colors represent low equivalent strains, while warm colors high equivalent strain values.

However, several failed regions in the upper part of MD1 appear in the simulations and the failure pattern is more difficult to distinguish in the models, see Fig. 4.36 (right). Nevertheless, similarities can be observed between DIC and FE simulations. Specimen MD2 suffers from deformation near the upper compression platen, which is not predicted in the simulations because we did not model compression platens nor its contact with the specimen. We simply applied a distributed load. An inclined failure pattern is detected by DIC and also predicted by the numerical model.

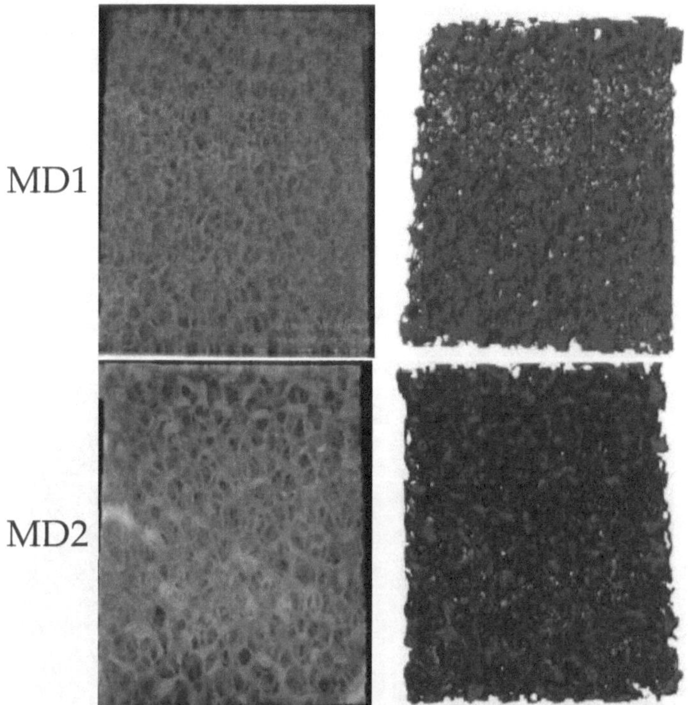

Figure 4.36: Representation of equivalent strain field for MD specimens using DIC (left) and FE results (right). Cold colors represent low equivalent strains, while warm colors high equivalent strain values.

DIC also detected high strains in the upper and lower surfaces of the low density specimens, Fig. 4.37. The lower the volume fraction, the greater the deformations suffered by the specimen at the platen-specimen interface. Again, a match between DIC and finite element predictions can be observed. Specimen LD1 presents some inclined fracture planes. These are maximum shear planes at 45° with respect to the applied compressive load. The fracture pattern is similar in specimen LD2, presenting also inclined fractures. It can be noted that volume fraction has an influence on the fracture shape. In our results, the high density foams showed a flat central fracture area, while medium and low density specimens presented more inclined fracture patterns

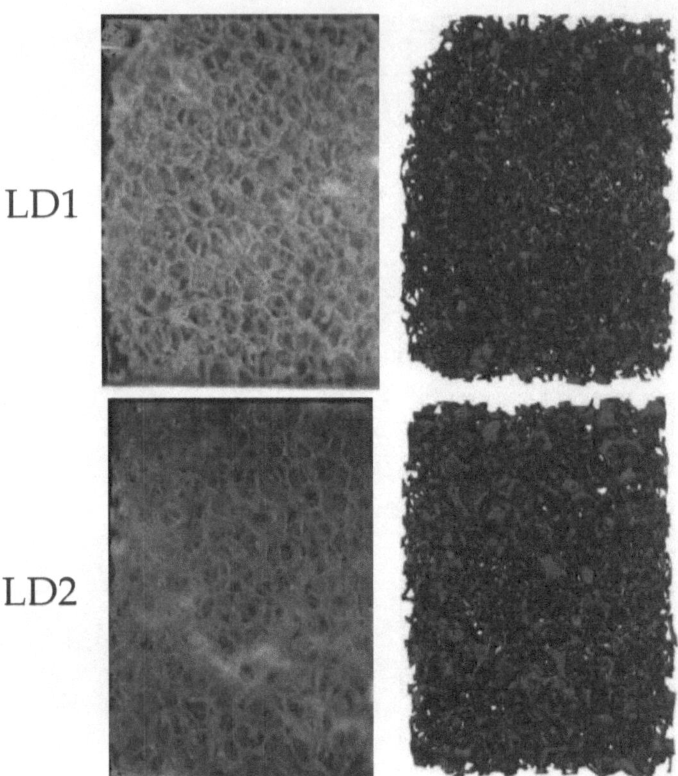

Figure 4.37: Representation of equivalent strain field for LD specimens using DIC (left) and FE results (right). Cold colors represent low equivalent strains, while warm colors high equivalent strain values.

due to planes of maximum shear.

The application of DIC to detect compression failure patterns in open cell polyurethane foams has allowed the validation of our FE models to predict failure response. Our model accurately predicts the failed regions observed experimentally and supports the idea that failure in foams is controlled by strains. In addition, microstructure has an influence on the elastic and fracture behavior, which vary among specimens, even for the same foam density.

4.9 Conclusions

In this chapter, we have characterized open cell polyurethane foams of three different densities from morphometric and mechanical perspectives. The morphometric characterization was performed on 6 specimens scanned by micro-CT and aims at evaluating each sample considering its microstructure. The three foam densities analyzed were distinguishable by any of the morphological parameters analyzed. Furthermore, the study of slices of 5 mm thickness revealed different morphometry evolution across the sample thickness according to density. The inhomogeneities were higher for the high density (HD) foams, which concentrate more material near the top and bottom surfaces. Morphometry varied according to that material distribution: for example, a lower volume fraction, foam surface to volume ratio or mean trabecular thickness were measured in the central region of HD samples. For some parameters, the inhomogeneities were high, like volume fraction, which varied from 40 % near the surfaces to about 20 % in the middle. Other parameters, like fractal dimension or connectivity density presented little changes within HD grade. MD foam grade is more homogeneous than HD, but presents similar trends about morphometry variation within a specimen, though of a much lower degree. In case of LD foam grade, the specimens are the most homogeneous. These analyses may be used to choose between cancellous bone surrogates according to the homogeneity needed for the experiments.

Moreover, the morphometry results of the whole specimens were used to analyze morpho-mechano dependencies through the calculation of linear regressions. Some parameters, like FV/TV, FS/FV, Str.Th, Str.N and D showed correlation to the elastic modulus, yield and ultimate stresses and yield strain measured in the experiments.

As regards the mechanical characterization, we measured the elastic response along the three main directions and up to failure along the direction defined as the main one. Three different axial stiffnesses were measured for each foam grade, but two of them were quite similar, so the specimens presented an orthotropic material behavior, close to transversely isotropic. In case of HD specimens, the lower material disposition in the central part makes the block thickness (we called it axial) direction less stiffer than the transversal ones. In case of MD and LD specimens, the axial direction is stiffer than the transversal ones, but at a lower degree. Therefore, MD and LD specimens are more homogeneous regarding the stiffness about the three main directions.

A linear relationship between strength (yield stress and ultimate stress) and stiffness was captured from the experiments, so the stiffer a sample is, the higher the strength at failure. Yield strains (ε_y) were relatively constant (HD foams had a mean value of 1.5 %, MD 1.6 % and LD 1.8 %) and more scatter was found for the ultimate strain (ε_f) (mean values of 1.9 %, 2.1 % and 2.5 % for HD, MD and LD specimens). It indicates that the less dense the foam is, the greater the failure strain.

Moreover, we applied DIC to images acquired during testing to evaluate failure strains at the fractured regions and compare the failure pattern prediction between DIC and experiments. An analysis about some DIC parameters was conducted, which allowed to estimate the variation of the strain at failure prediction as a function of the setting parameters whose variation had a significant effect on the estimation of the failure pattern and failure strain estimation.

DIC permitted to estimate failure strains in the fractured regions. Similar yield strain values were measured for each foam grade, which supports the idea that foams failure is strain-controlled. A mean value of 0.078 was estimated for HD, 0.062 for MD and 0.077 for LD specimens. With regards to the ultimate strain values, the mean value for each density grade was quite constant: 0.12 for HD, 0.11 for MD and 0.13 for LD group.

As regards the numerical characterization of the compression failure behavior, we calculated the elastic properties from two approaches. The elastic properties of the tissue were estimated using finite element models with a high level of discretization to define morphology and boundary conditions that match the experimental ones, combined with the experimental response curve. A mean tissue Young's modulus of 3 GPa was estimated for HD, 2.7 GPa for MD and 1 GPa for the LD foams.

The model detected the failure experimental pattern with high accuracy, which matched DIC failure prediction results. Hence, DIC was successfully used to validate the numerical approach to model compression fracture through the detection of fractured regions.

The apparent elastic behavior of each specimen was also assessed from a homogenization approach, that permitted to characterize each specimen through its complete stiffness matrix. The estimations are in line with the experimental observations: HD foams presented higher axial modulus for the transversal directions, while for MD and LD foams the axial modulus was lower for the transversal directions. Other engineering constants, like shear stiffness and Poisson's ratios were also calculated but could not be compared to experimental results.

Yield and ultimate strains back-calculated combining experiments and finite element modeling led to values approximately constant over the density grades analyzed. HD specimens presented a higher yield strain (0.045) than MD and LD specimens (0.03), which may be related to the inclusion of more structural fillers in the high density group. The ultimate strain properties estimated showed little variation between samples, with a mean value close to 0.07.

The information provided in this work is not reported in manufacturer's data sheets and it is relevant for a more accurate mechanical characterization needed in cement augmentation analyses or orthopedic implants assessment. The thorough morphometric analysis reported here provides information about its local variation and its relationship to mechanical behavior.

Chapter 5

Application of bone failure models for the evaluation of fixation techniques for scoliosis treatment

5.1   Introduction

The development of this chapter was motivated by the four months research stay at the Technique University of Eindhoven (TU/e) under the supervision of Prof. Bert van Rietbergen. This chapter is framed in a project about different procedures to treat scoliosis, specially for early onset scoliosis (EOS).

Scoliosis is a spine condition characterized by 3D abnormal deformity of importance prevalence at a wide range of ages [181]. Depending on its severity, different treatments may be applied and surgery may be necessary. Early onset scoliosis (EOS) is identified when the condition appears before the age of ten years old and surgery is reported at 56 % of cases [181]. The gold standard for scoliosis surgical treatment is spinal fusion using pedicle screws and rods, used to guide spine position, but it is not suitable for EOS because it may imply severe complications [181], and subsequent operative procedures and hospitalization are often necessary [182]. Moreover, those patients may suffer from great spinal growth alterations and other related diseases, such as

restrictive pulmonary disease due to the highly invasive pedicle screw fixation
[181]. Systems that permit spinal growth have been introduced in the clinical
practice, like expandable rods, that can be sorted as distraction-based implants and magnetically expandable growing rods [181]. However, the first of
those systems requires for surgeries to lengthen the rods at intervals of about 6
months, so it has high economic and psychosocial costs, while the second system reduces the need for further surgeries but instrumentation complications
have been reported to a higher degree than conventional rods [181]. Moreover,
pedicle screw pull-out strength has been reported to diminish for decreasing
bone mineral density, so this type of fixation may not be the best option for
osteoporotic patients [180].

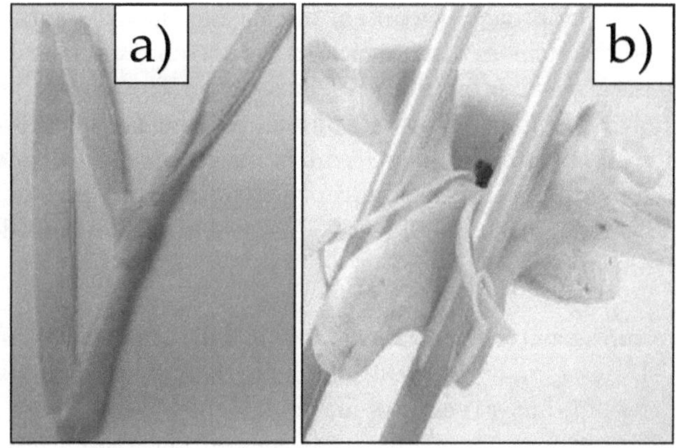

Figure 5.1: a) Radiopaque UHMWPE sublaminar wire and b) sublaminar fixation system
b), adapted from [180].

Less invasive fixation techniques that reduce the need for further surgical
interventions and that permit spinal normal growth are of great research interest. Polymeric sublaminar cable systems were introduced in the last decade,
including a flat shape that adapts better to the lamina morphology and improves load bearing thanks to the greater contact area [180]. Sublaminar wires
also permit spinal growth and may be applied in growth-guidance constructs
for EOS [181, 182]. Moreover, sublaminar wiring failure strength is relatively
constant for varying bone mineral density [180]. In this context, ultra-high

molecular weight polyethylene (UHMWPE) cables appear with high potential. Recently, Roth et al. [180] developed a radiopaque UHMWPE cable (Fig. 5.1), which contains bismuth oxide (Bi_2O_3), that enhances the contrast of the fixation system by imaging, so permits to control its stability and integrity during its use [182].

The results presented in this chapter deal with two different approaches to evaluate fixation techniques for scoliosis treatment: First, we evaluate two fixation constructs, pedicle screw (PS) and sublaminar tape (ST), using density-based finite element models at clinical CT resolution. Secondly, we use micro-finite element models based on micro-CT images for the estimation of the pull-out strength of a pedicle screw inserted in a vertebra.

Within the first approach, we aim at evaluating the differences in the pull-out strength and the stresses distribution in the vertebra between pedicle screw and sublaminar tape spine fixation configurations. This comparison can give insight into how each fixation system influences the failure modes observed experimentally. The finite element models based on density measurements simulated the experimental tests conditions to investigate both configurations in the same specimen. A simple linear failure criterion was considered to predict pull-out failure.

Regarding the second approach, we aim at validating micro-finite element models (μFEM) based on high resolution images acquired by micro-CT, for the prediction of the pull-out strength of an implant inserted in three porcine vertebrae. In the literature, it is claimed that the pull-out strength is determined by the quality of the bone next to the implant, density and osseointegration [148, 184, 185, 186, 187]. The objective is to evaluate the first hypothesis by estimating the dimensions of the volume of interest to be included in the simulations. Cancellous bone morphometry is also analyzed and its influence on the mechanical response is explored. The μFEM were validated against experiments performed on each vertebra. The pull-out strength was estimated from the force-displacement response in the experimental tests and using μFEM and Pistoia criterion [125].

The screw-bone interface was modeled as full-contact. To define the contact interface, different virtual screw placements were studied, analyzing the resulting stress field to optimize the load bearing, considering just the stress transfer through the screw-thread side against the displacement imposed. The effect of the screw depth insertion was also assessed through simulations.

For each approach analyzed, we will first describe the procedure followed, then we will present the specimens used, the imaging protocol followed, the experiments carried out and the finite element model generation. Finally, the results will be presented and discussed and some conclusions will be stated.

5.2 Fixation constructs evaluation by means of density-based finite element modeling and experimental testing

Our main goal in this section is to evaluate pedicle screw (PS) and sublaminar tape (ST) constructs as spine fixation systems using a vertebra and finite element models generated using images at CT resolution (0.5 mm). This comparison may give insight into how each fixation configuration influences the failure locations observed experimentally. PS configuration consists of the vertebra and screws inserted in the pedicles, while ST construct involves the vertebra, UHMWPE radiopaque wires and guidance rods, Fig. 5.2. These configurations were tested out experimentally until failure and modeled using finite elements.

Pull-out experiments were carried out bilaterally, using a custom configuration which is closer to *in vivo* situation than conventional axial pull-out tests. Bilateral pull-out consists in applying the load through a bending moment (Sec. 5.2.3). The experimental study was carried out at Maastricht UMC+ by A K Roth and R J P Doodkorte. We will focus on the numerical models generated, and detailed further explanation of the tested specimen, testing protocols and experimental results can be found in Doodkorte et al. [247].

The finite element models generated take into account the vertebra, where material properties are defined according to density measurements, pedicle screws and sublaminar UHMWPE wires. The experimental setup is modeled and full bonding is considered at the screws-bone or wire-bone interfaces. A comparison between the effect of considering each configuration on the stress distribution is carried out and the failure load is estimated using a linear tensile yield stress criterion.

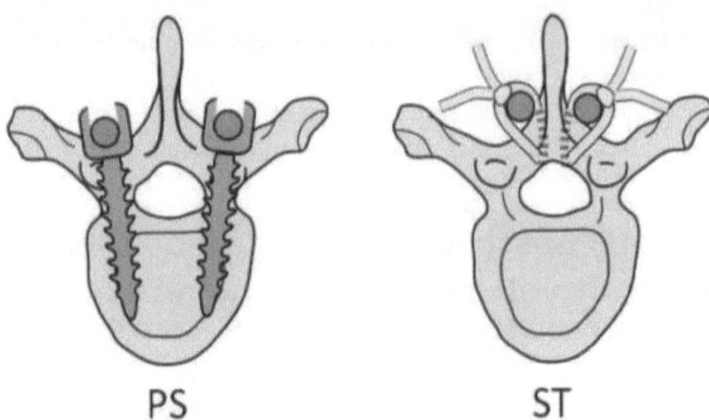

Figure 5.2: Scheme of the pedicle screw (PS) and sublaminar tape (ST) configurations evaluated in this chapter. Figure adapted from Doodkorte et al. [247].

5.2.1 Specimen description and instrumentation

A human vertebra (T9 level) was used to evaluate the pedicle screw (PS) and sublaminar tape (ST) configurations using finite elements. The human vertebra belonged to a 96 year old male and was dissected out at the Department of Orthopedic Surgery (Maastricht UMC+, Maastricht, the Netherlands).

The vertebral body was embedded in polymethyl methacrylate (PMMA) in a custom made device to ensure a perfect alignment between subsequent micro-CT scanning. The vertebra was first instrumented for ST configuration image acquisition. UHMWPE tape was included bilaterally and attached to surrogate rods to position the construct as in the experiments. After its scanning, a surgeon from Maastricht UMC+ instrumented the vertebra for PS configuration and inserted an implant through each pedicle. The construct was then scanned to determine the position of the screws in the vertebra. Both configurations are represented in Fig. 5.3.

Other 17 human thoracic or lumbar vertebrae were used for the experimental study and were randomly selected for PS and ST groups.

5.2.2 Micro-computed tomography images acquisition and segmentation

The vertebra used was scanned by micro-computed tomography (microCT100, SCANCO Medical, Switzerland) at a 34.2 μm spatial resolution (70 kV, 200 μA, 300 ms, Al 0.5 mm filter) at the Technique University of Eindhoven (TU/e) facilities and was then downscaled to clinical computed tomography resolution (0.5 mm) to make it feasible to simulate the whole fixation construct. In order to avoid image artifacts due to the different absorption coefficients of the materials used for PS and ST constructs, three scans were performed using the aforementioned settings and using a custom holder to scan each configuration at the same position. This enables to overlay the images between subsequent scans and add the PS and ST materials to the vertebra digitally. The first scan comprised the vertebra, the second one the vertebra with the sublaminar tape and rods to define its position in the experiment, and the last one the vertebra with the pedicle screws inserted.

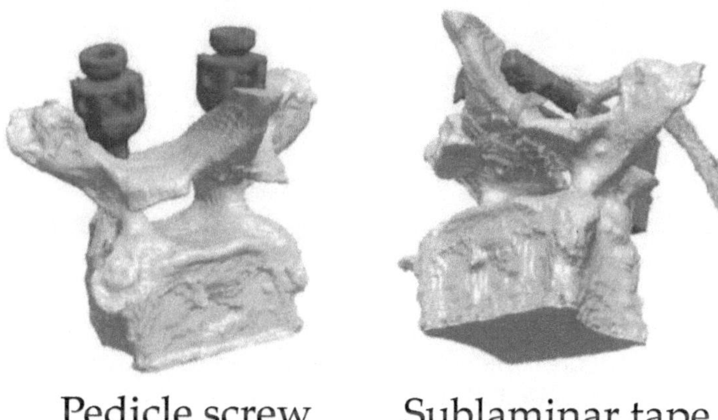

Figure 5.3: 3D reconstruction of the segmented masks of the pedicle screw (PS) and sublaminar tape (ST) constructs.

The downscaled images of the vertebra were segmented according to mineral content measurements, considering in the model tissues from 170 to 1085 mg HA/cm^3. Pedicle screws and sublaminar tape were segmented by manual

thresholding following visual inspection and the subsequent masks were overlapped to the images from the vertebra-only acquisition. A 3D reconstruction
of the resulting segmented models is depicted in Fig. 5.3.

5.2.3   Testing of fixation configurations

The experimental work was performed by A K Roth and R J P Doodkorte at
Maastricht UMC+ and we just present here the methodology and the results
to compare them to our simulations.

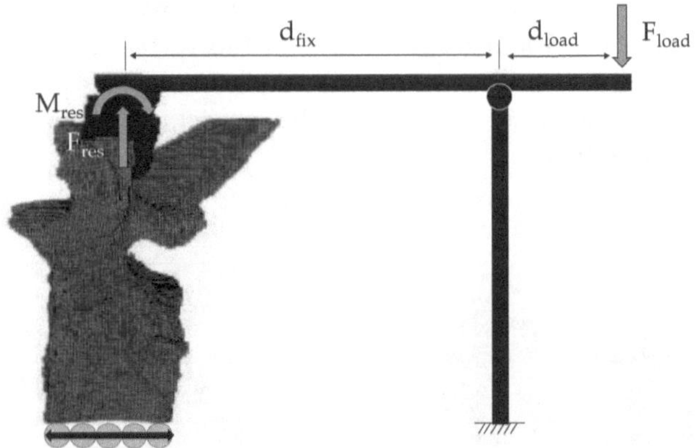

Figure 5.4: Scheme of the pedicle screw testing configuration model. The black rectangle
represents the column used to apply a bending moment.

The vertebrae were embedded in PMMA and mounted on a sliding car-
riage with sleeve barriers. Spinal rods were positioned bilaterally and cross-
links were used to stabilize rods during testing. Displacement was applied at
10 mm/min using a universal testing machine (Instron E3000, Instron, USA).
Fixation was tested by the reverse application of a bending moment, resulting
in a force (F_{res}) in the fixation, as depicted in Figs. 5.4 and 5.5. In case of
pedicle screws, a moment (M_{res}) is applied at the screw heads, which does
not appear for ST configuration. The distance between fixation and rotation
point was kept constant (d_{fix}=75 mm) as well as the distance between the load
application and rotation points (d_{load}=25 mm). The stiffness of each configuration was estimated between 100 and 500 N from the force-displacement

curve.

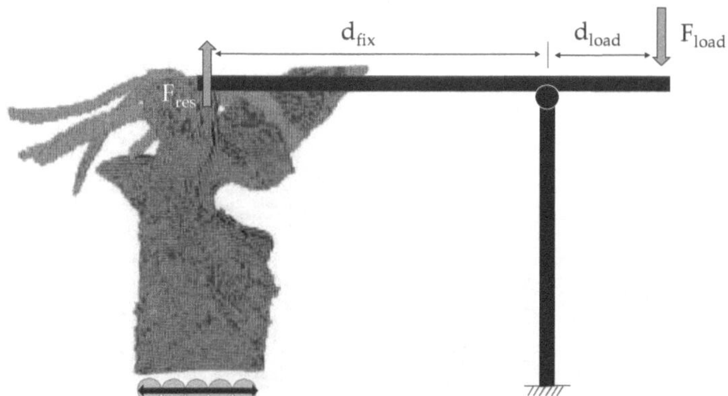

Figure 5.5: Scheme of the sublaminar tape testing configuration model. The black rectangle represents the column used to apply a bending moment.

A mean failure load of 2,678 ± 827 N was registered for the pedicle screw configuration, while sublaminar tape failed at a mean load of 3,563 ± 1,428 N. Besides, a lower stiffness was found for ST (638 ± 135 N/mm) than for PS (794 ± 168 N/mm). Different failure modes were observed: PS failed by screw pull-out or by pedicle fracture, whereas ST failed by pedicle fracture or by lamina fracture.

5.2.4 Generation of finite element models based on density measurement

Finite element models of each fixation construct were developed from the micro-CT images segmented using Abaqus (6.14, Dassault Systems, US). Two meshes were used: the first one is a voxel mesh, generated through a direct conversion from voxels to finite elements (element type C3D8 coded in Abaqus), while the second one is a tetrahedral fine mesh (element type C3D4 coded in Abaqus) which avoids the sharp corners of the voxel-based mesh and permits smooth surfaces, Fig. 5.6. A total of 211,630 voxel elements and 333,611 nodes, in case of the voxel mesh, or 2,221,436 tetrahedral and 591,859 nodes, in case of the tetrahedral mesh, compose the PS finite element model, while

223,466 voxel elements and 363,916 nodes or 2,504,885 tetrahedral elements and 682,117 nodes integrate the ST configuration models.

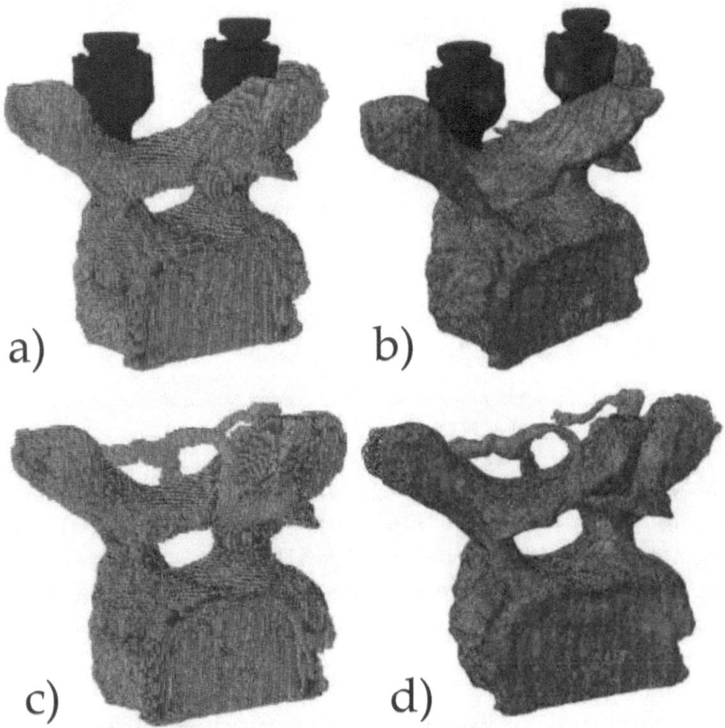

Figure 5.6: Finite element meshes generated for pedicle screw and sublaminar tape configurations: voxel meshes a) c) and tetrahedral meshes b) d).

A density-based FE model was made for the vertebra and a power law relationship was used in order to assign a Young's modulus dependent on the element density, which was obtained by Morgan et al. [130] for human vertebral tissue (E(GPa) $= 4.73\rho_{\text{app}}^{1.56}$). This relationship lead to elastic properties of the vertebra ranging from 1 to 11 GPa. On the other hand, a Poisson's ratio of 0.3 was defined for bone tissue. In case of SP configuration, isotropic elastic properties were considered for screw Titanium material (E=110 GPa, ν=0.3).

On the other hand, ST configuration model takes into account the bilateral spinal rods through a beam connector and the sublaminar tape (UHMWPE: E=19 GPa, ν=0.3 [181]).

Linear elastic simulations were carried out and a load of 1,000 N was applied bilaterally for both configurations to compare the load bearing and strain distribution between fixations. Boundary conditions were defined to mimic the experiments, that is, displacements in the roller direction were left free, while the other two orthogonal directions were constrained. A beam connector was defined, rotating at a distance (d_{fix}) from the construct connection, Figs. 5.4 and 5.5. Besides, full-bonding contact was assumed at the components interface. Moreover, failure load was estimated for each fixation construct as the load at which the maximum tensile principal stress exceeds the cancellous bone yield stress (115 MPa [73]).

5.2.5 Results and discussion

The finite element models permit to estimate stresses and strains for PS and ST configurations due to bilateral testing, Figs. 5.7 and 5.8, respectively. In both figures, a strain threshold of 0.7 % strain was selected to define yielding onset at the tissue level [73]. In case of PS construct, a bending moment of 25.05 Nm was applied to the screws head for a 1,000 N applied load, which produced high stresses and strains areas in the pedicles, Fig. 5.7 (right and centre). Trabecular regions surrounding screw and near the cortical cortex also suffer from greater deformations, leading to strain values around cancellous bone yield strain values for the 1,000 N applied load, Fig. 5.7 (left). Those highly loaded areas at the screw thread and the pedicles show that pull-out failure or pedicle fracture may occur. This results are consistent with the failure locations observed experimentally. Both finite element meshes lead to very similar stress and strain distribution results, except for the peak values, which were higher for the tetrahedral mesh (about a 50 % in terms of maximum principal stress) (Fig. 5.7).

ST configuration simulation lead to different strains and stresses distribution than PS, presenting higher values in the lamina, pedicles and in the contact areas between sublaminar tape and vertebra, Fig 5.8. In this case, the lamina transmits the load to the vertebral body, and is then distributed to the cortical cortex and the trabeculae, Fig. 5.8 (left). The failure locations observed experimentally are also consistent with the highly loaded regions predicted by the FE model. The high stresses and strains in the lamina may result in its fracture, Fig. 5.8 (right), while highly loaded pedicles are also detected by the numerical model, Fig. 5.8 (centre). In case of ST configuration, less differences on the peak values (13 % in the case of maximum principal stresses) between the voxel and tetrahedral meshes are found, compared to the results of the pedicle screw construct, Fig. 5.8.

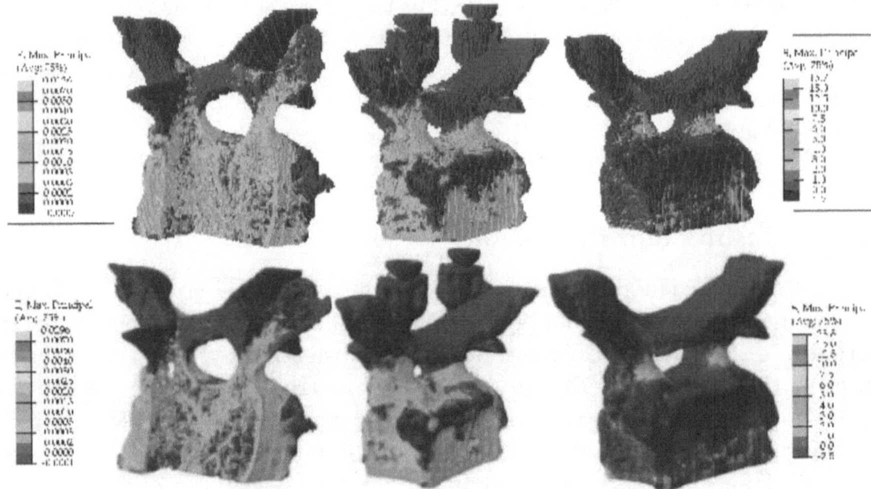

Figure 5.7: FE results for PS construct considering a 1,000 N applied load using the voxel mesh (top) and the tetrahedral mesh (bottom). Higher strains are present in the inner trabecular regions surrounding the screws (left) and in the pedicles (centre). Stresses are concentrated at the pedicles, lamina cortex and surrounding the screw (right).

Table 5.1 presents the estimation of the failure load for pedicle screw and sublaminar tape configurations, calculated as the load at which the maximum principal stress exceeds a tensile yield stress value of 115 MPa [73]. The results for the voxel mesh show important differences between configurations, predicting a higher failure load for PS. However, it is influenced by the presence of the lower peak stress values for PS in the voxel mesh, whose differences with the tetrahedral mesh results may indicate mesh dependence.

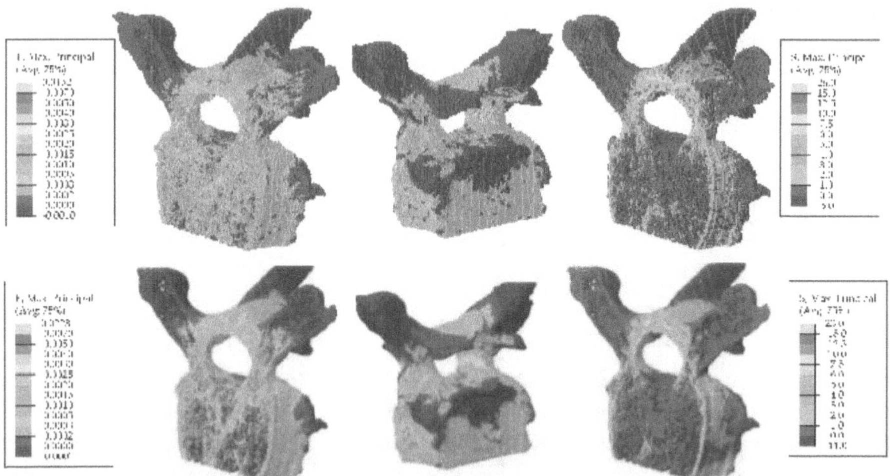

Figure 5.8: Sublaminar tape simulation results for the voxel mesh (top) and the tetrahedral mesh (bottom) for a 1,000 N applied load (F_{load}). FE results high strain areas are consistent to the failure locations observed experimentally for ST construct. The lamina and pedicle regions suffer from high strains (left, centre). The cortical cortex in the lamina and the pedicles transmits the loads to the vertebral body (right).

Table 5.1: Failure load for each configuration and mesh estimated as the load at which the maximum principal stress exceeds the cancellous bone yield stress, considered it as 115 MPa [73].

Failure load (N)	Pedicle screws (PS)	Sublaminar tape (ST)
Voxel mesh	8,110 N	4,974 N
Tetrahedral mesh	4,838 N	5,004 N

On the other hand, the failure load estimation for the tetrahedral meshes reveals very similar values between configurations, being slightly higher for sublaminar tape (3.4 % higher). Therefore, the fine tetrahedral mesh predicts a failure load to a certain degree higher for ST configuration, which is also a less invasive fixation system for the patient.

The experimental setup was modeled considering density-based FE for both PS and ST groups, which allowed the estimation of load bearing within the vertebra for each construct during its bilateral testing. Further, the regions of higher strains were consistent with the failure locations observed experimentally for PS and ST configurations. PS model presented higher strain values around the screw, which is related to pull-out failure mode, and at the pedicles due to the induced moment, which may result in fracture at this region. On the other hand, ST construct shows high strain values in the contact area between sublaminar tape and vertebra and in the pedicles. Moreover, if we compare the strain values between PS and ST configurations, similar peak values are found for the same applied load, while differences are on the high strained areas location.

The FE models developed have some limitations that need to be mentioned. First, we superimposed the segmented masks of vertebra and instrumentation. In case of sublaminar tape, it is not problematic because it does not modify vertebral morphology. However, for pedicle screws, they were directly included in the microstructure so the model does not take into account the damaged tissue due to pedicle screw insertion. However, this approximation may not be far from reality because the screw location is defined accurately and it is said that screw fixation depends on the quality of bone around the screw [148, 184, 185, 186, 187].

On the other hand, an isotropic elastic material model was assumed, while bone is reported to be non-isotropic and viscoelastic. Linear-elastic simulations were carried out, so non-linear behavior associated to yielding and post-yielding is not modeled in this work, but we consider a 0.7% threshold as yield strain to point out yielded areas [73, 125]. Besides, we considered full bonding contact at the screw-vertebra and sublaminar tape-vertebra interfaces, so a more complex model accounting for the contact forces at the interface would be needed to analyze more local failure effects.

Furthermore, downscaling the micro-CT images to CT resolution causes that trabecular microarchitecture tends to vanish. Therefore, a lower threshold was selected to account for those regions averaged with bone marrow. Moreover, we estimated the failure load as a linear approximation, considering failure as the load that exceeds the tensile yield stress. More complex models would be necessary to perform more accurate predictions. In that sense, the models developed in this section give an idea of how load for each configuration is transfered and the location of highly loaded regions rather than predicting failure load accurately.

5.3 Prediction of the pull-out strength of a screw inserted in a vertebra using micro-FE

Here, we aim at validating image-based numerical models to estimate the pull-out strength of a *Stryker Xia 3 Titanium Poliaxial* pedicle-screw (Fig. 5.9) inserted in the vertebral body of three porcine vertebrae. We would like to point out that, although in clinics the spine fixation is done on the pedicles, we chose to fix it in the vertebral body for the pilot study on animals. A general overview of the procedure followed in this chapter can be found in Fig. 5.10. The vertebrae under study were scanned using micro-CT before and after the screw insertion, in order to know its exact position to insert it virtually, avoiding the image artifacts surrounding the screw in the post-insertion micro-CT acquisition. Those image artifacts are result from the differences in the absorption coefficient of bone and screw. The virtual placement of the screw in the numerical model consisted in two stages: a 3D registration of the models pre- and post-screw-insertion and a model transformation step that allows translations and rotations to place the screw accurately.

Stryker Xia 3	
Outer diameter (mm)	5.5
Length (mm)	40
Material	Titanium alloy
E (GPa)	110
ν	0.3

Figure 5.9: Stryker Xia 3 (left) and its general geometric and material features (rigth).

We carried out axial pull-out test on each vertebra, recording the force-displacement response of the screw head. To mimic the experimental tests, micro-FE models were generated from the micro-CT images. Different finite element analysis were conducted: first, we estimated the volume of interest (VOI) dimensions of the problem under analysis. Secondly, we studied the influence of the screw depth insertion on the reaction force. Finally, we estimated the pull-out strength using Pistoia criterion [125] to estimate failure and we analyzed the critical strain and volume parameters that minimize the failure load prediction error. Further, the morphometry of the cancellous bone surrounding the implant was analyzed and a positive correlation was found between some parameters and the pull-out strength and stiffness.

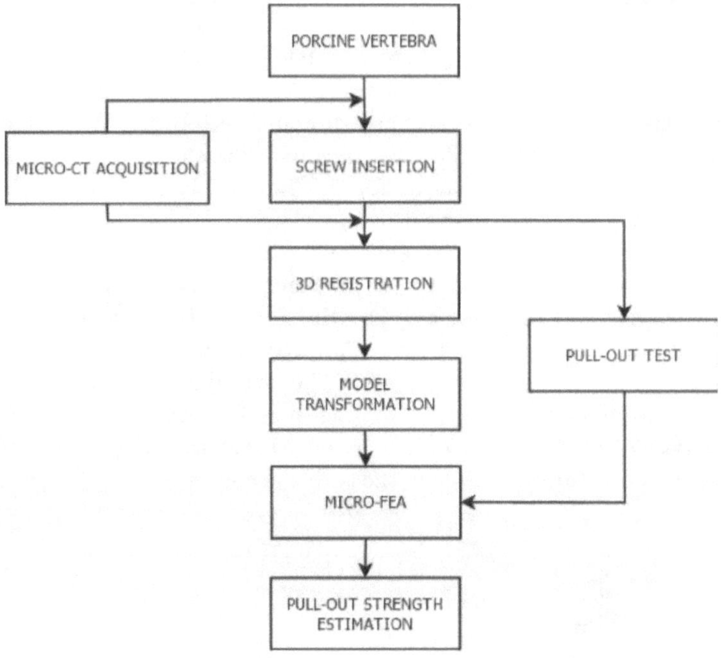

Figure 5.10: Scheme of the procedure followed to estimate the pull-out strength.

5.3.1 Specimen description

Three porcine vertebrae were used in this study. No information about age, gender or weight was provided. The vertebrae were embedded in PMMA to facilitate its gripping during the pull-out test, as depicted in Fig. 5.15, while the vertebral body was left free to allow the screw insertion, see Fig. 5.11. Specimens were kept frozen at -20 °C and thawed at room temperature prior its scanning and testing.

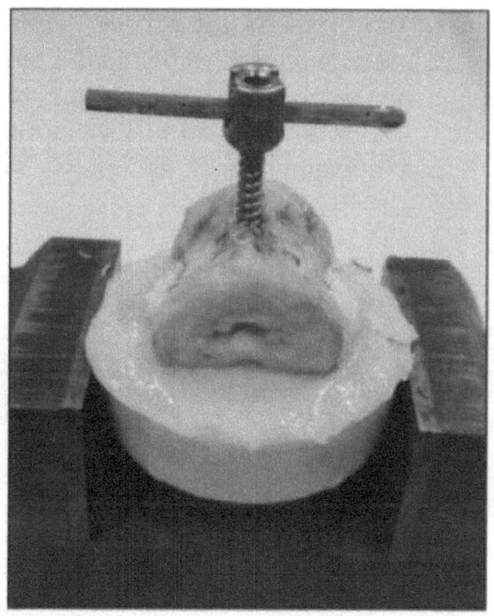

Figure 5.11: Specimen #1 embedded in PMMA during screw insertion.

The implant we used is a *Stryker Xia 3 Titanium Poliaxial* pedicle-screw, designed to treat vertebral degeneration, trauma and deformity correction applications including adolescent idiopathic scoliosis [248]. In Fig. 5.9, the *Stryker Xia 3* pedicle-screw is depicted together with its general material and geometric features [248].

5.3.2 Micro-computed tomography images acquisition, segmentation and morphometric analysis

The vertebrae were scanned by micro-computed tomography using micro-CT (microCT100, SCANCO Medical, Switzerland) in the Technique University of Eindhoven (TU/e) facilities at a resolution of 45 μm (integration time= 300 ms, energy= 70 kVp, intensity= 200 μA, Al 0.5 mm filter). The resolution of the scans allowed to describe cancellous bone microstructure.

Each vertebra was scanned before and after the screw insertion in the vertebral body. Due to the differences between the absorption coefficient of implant and bone, image artifacts appeared around the screw in the images acquired after screw insertion. Those image artifacts modified the gray values surrounding the screw and were only used to define the position of the screw in the FE model, while bone geometry was defined from the pre-insertion scan. Therefore, the numerical models developed in this chapter do not account for the induced damage resulting from screw insertion.

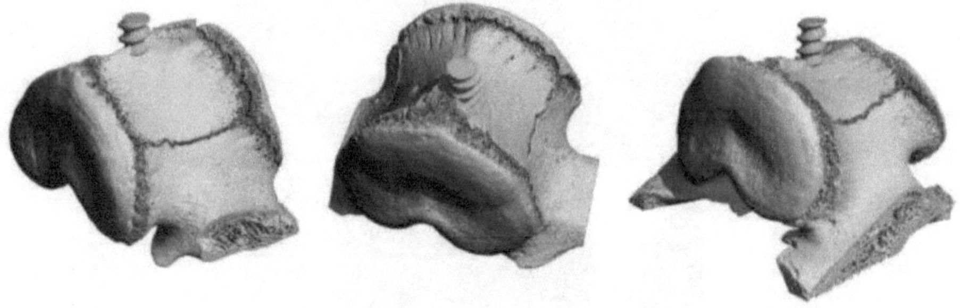

Figure 5.12: 3D reconstruction of samples #1 (left), #2 (centre) and #3 (right).

The micro-CT images were segmented using a Gauss-filtered thresholding method [249]. A 3D reconstruction of the segmented models including the screws is shown in Fig. 5.12, where growth plates are visible and we assumed them to be closed. In order to investigate the influence of bone microstructure on the pull-out strength, a morphometric analysis of the bone surrounding the screw was performed, estimating the bone volume fraction (BV/TV), mean trabecular thickness (Tb.Th), mean trabecular separation (Tb.Sp), trabecular number (Tb.N), bone surface to volume ratio (BS/BV) and the degree of anisotropy (DA) based on the estimation of the mean intercept length (MIL_{3D}) parameter [91]. All parameters were calculated using the SCANCO software to analyze cancellous bone because it was available at TU/e. Mean tissue density was also estimated for each vertebra from the scans, calibrated for that purpose, as the mean gray value of the segmented mask of each vertebra, see Table 5.2.

Table 5.2: Mean tissue density estimated from the segmented masks for each vertebrae.

	Vertebra #1	Vertebra #2	Vertebra #3
Mean density [mg HA/cm^3]	715.95	711.18	711.54

5.3.3 Screw insertion

The vertebral bodies were drilled before the insertion of the screw, generating a 2 mm diameter hole. Then, the screw was inserted manually using the drilled hole as a guide (see Fig. 5.11), until a depth of around 20 mm, with no intention of overtaking the cortex at the other side of the vertebral body and tended to avoid growth plates on the vertebral bodies.

The virtual placement of the screw followed the steps summarized on Fig. 5.13. After the screw insertion, each vertebra was scanned using micro-CT to receive information about its position. A 3D registration was then performed between the segmented models pre- and post-screw insertion. It allowed for the estimation of the transformation matrix that needs to be applied to the post insertion model to get the best mask overlap to the pre-insertion model. The algorithm searches for rotations and translations that minimize the difference between the first and the second models after applying the transformation. To avoid local minimum results, we used a multiscale approach where the registration is estimated first in downscaled models (with lower resolution) and the results are used in the next level till reaching the original resolution level. This approach permits to save CPU time and improves the convergence of the estimations [249].

The result of the 3D registration for sample #1 is shown in Fig. 5.14, where we can distinguish overlapping zones (in blue) and non-overlapping zones after the transformation of the post-insertion model (in red: bone present in pre-insertion model, in green: material present in the post-insertion model but not in the initial one).

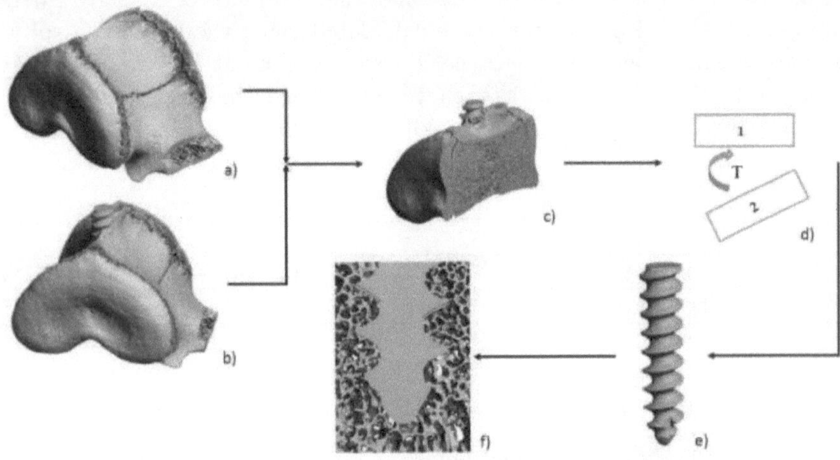

Figure 5.13: Virtual screw insertion scheme. Reconstruction of a) pre-insertion model, b) post-insertion model, c) 3D registration, d) model transformation, e) screw segmentation after model transformation and f) screw positioning in the pre-insertion vertebra (in red, non contact region interface).

In Fig. 5.14 (enlarged view), it can be noted the accuracy of the registration, as the bone microstructure is maintained (in blue). The differences that can be noticed (in red), are due to the differences in the segmentation parameters between the models, whose selection was not considered relevant for the registration step. The segmentation threshold chosen within this approach may be slightly different but, as the microstructure morphology is maintained, the 3D registration is accurately estimated.

The transformation matrix was then applied to the post-insertion model, to position the screw in the pre-insertion model. Then, the screw was segmented and overlapped to the pre-insertion model. Full bonded contact is considered in the simulations and we modeled the bone reaming which resulted from implant insertion (marked in red in Fig. 5.13 f) to disconnect screw and vertebra in the screw voxels that do not bear load. First, a bone mask erosion was performed moving down the screw mask a certain distance. After reaming the bone mask, the implant was placed back to its original position, resulting in a loss of contact in the screw voxels that do not transfer load in the screw pull-out. Due to the use of a voxel mesh, the bone reaming used to define

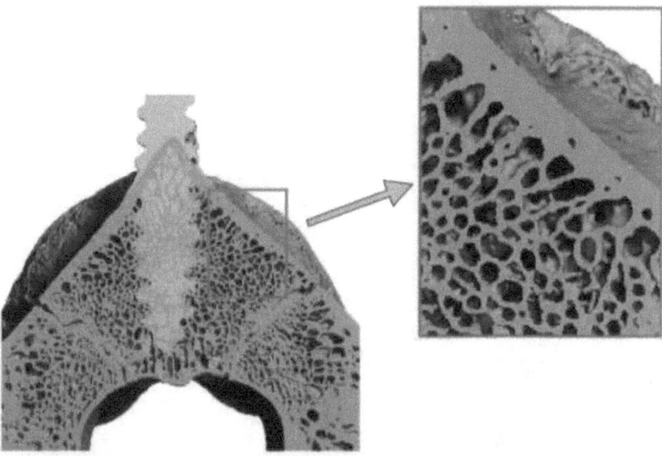

Figure 5.14: 3D registration of the models pre- and post-insertion. In the detail, (in blue) we can distinguish the overlapping after the model transformation. The differences (in red) result from the different threshold segmentation.

the contact zone needs to be studied. Through this approach, node to node contact (between voxel corners) may still occur, so we studied different mask translations (or bone reaming) in a range of [45–270] μm, corresponding to 1 to 6 pixels distance reaming to control load bearing.

5.3.4 Pull-out test

Pull-out tests were carried out on each sample using an Instron (E3000) testing machine at Maastricth University (UMC+) facilities. The fixtures used to position the samples in the experimental tests allow the rotation in different planes to ensure the alignment during uniaxial testing, see Fig. 5.15. A linear response is expected in the pull-out test until the progressive damage and failure occurs. We define the pull-out strength (F_{po}) as the peak value of the force-displacement response while the stiffness K (N/mm) is defined as the slope of the linear response.

The test fixtures were positioned to perform an uniaxial tension test and a displacement ratio of 60 mm/min was defined with a data acquisition frequency of 10 Hz. A pre-load of 45 N was defined for each test.

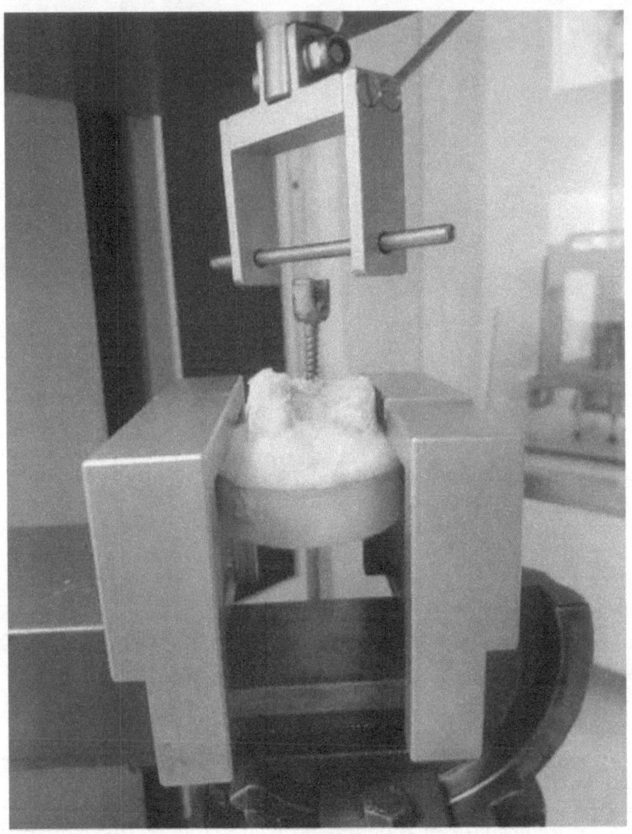

Figure 5.15: Pull-out test montage. It can be distinguished the rotative device to ensure uniaxial test conditions.

The force-displacement response of the experimental tests is used to validate the finite element models for failure strength prediction. The displacement recorded in the pull-out test takes into account the displacement of the entire assembly and was measured using the load cell displacement, so we hypothesize that the local relative displacement between screw and vertebra is lower than the recorded one.

5.3.5 Finite element modeling

Finite element models voxel-based were generated from the segmented micro-CT images, using the voxel to finite element conversion of SCANCO software. This approach has been extensively used and validated to model the elastic response of bone tissue [48].

Due to the size of the samples and the resolution of the images, it was not feasible to simulate the whole vertebra within an acceptable calculation time. This motivated us to calculate the dimensions of the volume of interest to reduce the computational resources needed. Furthermore, the FE models were also used to analyze the influence of the screw depth insertion and the pull-out strength.

Regarding the material properties of each component, we defined two different linear elastic isotropic materials: Titanium alloy ($E_{Ti} = 110$ GPa, $\nu_{Ti} = 0.3$) and bone ($E_{bone} = 10$ GPa, $\nu_{bone} = 0.3$) [250].

The boundary conditions consist in the application of a displacement in the top face nodes of the screw and the constraint of the nodes of bone at the lateral faces, while the nodes at the bottom face were left free.

5.3.5.1 VOI dimensions estimation

Few works in the literature have addressed explicitly the estimation of the volume of interest (VOI) dimensions when studying the pull-out strength [199, 201, 251]. In [201], the authors analyze what they call global and local VOIs. The global VOI is a cylinder of 26.5 mm diameter and 9.3 mm height, while the local VOIs are cylinders of 7 mm diameter and 9.3 mm height. In [251], a parallelepiped VOI of 12x12x18 mm is studied, while [199] analyze a cubic VOI of 17 mm side beam-lattice model. In the case of Gabet et al. [184] the VOI used to perform morphometric analysis accounted for 0.9 mm from the implant surface. However, the dimensions considered seem to be arbitrary or at least the authors did not mention any reason.

We carried out a convergence study to estimate the VOI dimensions from a morphometric and mechanic perspectives. We consider the VOI to be parallelepiped-shaped and centered on the screw. Different VOI dimensions are analyzed, from 8 to 23 mm parallelepiped side, maintaining constant the

VOI height. The morphometric approach consists in the analysis of morphology evolution for increasing VOI side size, while the numerical simulation approach consists in performing linear elastic simulations of different VOI sizes and evaluate the reaction force from the simulations to assess the distance limit at which cancellous bone bears loading.

5.3.5.2 Screw depth insertion study

We found few studies dealing with the study of the influence of the depth insertion on the pull-out reaction force [196, 197]. In these studies, the authors conducted pull-out tests on synthetic cancellous bone of different apparent densities, trying to mimic either healthy or osteoporotic cancellous bone. They analyzed the influence of different factors such as density, insertion angle or insertion depth both alone and combined, proposing a surrogate model to estimate the pull-out strength.

In our study, the influence of the screw depth insertion on the pull-out strength was assessed using finite element models. A range of depth insertion between 5 to 20 mm is analyzed.

5.3.5.3 Pull-out strength estimation

Our numerical approach to estimate the pull-out strength is based on Pistoia criterion, that evaluates high strained volumes inside the VOI [125].

Fig. 5.16 shows a scheme of Pistoia criterion. Bone failure is assumed to happen when a significant volume tissue is overloaded. Specifically, the overloading is considered as exceeding a critical limit of effective strain, defined as $\varepsilon_c = 0.7\%$ in the literature. However, we analyze critical strain to vary in a range of values reported in the literature for yield strain [0.6-0.9] % [72, 73, 75]. In the analyses, the effective strain at the tissue level is dependent of the strain-energy density U and the Young's modulus E (Eq. 5.1).

$$\varepsilon_{\text{eff}} = \sqrt{\frac{2U}{E}} \tag{5.1}$$

Pistoia et al. [125] investigated the critical volume threshold that lead to best prediction. Similarly, we performed a parametric analysis about critical volume, varying it between 0.5 and 6 %.

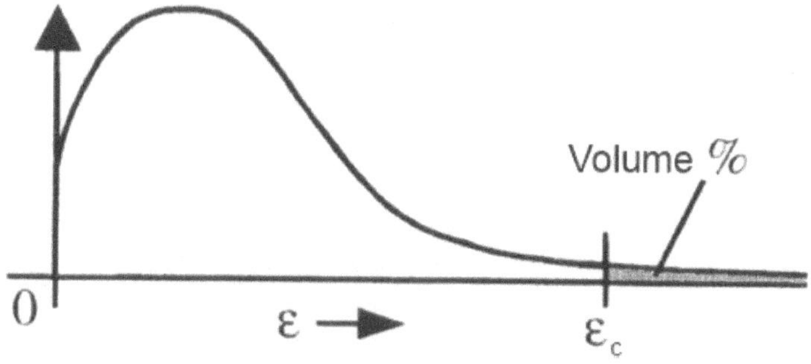

Figure 5.16: Pistoia criterion scheme: Failure occurs when a percentage of the volume under analysis reaches a critical strain value (ε_c).

The calculation method of the pull-out strength may be explained as follows: for a force-displacement simulation, the effective strain distribution for the vertebra is represented using an histogram. This histogram can be scaled for other force magnitudes. The pull-out strength is calculated as the one that makes the histogram to match Pistoia criterion critical values. Then, we calculate the percentage differences between the numerical prediction and the experimental results for each pair of critical parameters, computing the overall estimation error, Eq. 5.2, where E_i is the percentage difference between prediction and estimation and N is the number of samples in our data set.

$$E_{estimation} = \sqrt{\sum_{i=1}^{N} E_i^2} \tag{5.2}$$

5.4 Results and discussion

5.4.1 Pull-out test

The force-displacement response recorded in the pull-out tests for the three samples is shown in Fig. 5.17. The responses show high reproducibility and a linear behavior followed by a rapid decrease, corresponding to the appearance of damage prior to complete pull-out failure. In Table 5.3, a summary of the stiffness and the pull-out strength for each tested sample can be found, estimated from the force-displacement experimental data.

Table 5.3: Pull-out strength and stiffness of the three porcine vertebrae estimated from the experimental response data

Sample	K [N/mm]	F_{po} [N]
Vertebra #1	557.55	1550
Vertebra #2	575.54	1600
Vertebra #3	538.76	1390

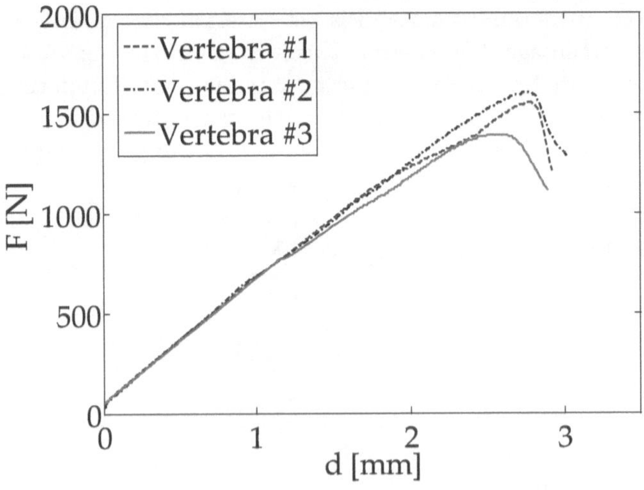

Figure 5.17: Force-displacement response of the three porcine vertebrae in the pull-out test

5.4.1.1 Morphometric analysis

The following morphometric parameters were estimated for different VOI sizes for vertebra #1: BV/TV, BS/BV, Tb.N, Tb.Th, Tb.Sp and DA. As expected, it can be noted that the values of the microstructural parameters tend to converge as we increase the VOI dimensions, Fig. 5.18. If the morphometry affects the pull-out strength, it is important to know the amount of bone to be considered around the implant for the analysis. The VOI dimensions for which convergence is achieved are similar to the obtained in the numerical convergence analysis of section 5.4.2.3, around 17 mm.

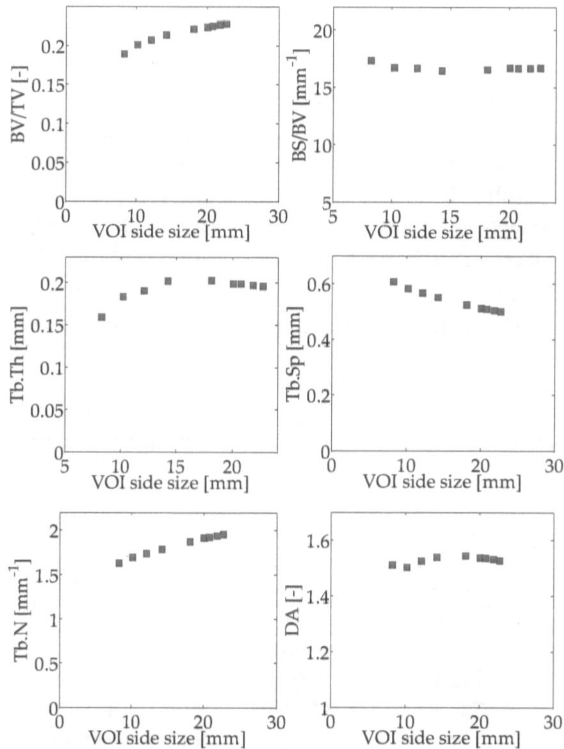

Figure 5.18: Microstructural parameters estimated varying VOI dimensions. The values tend to converge for increasing VOI size.

Table 5.4: Microstructural parameters estimated for each vertebra in a VOI of 17 mm side.

Sample	BV/TV [-]	BS/BV [mm^{-1}]	Tb.N [mm^{-1}]	Tb.Th [mm]	Tb.Sp [mm]	DA [-]
Vertebra #1	0.218	16.56	1.81	0.1208	0.432	1.545
Vertebra #2	0.261	15.32	2.00	0.1306	0.369	1.521
Vertebra #3	0.219	14.80	1.62	0.1351	0.483	1.636

We estimated the microstructural parameters for a VOI of 17 mm side for each vertebra, Table 5.4. The morphology analysis aims at exploring regressions between the parameters that define the VOI microstructure and the measured pull-out strength and stiffness. Some of the parameters are similar between samples so the conclusions extracted from the regressions are limited and should be confirmed with extended data sets.

The results obtained for the relationships between morphometry and pull-out strength (Table 5.5) and stiffness (Table 5.6) show that some parameters have a significant influence on them. For example, anisotropy degree (DA) is the parameter that better correlates to the pull-out strength ($R^2 = 0.999$) for the 3 points available. Further, mean trabecular separation and trabecular number correlate well to the pull-out strength, Table 5.5. Those significant tendencies are depicted in Fig. 5.19. Nevertheless, we would like to emphasize that both the correlation and the lack of correlation are limited to only 3 points, so some of them may be spurious while other may be more significant than reported.

Table 5.5: Parameters defining the regressions between microstructure and the pull-out strength estimated experimentally. Linear regressions in form $F_{\text{pullout}} = A_x x + B$. The correlation coefficient (R^2) for each case is reported.

$F_{\text{pullout}}(param)$	A_x	B	R^2
BV/TV	3014.1	811.55	0.462
BS/BV	66.791	474.15	0.3034
Tb.N	546.48	524.6	0.913
Tb.Th	-8551	2615	0.325
Tb.Sp	-1800.4	2284	0.877
DA	-1799.9	4334.3	0.999

On the other hand, we also estimated regressions between microstructural parameters of each sample and the stiffness from the experimental pull-out

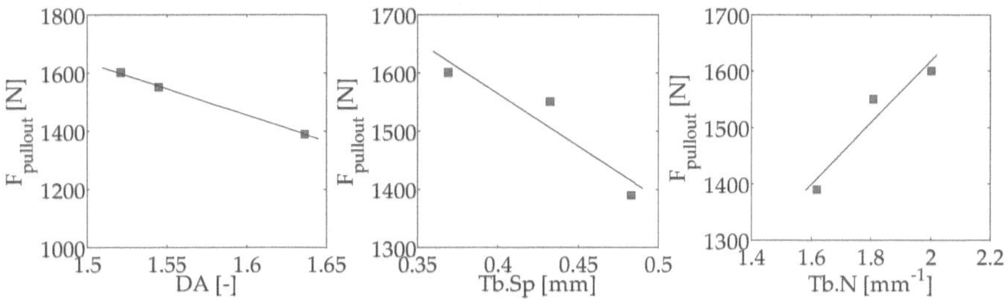

Figure 5.19: Significant linear relationships calculated between morphometry (DA, Tb.Sp and Tb.N) and pull-out strength.

tests. The most significant linear relationships were found to trabecular number (Tb.N), mean trabecular separation (Tb.Sp), degree of anisotropy (DA) and bone volume fraction (BV/TV), depicted in Fig. 5.20. Moreover, the regression results for all the morphometric parameters are summarized in Table 5.6. It is noteworthy that only three samples (n=3) were used in the study, so the results obtained need to be confirmed in larger datasets.

Table 5.6: Parameters defining the regressions between microstructure and stiffness, estimated from the force-displacement response in the pull-out tests. Linear regressions in form $K = A_x x + B$.

$K(param)$	A_x	B	R^2
BV/TV	636.71	409.04	0.7336
BS/BV	6.0533	463.1	0.0886
Tb.N	95.871	383.83	0.9997
Tb.Th	-804.32	660.91	0.1023
Tb.Sp	-321.32	694.83	0.9941
DA	-287	1007.1	0.9035

In the literature, there is no consensus about which morphometric parameters affect at a higher degree to the stiffness and strength on an implant inserted in a vertebra. Some of the results are contradictory, so deeper analysis are needed to extract more robust conclusions. For example, in [184], it is claimed that the parameters that better correlate to the pull-out strength are mean trabecular thickness and bone volume fraction. We also found correla-

tion between stiffness and BV/TV, but not between strength or stiffness and
Tb.Th. A work from Wirth et al. [201] found some parameters to correlate,
such as BV/TV, Tb.Th, Tb.Sp, and Tb.N, but they did not for every sample
in their study. Therefore, a more accurate strength prediction may depend on
a combination of parameters that define mechanical competence.

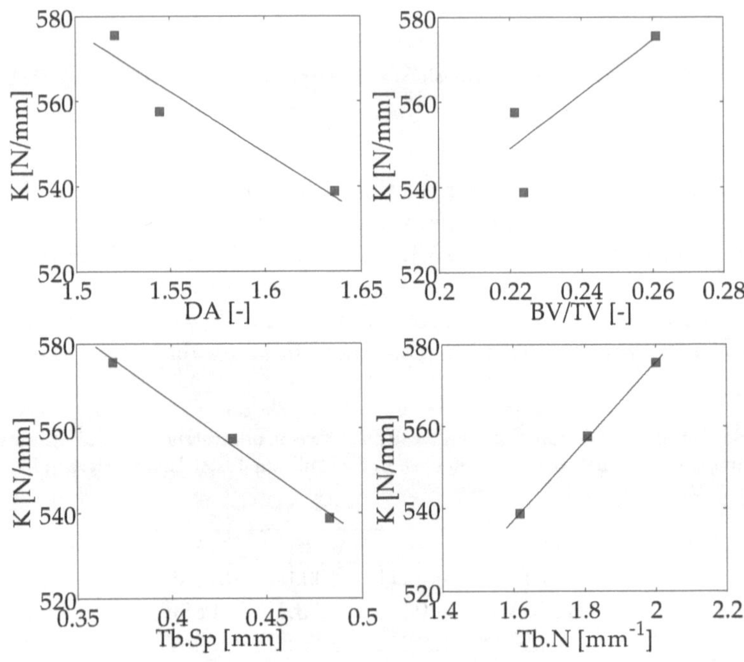

Figure 5.20: Regressions with a significant correlation between bone-screw stiffness and
anisotropy degree (DA), bone volume fraction (BV/TV), mean trabecular separation (Tb.Sp)
and trabecular number (Tb.N).

5.4.2 Finite element modeling

Finite element models of 45 μm resolution were generated to predict the pull-out strength of a screw inserted in the vertebral body of three porcine vertebrae. To achieve the goal, other objectives emerged, like the estimation of the VOI dimensions, the influence of screw placement configuration or its depth insertion.

Linear elastic simulations were carried out. In Fig. 5.21, the effective strain distribution of the screw pull-out simulation for each sample is shown in a cut containing the screw. It can be noted that the load bearing is produced in the cortical cortex and in cancellous bone up to a certain distance from the implant. Depending on the morphometry and the contact regions, the load bearing changes, see Fig. 5.21.

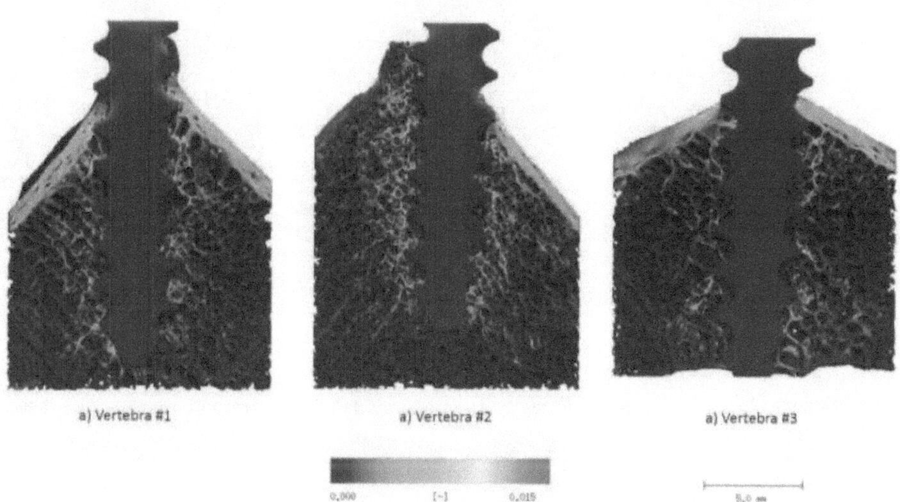

Figure 5.21: Finite element results of the effective strain contours in the mid-plane of the screw-bone model.

Load bearing is even more clearly distinguished in Fig. 5.22, where the strain contours for each VOI are presented without the implant. Vertebrae #1 and #2 show high strained areas in the screw thread contact in the cortical and cancellous regions, while the high strained areas are less in case of Vertebra #3, and almost appear in the cortex only. This situation correlates to the pull-out strength measured experimentally and indicates that the amount of bone in contact to the implant and the trabecular architecture have a major importance on the load-bearing and thus in the pull-out strength.

On the other hand, as discussed in section 3.2.1, reaming the bone mask to define contact and considering full bonding on the interface may be realistic from the point of view that it represents a fully osseointegrated implant and assuming that screw-bone interlocking dominates other modes like friction within pull-out [201]. Further, much less computational resources are needed than when considering the non-linearities associated to this problem.

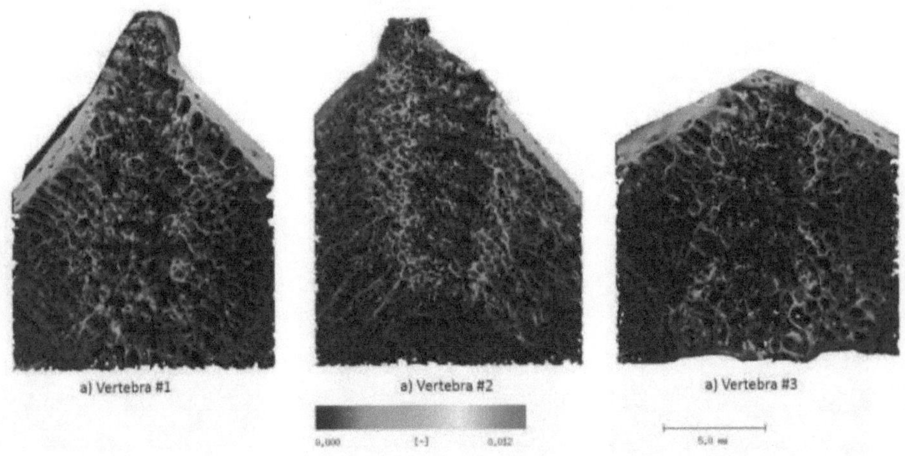

Figure 5.22: Effective strain contours on the bone model. High strained areas can be distinguished as result of the pull-out simulation

5.4.2.1 Screw virtual placement

We inserted the screw virtually in the bone mask in order to avoid image artifacts from the post-insertion micro-CT acquisition. To perform more realistic simulations, we considered bone reaming resulting from implant insertion by eroding bone mask after the translation over a distance in the insertion direction. The voxel characteristics of the finite element mesh made necessary to analyze the effect of the reaming distance to avoid contact on the screw thread reaming side, that would lead to less realistic load bearing, Fig. 5.23.

Then, we performed analysis to evaluate bone reaming effect over a range of [1-6] pixels displacement from its original position, corresponding to between 0.045 and 0.27 mm reaming displacement. Fig. 5.23 shows the image-based finite element models for reaming between 1 to 4 pixels. It can be noted, in red, contact regions in the reaming thread side that, as the reaming distance increases they detach, a loss of contact occurs and load transmission is more realistic, see areas marked in yellow in Fig. 5.23.

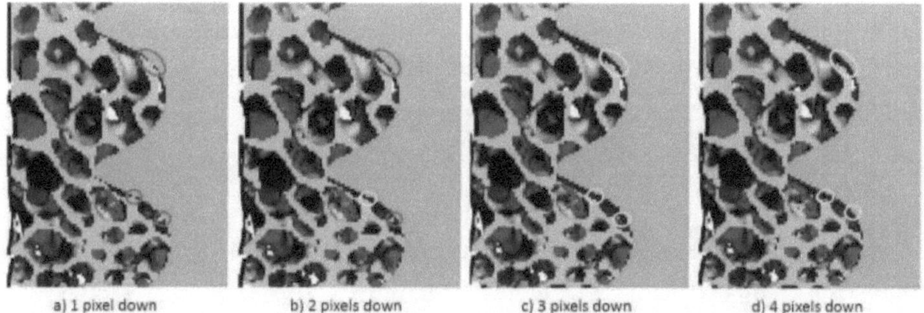

Figure 5.23: Detail of the contact zones after the virtual screw placement modeling bone reaming due to screw insertion over a number of pixels: a) 1 pixel, b) 2 pixels, c) 3 pixels and d) 4 pixels. In red, contact zones in the screw reaming side that should be avoided. In yellow, detachment occurs after reaming bone mask a certain distance, making load transmission more realistic.

Stress distribution results for bone reaming distances of 1 to 4 pixels are shown in Fig. 5.24. For some of the configurations, the bone-screw contact cannot be avoided in the reaming side of the thread, marked in red in Fig. 5.24. Increasing the reaming distance permits to disconnect those nodes, marked in yellow. However, as can be seen in Fig. 5.24 d) (in red), this screw placement approach cannot avoid node to node contact on the screw thread tips.

Moreover, we analyzed the bone reaming influence to place the implant on the variation of the reaction force from the simulations for a VOI side size of 8 mm, Fig. 5.25. Reaming effect is significant so it influences around a 14%

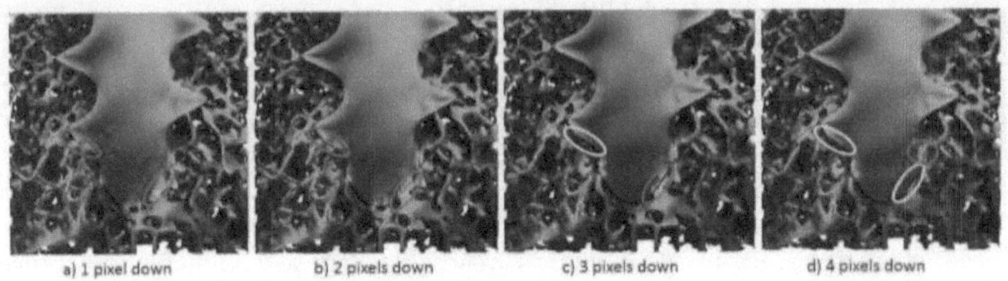

Figure 5.24: von Misses stress distribution after the virtual screw placement, considering bone mask reaming over a distance of a) 1 pixel, b) 2 pixels, c) 3 pixels and d) 4 pixels. In red, none realistic contact regions. In yellow, contact detachment areas after reaming.

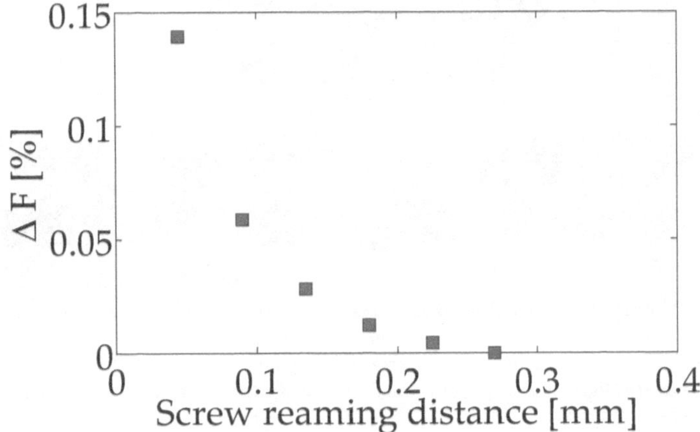

Figure 5.25: Reaming distance influence on the variation of the reaction force. A maximum reaming distance of 0.27 mm corresponds to 6 pixels.

for a reaming distance of 0.045 mm and it converges for a distance of 0.27 mm, corresponding to 6 pixels reaming distance. We also quantified this effect varying the VOI side size dimensions between 8 to 22.4 mm, Table 5.7. As expected, the influence is greater for lower VOI side sizes and it also tends to converge to about a 6 % influence on the reaction force for a VOI side size of around 22 mm, Table 5.7.

Table 5.7: Influence of the screw virtual placement configurations (corresponding to 1 and 6 pixels down movements) on the numerical estimation of the failure force.

VOI size side [mm]	Δ_{1-6} Failure force [%]
8	-13.9
10	-11.6
12	-10
14	-8.8
17.1	-7.6
19.8	-6.8
20.6	-6.6
21.6	-6.5
22.4	-6.2

5.4.2.2 Screw depth insertion study

In Fig. 5.26, we present the numerical results of the influence of the screw depth insertion on the reaction force from the simulations. As was expected, a decreasing load is obtained as the depth insertion decreases. The lower the screw depth insertion is, the lower is the stress transmission to the cancellous lattice, while the load bearing to the cortical cortex is equivalent. Therefore, the results in Fig. 5.26 reflect cancellous bone load-bearing capacity, which seems to be non-linear. To evaluate it, we explored linear and non-linear regressions.

Different regressions were checked out: linear, quadratic and logarithmic. All of them lead to high correlations but a quadratic relationship ($F_{po} = -1.42d^2_{screw} + 73.8d_{screw} + 743.3$, $R^2 = 0.9982$) was found as the best descriptor of the screw depth insertion influence, compared to linear ($F_{po} = 37.9d_{screw} + 943.4$, $R^2 = 0.9766$) and logarithmic ($F_{po} = 437.6ln(d_{screw}) + 344.3$, $R^2 = 0.9941$) relationships. However, the high correlation coefficient of the linear regression makes it a good approximation for studying this effect according to our data.

Our results about screw depth insertion are in line with others in the literature [196, 197], where the authors found higher pull-out force as the depth insertion increased, but they did not estimate regression models. Anyway, the force evolution in their study is very similar to our numerical estimation with a quadratic/logarithmic shape.

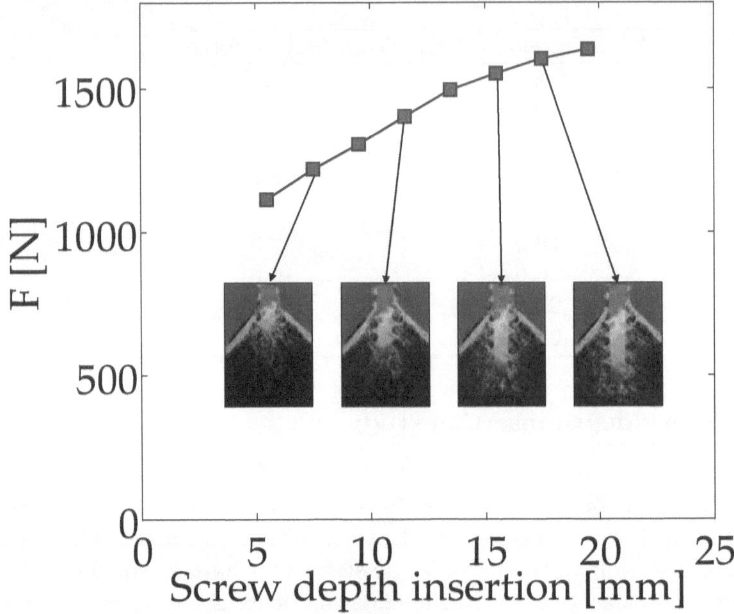

Figure 5.26: Effect of the screw depth insertion on the reaction force for Vertebra #1.

5.4.2.3   VOI dimensions estimation

We analyzed how reaction force is affected by the dimensions of the VOI. The results for the analysis for Vertebra #1 are depicted in Fig. 5.27. Similar results were obtained for Vertebrae #2 and #3. The results point out that pull-out has influence not only on the bone in contact to the implant but also on the bone at a certain distance. The reaction force decreases and converges to a value as the VOI side dimensions increase. Therefore, based on these results, we may define a VOI of 22 mm diameter to estimate the pull-out strength numerically. Our results are in line with other VOI dimensions defined in the literature for an analogous situation[201, 251]. However, this study is limited because of the screw insertion location. In the clinical practice, the implant is inserted in the pedicles and there is not such amount of cancellous bone to be considered in the models, so the whole pedicles should be included in the analyses.

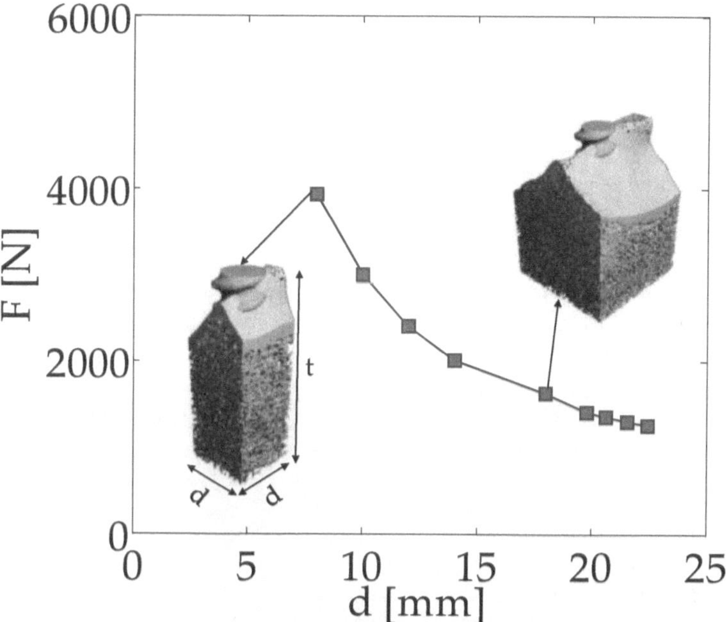

Figure 5.27: VOI dimensions estimation. The reaction force decreases for increasing VOI side size, which highlights that load bearing includes bone up to a certain distance.

5.4.2.4 Pull-out strength estimation

We used Pistoia criterion to predict failure as the load at which a critical volume exceeds a critical strain. It involves two parameters: critical volume and critical strain. When it was proposed, the authors considered a critical strain of 0.007 as the compression yield strain [125], and studied the critical volume that led to best failure load prediction, which was 2 % of the volume. Similarly, we developed a parametric analysis about those two variables within the following ranges: in case of critical strain, some works report values between 0.006 and 0.009 (Table. 1.4), while we varied the critical volume from 0.5 to 6 %.

The results of the parametric study about failure criterion are presented as pullout force prediction error as a function of failure parameters, shown in Fig. 5.28. We can clearly distinguish a part of the surface where the estimation error is larger. For example, errors from 50% to 200% on the pull-out strength estimation can be found when considering a critical strain equal or greater than 0.008 and critical volumes larger than 2 %.

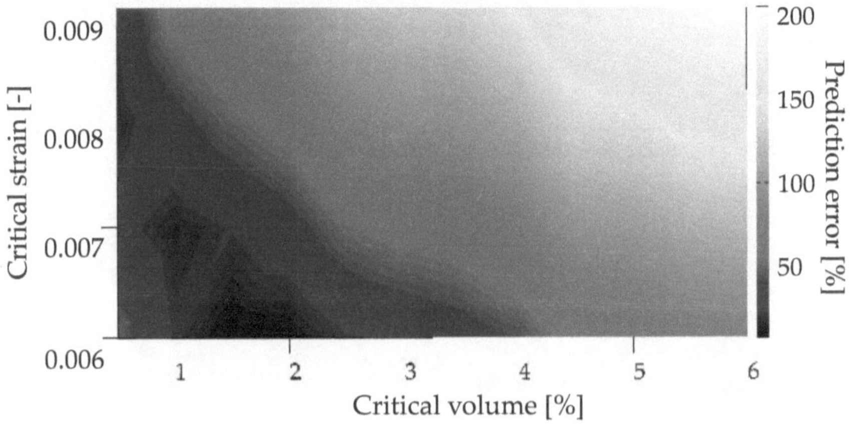

Figure 5.28: Strain distribution for each sample under study.

On the other hand, the region defined by critical strains between 0.006 and 0.008 and critical volumes between 1 to 3 % presents errors lower than

20%, Fig. 5.28. Within this area, a minimum estimation error is achieved considering a critical volume of between 1 and 2% and a critical strain of between 0.006 and 0.007, leading to around 8% error on the estimation of the pull out strength for our data set.

Pull-out strength values, estimated through finite element models and experiments are summarized in Table 5.8. We defined a critical volume of 1%, and a critical strain of 0.007 for the results presented in Table 5.8. A good level of accuracy is found on the failure strength prediction using those critical values, Fig. 5.29.

Table 5.8: Pull-out strength of the three porcine vertebrae estimated from experimental tests ($F_{\text{PO,exp}}$) and on an adaption of Pistoia criterion ($F_{\text{PO,predicted}}$).

Sample	$F_{\text{PO,exp}}$ [N]	$F_{\text{PO,predicted}}$ [N]
Vertebra #1	1550	1580.4
Vertebra #2	1600	1514.8
Vertebra #3	1390	1240.2

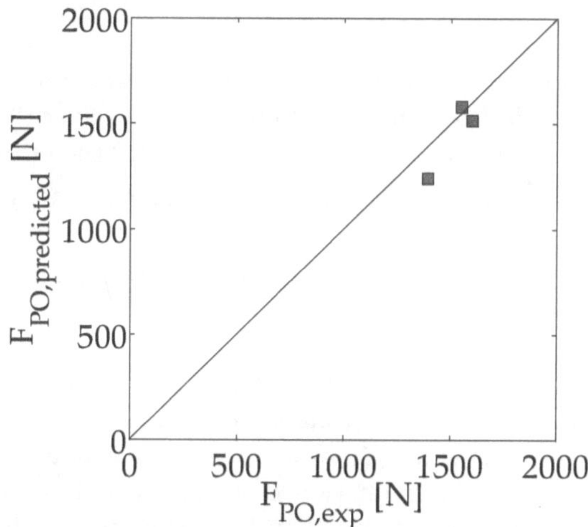

Figure 5.29: Comparison between pull-out strength prediction using micro-FE and Pistoia criterion and experimental measurements.

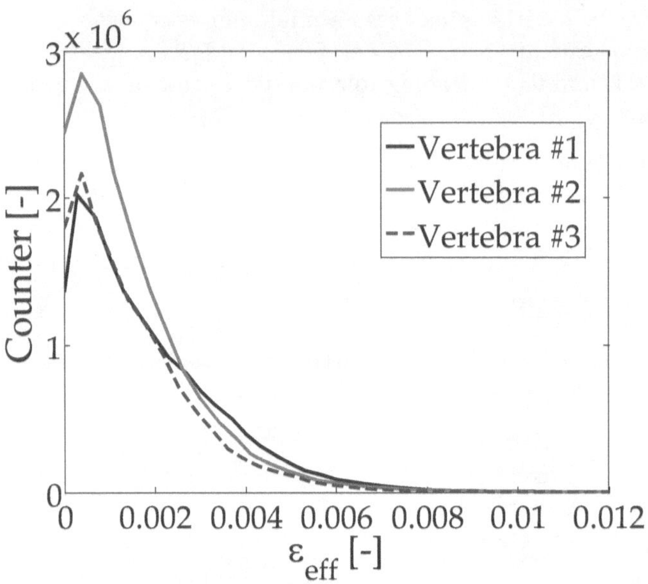

Figure 5.30: Strain distribution for each sample under study.

The failure criterion considered in this study takes into account the percentage of volume suffering from strains greater than the critical strain. Thus, the selection and definition of the VOI is relevant for the criterion.

In Fig. 5.30, the effective strain distribution for a VOI of 17 mm side is shown for each vertebra. We can notice how Vertebra #1 shows a higher stressed area than Vertebrae #2 and #3 in the strain histogram. This leads to a higher pull-out strength estimation.

Based on our results, we can state that a simple linear criterion that takes into account a high strained bone volume permits to achieve enough accuracy to estimate the pull-out strength of a screw inserted in a vertebral body. This way, a quick first approximation of failure load is performed and less computational resources are needed than if considering non-linearities.

In the literature, Niebur et al. [72] reported that at the apparent compressive yield point, 2.5 % of cancellous bone tissue had exceeded the tissue yield strain, which is a similar critical volume threshold than our estimation.

Other works have addressed the problem in an analogous way [200]. They performed a parametric study about the critical volume fraction and the VOI dimensions on the pull-out strength estimation and found that for a VOI of 4.7 mm radius around the implant, a critical volume of 84 % led to the best correlation. This high strained volume is much higher than the one we considered and highlights the importance of VOI dimensions estimation. The VOI dimensions we proposed are larger than those but the failure load prediction was notably accurate. On the other hand, a work from Wirth et al. [201] pointed out the importance of microstructural features variability for the evaluation of screw-bone constructs stiffness. Furthermore, they claimed that not all the same morphometric parameters were suitable for failure prediction for different samples, so it may be a combination of microstructural parameters which are responsible of an accurate prediction. Nevertheless, parameters like BV/TV, Tb.Th, Tb.Sp and Tb.N were suitable for failure prediction for some of the samples [201].

We acknowledge some limitations in this study. First, we analyzed three samples, so our conclusions are limited to them and should be confirmed in larger data sets. Secondly, the location of the screw did not follow clinical guidelines. Spine screw fixation is performed through the pedicles and we inserted them in the vertebral body. This conditions the conclusions about the VOI dimensions estimation because there is not much bone around the screws when inserted in the pedicles, so the whole bone pedicles region may be needed in the models. The image resolution used for the finite element models generation is on the limit to properly define cancellous bone microstructure and it is possible to have few elements along the tissue thickness, so the strain calculation in some points may be inaccurate. However, the strain distribution histogram was demonstrated not to be much affected by those errors [125]. Furthermore, the virtual screw placement did not account for the damage induced during insertion and we also considered perfect bonding in the screw-bone interface. Full bonding would represent a fully osseointegrated implant, neglecting friction or peri-implant damage. However, this approximation may be appropriate as screw-bone interlocking dominates frictional and detachment phenomena [201]. Moreover, we carried out linear elastic simulations to predict failure, which is a non-linear event, so more complex models would be needed to perform more accurate predictions of local failure effects.

5.5 Conclusions

In this chapter, we have evaluated spine fixation techniques for scoliosis treatment from two different approaches. The first one consists in the development of density-based finite element models of clinical images resolution of two fixation techniques: pedicle screws and sublaminar tape. The second approach is based on the generation of micro-FE models of a bone-screw construct to predict its pull-out strength.

With regards to the first approach, a human vertebra was scanned by micro-CT at clinical resolution and was used to compare the stress distribution resulting from each configuration from numerical simulations. The models reproduce bilateral pull-out bending tests conducted on other specimens, where pull-out load is applied through a bending moment, which is closer to the *in vivo* fixation situation. Material properties were assigned at the tissue level as a function of density measurements from micro-CT and two meshes were generated: a coarse voxel mesh and a fine tetrahedral mesh.

The models allowed to estimate the load bearing through the vertebra for each fixation construct. Pedicle screws induce a bending moment in the testing configuration, that does not occur in the sublaminar tape configuration. Highly loaded regions in PS were found in the pedicles, where the induced moment was relevant for the deformation state, in the cortical cortex and in the trabecular lattice around the screw. The implants affect a large region of cancellous bone in the vertebral body and are much more invasive than sublaminar tape configuration.

On the other hand, sublaminar tape induces high strains in the lamina, due to wires attachment, in the pedicles as reaction from the wires anchorage and in the cortical cortex, which bore some of the loading. The highly loaded regions predicted by the finite element models match the experimental observations of failure modes and location for the two fixation configurations analyzed.

Furthermore, failure load was estimated using a simple linear criterion that considers failure as the load at which the tensile yield stress is exceeded and similar values were obtained for both configurations, but significantly higher for the sublaminar tape (around a 3.5 %). Therefore, sublaminar tape provides a similar and significantly higher pull-out strength than pedicle screws and is much less invasive because it requires much less surgical interventions and permits its use with growth-guidance systems, particularly relevant for early onset scoliosis treatment.

Regarding the second approach, we analyzed pedicle screw fixation in three porcine vertebrae using micro-FE to predict pull-out strength. Morphometry was also studied to relate pull-out strength and stiffness from experiments to the underlying microstructure. Parameters like anisotropy degree (DA), mean trabecular separation (Tb.Sp) and trabecular number (Tb.N) correlated to pull-out strength and stiffness. Also, bone volume fraction (BV/TV) correlated to the pull-out stiffness. However, our regressions were calculated using only three points, so they need to be confirmed with extended datasets.

The morphometry was also estimated for different VOI side sizes in order to evaluate cancellous bone homogeneity within a vertebral body and we found that a volume around the implant of about 17 mm was representative in terms of morphometry. VOI side size was also estimated from numerical models, analyzing the reaction force variation for increasing VOI side size, and that force converged for a VOI of around 22 mm. Then, the morphometry and FE approaches lead to similar VOI side size results.

On the other hand, we explored the bone reaming effect that results from screw insertion on the variation of the reaction force. Specifically, we aim at finding more realistic load bearing for full bonding contact simulations, and we studied bone reaming distances between 0.045 to 0.27 mm. A bone reaming distance of 0.23 permits to avoid load transmission through the reaming thread side of the screw. Reaming has a different contribution according to VOI dimensions. It decreases for increasing VOI size until a difference of 7 % for a VOI side size of about 20 mm compared to a reaming distance of 0.045 mm.

Screw depth insertion was also important for the pull-out strength. The deeper it is, the larger the force, as it could be expected. The load transmission to the cortical cortex was equivalent between insertion depth, so the differences could be attributed to cancellous bone load bearing, which obviously decreases for a lower insertion depth. The relationship obtained could be approximated with a second order polynomial or with a linear regression, with high accuracy for both cases.

Finally, we predicted pull-out failure using a high strained volume criterion, known as Pistoia criterion. It considers failure to occur when a percentage of volume exceeds a strain threshold, usually the compression yield strain. It is a simple criterion that has been used as an approximation in several works in the literature with pretty good performance. We analyzed the pull-out strength estimation in a parametric study over the critical strain and the critical volume. The results show that the best predictions were performed for a critical strain of between 0.006 and 0.007 and a critical volume between 1 and 2 %. The compressive yield strain values reported in the literature match those values. The failure criterion values results show that a low percentage of volume that undergoes strains greater than the yield strain is enough to produce pull-out failure. Using those parameters, we predicted the pull-out strength of the three samples tested with a good accuracy and differences less than 8 %. Therefore, a simple failure criterion that accounts for high strained regions over the VOI may be enough as an approximation to predict pull-out failure.

Chapter 6

book conclusions and main contributions

6.1 Conclusions

In this book, we have addressed the problem of mechanical and morphomet-ric characterization of cancellous bone tissue and surrogates. The mechanical characterization was conducted from experimental and numerical approaches, while the morphometry was assessed by analyzing cancellous bone images acquired by micro-computed tomography. Moreover, we studied how microstructure influences the mechanical performance of cancellous bone-like structures.

Morphometry and segmentation

With regards to morphometry characterization, the following parameters were estimated: BV/TV, BS/BV, BS/TV, Tb.Th, Tb.Sp, Tb.N, D_{2D}, D_{3D}, $DA_{MIL,2D}$, $DA_{MIL,3D}$ and Conn.D. Morphometry estimation depends on image segmentation and we studied its influence for three cancellous bone specimens of different volume fraction.

A segmentation threshold variation of $\pm$ 15 % produced changes in the microstructure as a function of the BV/TV of the sample. This may result in the disruption of trabecular microstructure for low BV/TV samples, while for samples of higher volume fraction is less critic. Then, segmentation threshold has a greater importance for the analysis of osteoporotic samples because it may cause the loss of connectivity and a wrong morphometric characterization.

Some parameters were little influenced by segmentation threshold variation, such as anisotropy degree, with a maximum effect of 4 % for a 15 % threshold increment. Other parameters were linearly influenced, such as BV/TV and Tb.Th, presenting variations for the limit segmentation threshold values of -64 % to 55 % for BV/TV and of -20 % to 24 % for Tb.Th.

Other parameters showed a non-linear influence for segmentation variation, such as BS/BV, BS/TV, Tb.Sp, Tb.N, Conn.D and fractal dimension, and that non-linear effect was greater for samples of lower BV/TV. For example, connectivity density (Conn.D) increased for a greater threshold up to a point that defined the beginning of trabecular connections disruption.

On the other hand, we also evaluated segmentation influence on the apparent modulus estimated using finite element models developed from segmented masks. We report variations of between 45 to 120 % for the limits that we considered for threshold variation, which shows the importance of an accurate segmentation. Furthermore, this study permitted to obtain a power relationship between apparent modulus and bone volume fraction, in agreement with the literature.

Mechanical characterization

With regards to the mechanical characterization, we followed experimental and numerical approaches. The first one includes compression testing and DIC application to images taken during testing, while the numerical analysis involves finite element modeling based on images acquired by micro-CT.

Quasi-static compression tests permitted to assess the elastic and failure behavior at the apparent or macro level. The specimens presented an orthotropic behavior with a direction of higher stiffness, aligned to the main trabecular orientation, while the other two directions showed similar stiffness but significantly different.

Furthermore, we estimated tissue elastic properties of cancellous bone from FE and a phantom-based approach. A tissue Young's modulus of 11.09 ± 1.69 GPa was assessed through a back calculation approach, while using a modulus-density relationship from Morgan et al. [130] provided similar estimations, about 10.45 ± 0.18 GPa.

The stiffness matrix was estimated for 5 of the cancellous bone specimens tested and the results were compared to the experimental measurements, finding accurate numerical prediction for the main trabecular orientation direction and numerical overestimation for the transversal directions. We hypothesize and confirmed for the main direction that the estimation about the transversal directions were performed under a strain range level lower than the one where stiffness is approximately constant, prior to failure onset, so the differences about that directions were explained.

We used digital image correlation to estimate surface displacements and failure strains on the fractured areas. First, we assessed the influence of DIC parameters variation on strain estimation at failure. Facet and step sizes have a relevant effect on the failure strain estimation, and an increment of both parameters reduce the strain estimation up to 40 %. Besides, several parameters combination lead to correct failure pattern detection, so values reported in the literature should be referred to the parameters used.

Furthermore, shear strain (γ_{12}), equivalent strain (ε_{eq}) and principal strain (ε_1) were evaluated as variables for failure pattern description and ε_{eq} emerged as the most accurate one. Finally, using a facet size of 125 pixels, 10 pixels of step size, normalized sum of squared differences pattern matching criterion, incremental correlation and a filter strain size of 15 pixels led to the estimation of a maximum equivalent strain at the apparent yield and ultimate points of 2.42 % and 3.66 %, respectively.

Our numerical approach to estimate cancellous bone failure strain properties consisted of a combination of elastic properties degradation, under a damage approach, and the elimination of finite elements at fracture conditions through the element deletion technique. The damage law used was suitable to reproduce the experimental force-displacement curve until the ultimate point and allowed the estimation of a tissue yield strain close to 0.7 %. In case of the ultimate strain ($\varepsilon_{f,c}$), more scattering was found and values in the range 2.8 to 5.25 % were calculated. The behavior of yield and failure strains estimated numerically supports observations reported in the literature that state that yield strain values are relatively constant, while ultimate strain values present a wider scattering.

Relationship between microstructure and mechanical response

We analyzed the dependence of mechanical parameters (E_{app}, σ_y, ε_y, σ_f and ε_f) measured in quasi-static compression tests to specimen-specific morphometric parameters. We have estimated single parameter linear regressions that have permitted to find which morphometric descriptors explain variations of mechanical properties. Specifically, bone volume fraction (BV/TV), bone surface to volume ratio (BS/BV), mean trabecular thickness (Tb.Th) and fractal dimension (D) presented the best linear correlations.

On the other hand, both the yield and failure strains did not show correlation to any morphometric parameter, except for the case of anisotropy degree calculated over the transversal plane (DA_{MIL2D} 3), which we considered as a spurious correlation because of the nearly isotropic values obtained for this parameter. Therefore, our observations regarding yield and failure strains confirm other results from the literature that claim that they are almost independent from density and microstructure.

A similar analysis was conducted relating the complete stiffness matrix of cancellous bone specimens and their microstructure. Some morphometric parameters, like BV/TV, BS/BV, Tb.Th and fractal dimension, presented linear correlation to the axial and shear stiffnesses, so their assessment may be used to estimate those properties which are difficult to measure experimentally. Moreover, multiple parameter linear regressions were proved to improve the correlation for the elastic properties prediction. For example, including BV/TV, BS/BV and fractal dimension improved the correlation for axial stiffness to R^2=0.9.

Both approaches, the experimental and the numerical one match as far as the parameters that showed influence on the mechanical properties are concerned. This enforces the conclusions obtained.

Cancellous bone surrogates analysis

Open cell polyurethane foams resemble cancellous bone microstructure. We characterized foams of three different densities from morphometric and mechanical perspectives.

Morphometry was characterized for 6 specimens scanned by micro-CT and aimed at evaluating each sample to give insight into the inhomogeneities within them. A different morphometry evolution across the samples according to density was observed. The inhomogeneities were greater for the high density (HD) foams, concentrating more material near the top and bottom surfaces. Morphometry varied according to that material distribution: for example, lower volume fraction, foam surface to volume ratio or mean trabecular thickness were measured in the central region of HD samples. Other parameters, like fractal dimension or connectivity density presented little changes within HD grade. MD foam grade is more homogeneous than HD, but present similar trends about morphometry variation within a specimen, but of a much lower degree. In case of LD foam grade, the specimens are the most homogeneous. These analyses may be used to choose between cancellous bone surrogates according to the homogeneity needed for the experiments.

With regards to the mechanical characterization, experiments and numerical elastic homogenization match regarding predicting an orthotropic, close to transversely isotropic, material behavior. In case of HD specimens, the lower material disposition in the central part makes the block thickness (we called it axial) direction less stiffer than the transversal ones. In case of MD and LD specimens, the axial direction is stiffer than the transversal ones, but at a low degree. Therefore, MD and LD specimens are also quite homogeneous regarding the stiffness about the three main directions.

Yield and ultimate stresses presented a linear relationship to the stiffness. Furthermore, yield strains were relatively constant over the foam densities studied, but a slightly decreasing yield strain was registered for increasing density. HD foams had a mean yield strain ε_y of 1.5 %, MD 1.6 % and LD 1.8 %. More scattering was found for the ultimate strain ε_f values but the trend was analogous to that of yield strain. A mean ultimate strain value of 1.9 %, 2.1 % and 2.5 % was registered for HD, MD and LD specimens. It indicates that the less dense the foam is, the greater deformations undergo prior to failure.

The influence of microstructure on the mechanical response was explored through linear regressions analysis. Similarly to for cancellous bone, parameters like FV/TV, FS/FV, Str.Th, Str.N and D showed correlation to the elastic modulus, yield and ultimate stresses and yield strain measured in the experiments. However, the regressions had only 6 points, so the correlations need to be confirmed in other data sets.

DIC permitted to estimate failure strains in the fractured regions. Similar yield strain values were measured for each foam grade, which supports the idea that foams failure is strain-controlled and may be independent of density. A mean value of 0.078 was estimated for HD, 0.062 for MD and 0.077 for LD specimens. With regards to the ultimate strain values, the mean value for each density grade was quite constant: 0.12 for HD, 0.11 for MD and 0.13 for LD group.

Regarding the numerical characterization of the compression failure behavior, we calculated tissue elastic properties using finite element models with a high level of discretization to define specimens morphology and boundary conditions that match the experiment ones, combined with the experimental response curve. A mean tissue Young's modulus of 3 GPa was estimated for HD, 2.7 GPa for MD and 1 GPa for the low density foams.

Compression failure was modeled using finite elements, material properties degradation and the element deletion technique. The models allowed to estimate by inverse analysis yield and ultimate strains for each specimen. Failure strain properties were relatively constant over the density grades analyzed. However, HD specimens presented a higher yield strain than MD and LD specimens, which may be related to the inclusion of more structural fillers in the high density group. The ultimate strain properties estimated showed little variation between samples, with a mean value close to 0.07. The model proposed detected with high accuracy the failure compression experimental pattern, which matched DIC failure prediction results. Therefore, DIC was successfully used to validate the numerical approach to model compression fracture through the detection of fractured regions.

Evaluation of spine fixation techniques

We have evaluated spine fixation techniques for scoliosis treatment from two different approaches: density-based finite element models of clinical images resolution of two fixation techniques, pedicle screws and sublaminar tape, and micro-FE models of a bone-screw construct to predict its pull-out strength.

A human vertebra was scanned by micro-CT at clinical resolution and was used to compare the stress distribution resulting from each configuration by simulating bilateral pull-out bending tests that reproduce the *in vivo* fixation situation. The models allowed to estimate the load bearing through the vertebra for each fixation construct. We observed that pedicle screws induce a bending moment in the screw head that does not occur in the sublaminar tape configuration. Highly loaded regions in screws group were found in the pedicles, where the induced moment was relevant for the deformation state, in the cortical cortex and in the trabecular lattice surrounding the screw. The implants affect a large region of cancellous bone in the vertebral body and are much more invasive than sublaminar tape configuration. On the other hand, sublaminar tape induces high strains in the lamina, due to wires attachment, in the pedicles as a reaction from the wires anchorage and in the cortical cortex. The highly loaded regions predicted by the finite element models match the experimental observations of failure locations for the two fixation configurations analyzed.

Failure load, predicted from simulation results was similar for both configurations, but about a 3.5 % higher for sublaminar tape construct. Then, sublaminar tape is much less invasive, because it requires less surgical interventions, permits its use with growth-guidance systems and has a significantly higher pull-out strength, so it may be more suitable to treat disorders like early onset scoliosis.

Regarding the second approach, we analyzed pedicle screw fixation on three porcine vertebrae using micro-FE to predict pull-out strength. Morphometry was also studied to relate pull-out strength and stiffness from experiments to the underlying microstructure. Parameters such as anisotropy degree (DA), mean trabecular separation (Tb.Sp) and trabecular number (Tb.N) correlated to pull-out strength and stiffness. Also, bone volume fraction (BV/TV) correlated to the pull-out stiffness. However, our regressions were calculated using only three points, and they need to be confirmed with extended datasets.

The morphometry was also estimated for different VOI side sizes in order to evaluate cancellous bone homogeneity within a vertebral body and we found that a volume surrounding the implant of about 17 mm was representative in terms of morphometry. VOI side size was also estimated from numerical models, analyzing the reaction force variation for increasing VOI side size, and that force converged for a VOI of around 22 mm. Then the morphometry and FE approaches lead to similar VOI side size results.

On the other hand, we explored the bone reaming effect that results from screw insertion on the variation of the reaction force. Specifically, we aim at finding more realistic load bearing for full bonding simulations, and we studied bone reaming distances between 0.045 to 0.27 mm. A bone reaming distance of 0.23 permits to avoid load transmission through the reaming threat side of the screw. Reaming has a different contribution according to VOI dimensions. It decreases for increasing VOI side until a difference of 7 % for a VOI side size of about 20 mm compared to a reaming distance of 0.045 mm.

Finally, we predicted pull-out failure using a high strained volume criterion that considers failure to occur when a percentage of volume exceeds a strain threshold, usually the compression yield strain. The scattering of the compression yield strain values in the literature motivated us to analyze the combination of critical volume and strain that led to the best failure strength prediction, which were a critical strain between 0.6 and 0.7 % and a critical volume between 1 and 2 %. Those failure criterion values point out that a low percentage of volume that suffers from strains greater than the yield strain is enough to produce pull-out failure. Using those parameters, we predicted the pull-out strength of the three samples tested with a good accuracy and differences lower than 8 %. Therefore, a simple failure criterion that accounts for high strained regions over the VOI may be enough as an approximation to predict pull-out failure.

6.2   Main contributions of the book

- It has been shown that morphometry is highly dependent on image segmentation. This is of great importance for osteoporotic samples (low BV/TV) because a slight change of the segmentation threshold can produce the disruption of the trabecular mask lattice and a wrong morphometric characterization.

- Changes of the segmentation threshold have an important effect on the estimation of the apparent properties using image-based finite element models.

- Finite element models and the bone mineral density using image phantoms lead to very similar results for the estimation of cancellous bone Young's modulus at tissue level.

- DIC permits to characterize strain fields during testing and compression failure patterns using directly the cancellous bone microstructure as pattern for correlation (no need of speckle).

- DIC performs a reliable and quick validation of the failure model proposed using FE.

- The equivalent strain was the best descriptor of cancellous bone compression failure using finite elements and DIC.

- A combination of micro-CT scanning, experimental tests and finite element modeling is a reliable tool to estimate the tissue and failure properties of cancellous bone.

- Our FE results of cancellous bone failure strains are consistent with the hypothesis that yield strains are relatively constant over a range of densities, while failure strains present a wider range of variation.

- Four morphometric parameters such as bone volume fraction (BV/TV), bone surface to volume ratio (BS/BV), mean trabecular thickness (Tb.Th) and fractal dimension (D) presented the best linear correlations to the apparent stiffness (E_{app}) and the yield (σ_{y}) and ultimate stresses (σ_{f}).

- The estimation of axial and shear stiffnesses through homogenization was improved when the multiple regression included BV/TV, BS/BV and D.

- A linear relationship was found between the apparent stiffness and yield and ultimate stresses of the open cell polyurethane foams of different densities analyzed as cancellous bone surrogates.

- A detailed morphometric characterization of the three density groups of open cell foams is provided, that is not available in the manufacturer's data sheets.

- The morphometric parameters that presented the best correlation to the apparent stiffness (E_{app}) and the yield (σ_{y}) and ultimate stresses (σ_{f}) for the open cell foams match the ones of cancellous bone.

- Two spine fixation configurations, pedicle screw and sublaminar tape, have been evaluated using the finite element method. The highly loaded regions of the models match the failure regions observed experimentally.

- Pull-out strength was predicted with a high accuracy using Pistoia criterion.

- Some morphometric parameters, such as BV/TV, anisotropy degree (DA), mean trabecular separation (Tb.Sp) and trabecular number (Tb.N), presented a good correlation to the pull-out strength.

Chapter 7

Future work

Some future work may be derived from the investigations developed in this book.

With regards to cancellous bone morphometric characterization, segmentation is often performed on whole specimens and few works have addressed the problem of individual trabecular segmentation. We propose to use individual trabecular segmentation to enable a complete 3D description of trabecular lattice and estimate the local trabecular orientation. It could be then used to analyze failure at trabecular level and refer damage and fracture to modes about the local axis.

It may be interesting to study volumes within a sample and relate their inhomogeneities in morphology to variations on the mechanical behavior from a numerical approach. Also, a similar study could be performed *a posteriori* in fracture analysis and evaluate the morphometry in the failure regions.

Regarding experimental mechanical characterization, many works in the literature perform compression tests, but there is a lack of consensus and homogenization regarding the experimental protocols used in the literature.

On the other hand, it is known the major importance of microstructure on the mechanical behavior of cancellous bone and many works explore several morphometric parameters to be descriptors of the mechanical properties variation. However, a deeper analysis of large datasets is needed to propose accurate descriptors based on bone morphometry to elucidate why some parameters work for some specimens and not for others.

Machine learning and artificial neural networks (ANN) can be applied to large data sets of cancellous bone in order to propose models of the influence of microstructure on cancellous bone mechanical properties. These models can be used as fracture risk predictors and to find cancellous bone microstructures of great mechanical performance.

Also, it is unclear the dimensions of a specimen to be considered representative as a function of BV/TV and location. The non-repetitive cancellous structure and its heterogeneity among locations may mean that bone state and failure may depend more on inhomogeneities than the behavior of a homogeneous representative volume. Therefore, we propose to investigate the inhomogeneities to control failure and a representative volume to control the elastic behavior.

With regards to digital image correlation, there is controversy about proper settings to estimate local properties of a heterogeneous structure and the accuracy of the method to estimate them. Yield and failure at the tissue level do not occur at the apparent yield point so, a combination of finite element models and DIC may be used to determine the strain at failure at a specific trabeculae using the numerical results to assess the apparent strain at which failure happened.

Cancellous bone toughening mechanisms have not been completely modeled in the literature and their contribution in bone failure is relevant, so we propose to develop numerical models that account for some of the toughening mechanisms like bridging or crack deflection, which would be necessary to perform more accurate failure analysis. Those models could be used to analyze local effects of fatigue behavior in bone.

Regarding open cell polyurethane foams, the influence of microstructure on the overall behavior could be assessed through the estimation of the stiffness matrix of slices of few millimeters and estimate the contribution to the whole specimen behavior. Furthermore, DIC could be applied to slices of few millimeters of foam to distinguish local trabecular failure by imaging and estimate those failure properties at individual struts.

The evaluation of spine fixation techniques for scoliosis treatment aimed at simplicity and accurate predictions of the failure load. However, many approximations were considered. Contact modeling could be included in the models to evaluate the relative importance of screw-bone interlocking, friction and detachment. Also, the damage induced by implant insertion and its effect on anchorage and implant performance could be included in the models by scanning the samples without the implant after its insertion and performing a registration between the intact bone mask and the damaged one.

www.ingramcontent.com/pod-product-compliance
Lightning Source LLC
LaVergne TN
LVHW042351190726
843493LV00005B/973